BELMO
BELMO
1900 BE
NASHVILLE, TN 37212

D0909166

Therapeutic Lasers

For Churchill Livingstone

Publisher: Mary C. Law
Senior Project Controller: Neil A. Dickson
Project Controller: Nicky S. Carrodus
Copy Editor: Sukie Hunter
Sales Promotion Executive: Hilary Brown

Therapeutic Lasers
Theory and Practice

G. David Baxter TD BSc(Hons) Physiotherapy DPhil MCSP

Professor of Rehabilitation Sciences, School of Health Sciences, University of Ulster, Northern Ireland

with contributions by
Costas Diamantopoulos BSc(Hons) CEng FASLSM

Research Director, Omega Laser Systems Ltd, London

Sharon O'Kane BSc(Hons) DPhil

Research Officer, University of Manchester

T. Dolores Shields BSc(Hons) Physiotherapy DPhil MCSP

Chartered Physiotherapist, Private Practice, Northern Ireland

Foreword by
Jim Allen BSc(Hons) PhD CBiol FIBiol

Professor of Physiology, School of Biomedical Sciences, University of Ulster, Northern Ireland

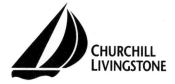

CHURCHILL
LIVINGSTONE

EDINBURGH LONDON MADRID MELBOURNE NEW YORK AND TOKYO 1994

CHURCHILL LIVINGSTONE
An imprint of Harcourt Publishers Limited

© Longman Group UK Limited 1994
© Harcourt Publishers Limited 1999

All rights reserved. No part of this publication may be reproduced, stored in a retrieval system, or transmitted in any form or by any means, electronic, mechanical, photocopying, recording or otherwise, without either the prior permission of the publishers (Harcourt Publishers Limited, 24–28 Oval Road, London NW1 7DX, UK), or a licence permitting restricted copying in the United Kingdom issued by the Copyright Licensing Agency Ltd, 90 Tottenham Court Road, London W1P 0LP.

First published 1994
  Reprinted 1995
  Reprinted 1999

ISBN 0-443-04393-0

British Library of Cataloguing in Publication Data
A catalogue record for this book is available from the British Library.

Library of Congress Cataloging in Publication Data
Baxter, G. David.
    Therapeutic lasers: theory and practice / G. David Baxter, Costas Diamantopoulos.
      p. cm.
    Includes index.
    ISBN 0-443-04393-0
    1. Lasers in medicine. I. Diamantopoulos, Costas. II. Title.
    [DNLM: 1. Lasers—therapeutic use. WB 480 B355c 1994]
    R857.L37B38 1994
    610′.28–dc20
    DNLM/DLC
    for Library of Congress   93-14226

Printed in China
GCC/03

203842
BELMONT UNIVERSITY LIBRARY

The
publisher's
policy is to use
paper manufactured
from sustainable forests

57
L37
338
994

ABC-3244

Contents

Foreword   vii

Preface   ix

Acknowledgements   xi

1. Medical lasers and photomedicine   1
   David Baxter

2. Laser physics   23
   David Baxter

3. Safety and good treatment practice   49
   David Baxter

4. Bioenergetics and tissue optics   67
   Costas Diamantopoulos

5. Laser photobiomodulation of wound healing   89
   Dolores Shields, Sharon O'Kane

6. Low-intensity laser therapy for pain relief   139
   David Baxter

7. Principles and practice of laser treatment   187
   David Baxter

8. Current developments and future directions   221
   David Baxter

Appendix I.   Key terminology   243

Appendix II. Guide to commercial systems   245

Index   255

Foreword

The use of laser and photodiodes at relatively low intensities has been promoted since the late 1960s as effective for the treatment of a variety of conditions including arthritis, soft tissue injuries and pain, as a result of which this therapeutic modality is gaining widespread acceptance within the clinical professions. 'Laser therapy' now forms a part of most if not all physiotherapy undergraduate training programmes within the UK, and it is increasingly rare to find hospital physiotherapy departments or private clinics without access to this modality. Yet there remains a considerable amount of ignorance and scepticism concerning laser's use and clinical efficacy. This is, at least in part, a consequence of the generally poor quality of the many original publications within the area and, until recently, the lack of critical scientific scrutiny of the many claims made for these devices. Happily this unacceptable situation is now being addressed and there are many recent high quality publications within the medical and scientific literature attesting to the clinical usefulness of these devices and quantifying their (apparently) many photobiological effects upon mammalian cells. It seems likely that, as the research progresses and laser's effects are further defined, laser therapy will find increasing use in the clinical setting. It is with this in mind that this book has been written. The text is aimed to be of use to undergraduate and postgraduate physiotherapy, nursing and medical students who need to be informed on the physics, biological effects and clinical usefulness of this modality, as well as to practising physiotherapists and other clinicians who wish to update their knowledge and make informed decisions upon appropriate treatment regimes. The book reviews important aspects of laser physics, biology and clinical applications and includes many references to original material of relevance to both the research scientist and practising clinician. It has been written and compiled by experts within the field and is a timely contribution to this important but, to date, relatively ignored area. I am confident that all who read it, regardless of their existing knowledge or expertise will gain significant benefit from its contents.

1993   J.M.A.

Preface

At the time of publication, the use of laser and phototherapy devices has become a routine component of physiotherapeutic treatment, at least in the British Isles. However, and in spite of such apparently wide acceptance, a recent survey among chartered physiotherapists[1] found that 94% of respondents were dissatisfied with the amount and quality of information on low-intensity laser therapy upon which to base their clinical practice. Apart from the lack of formal courses on the subject, respondents also identified the quality of manufacturers' literature and a lack of firm guidelines on treatment parameters/dosage etc. as the main causes of such dissatisfaction. However, and most relevant here, almost 70% complained about the lack of published articles and textbooks upon which to base clinical practice and application. Respondents also expressed confusion over conflicting advice given by different manufacturers and by the apparently contradictory results reported in the research literature. While this survey was the first of its kind, such findings were neither novel nor surprising to anyone within the field. Given such dissatisfaction, the primary objective of this book is to provide the reader with up-to-date critiques and reviews of the current literature, and an overview of the principles of treatment practice for those conditions which appear to be indicated for low-intensity laser therapy. In presenting this material together under one cover, the book is designed to fill what I perceive as an obvious gap in the literature, and consequently to satisfy the needs of busy clinicians who have limited time and resources to attempt comprehensive library searches. It is hoped therefore that the current text will help to resolve some of the apparent dissatisfaction on the part of the clinicians towards whom the current book is primarily directed. However, the book should also be of use to basic and clinical researchers within this field and thus, in this respect, I earnestly hope that the current text will in some way help to improve the quality of the research conducted on low-intensity laser therapy, both basic and applied.

I would also like to stress that no one modality or therapeutic intervention represents a panacea; this applies equally, and regardless of

---

[1]Baxter et al (1991) (see Ch. 1)

claims to the contrary, to low-intensity laser therapy. In order to produce therapeutic results, laser therapy, like any other modality, needs to be applied appropriately; this book will, I hope, serve to help promote more appropriate use of this modality.

Finally, I consider myself extremely fortunate to be at once a researcher and a clinician, with my experiences in one area complementing and extending my practice in the other. For those colleagues who devote all of their time to the treatment of patients, I hope that the contents of this book will help to better inform such treatments, and thus enable them to become more objective and reflective practitioners.

1993   G.D.B.

Acknowledgements

Many individuals, wittingly or unwittingly, contributed to the current text, and in a variety of ways; so many, indeed, that it is impossible to mention them all. However, I would like to identify in particular my colleagues in the research group at the University of Ulster, whose contributions ranged from proofreading unintelligible manuscripts to preserving my sanity by persuading me to go for coffee when all I really wanted to do was heave my Macintosh through the office window. They are, in alphabetical order: Dr Jim Allen, Mrs Jean Bell, Dr Bernie Hannigan, Ms Andrea Lowe, Mr Denis Martin, Mr Basim Mokhtar, Ms Sharon O'Kane, Dr John Ravey, Ms Dolores Shields and last, but certainly by no means least, Dr Deirdre Walsh.

Apart from my colleagues at Ulster, I would also like to record my thanks to my friends and associates at the Tissue Repair Research Unit at Guy's Hospital in London, particularly Mr Peter Bolton, who kindly supplied me with notes upon which to prepare the update on current research which features at the end of the book (Ch. 8).

I would also like to acknowledge the considerable help and support provided by the staff at Churchill Livingstone, especially Mrs Mary Emmerson-Law, Ms Dinah Thom and Ms Nicky Carrodus.

Finally, I would like to express my sincere thanks to Alice Louise, Susan Victoria, Marian Louise and Jennifer Michelle, not least for their patience.

1. Introduction: medical lasers and photomedicine

INTRODUCTION AND THE NEED FOR THE CURRENT TEXT

Laser is an acronym for Light Amplification by Stimulated Emission of Radiation. Such devices have, within a relatively short period of time, become part of our language and our everyday world. The applications of lasers are legion and span almost every field of human endeavour from medicine, science and technology to business and entertainment. At their extremes these applications range from the preservation of life (for example by the use of high-power medical lasers to excise cancerous lesions from the body) to patently military applications such as range finders and as weapons (as in the American 'Strategic Defence Initiative' (SDI) for example). Indeed, for most people, the association of lasers is with 'death rays' in science fiction novels and films. To this end, the SDI project almost confirms what most people always suspected: laser rays are ultimately a space age weapons system.

Thankfully for most of us, our contact with lasers is limited to their use in such devices as supermarket barcode readers, compact disk (CD) players, lecture theatre pointers and laser light shows. Among their many uses in medicine (some of which will be outlined in more detail below) the therapeutic use of lasers at relatively low power and energy densities for such things as the promotion of tissue healing and the reduction of pain has recently attracted a lot of attention, especially among chartered physiotherapists. The devices used in this application usually produce either infra-red or visible red radiation and, unlike the majority of other lasers used in surgery and medicine, are essentially athermic, producing no significant heating of tissue as a result of irradiation.

However, the claims made on behalf of laser therapy, particularly by some laser manufacturers, have been grossly exaggerated, if not actually misleading. Not surprisingly, this has caused a certain amount of scepticism in some quarters of the medical professions and has tended to confuse responsible clinicians who find it hard to separate the hype from the reality. Such scepticism has been reinforced by at least two factors, the first of which is the fact that most of the papers on therapeutic laser are published in foreign language journals, often without English abstracts.

1

Consequently these papers are often inaccessible or indecipherable to the majority of Anglophone researchers and clinicians. Secondly, the quality of a large proportion of the papers published on therapeutic laser (regardless of language!) is poor, often being no more than anecdotal reports of the authors' experiences of a particular type of laser system or the laser treatment of a certain condition or range of conditions. Basford (1986, 1989) has identified the most common weaknesses in published articles as follows:

1. Inadequate specification of laser irradiation/treatment parameters by authors: While a number of authors have indicated the ideal in reporting laser research (see Ch. 4), few published papers have met even the minimum acceptable standards. Indeed, in a (thankfully) small number of cases, authors have merely indicated that 'laser' was the therapeutic modality used, without even specifying the type of lasing medium and thus the wavelength of the therapeutic system employed as the basis of their report. As a result, it is often impossible to replicate reported research, or indeed to attempt to realise reported positive effects in the clinical setting.

2. Poor experimental design, especially lack of control groups: Reports frequently document uncontrolled trials, in which positive results are invariably reported. While such reports represent a large body of anecdotal evidence in favour of the continued clinical application of therapeutic laser, the dangers in unquestioning acceptance of results from this type of research are obvious.

3. The use of only limited blinding by researchers: Even in those studies where placebo groups have been used, trials are frequently only single-blind so that, while subjects or patients were unaware as to whether active or sham irradiation was performed, investigators were able to distinguish between data for placebo and treated groups. Consequently, experimenter bias cannot be discounted as one possible factor where positive results have been obtained in some such single-blind studies.

It might appear from the above that low-power lasers are of questionable therapeutic benefit, whose continued use by clinicians is based upon the exaggerated claims of some interested parties. Indeed, this has already been suggested by at least one guest editor for the journal *Pain* (Devor 1990). However, in spite of the criticisms levelled above, there is a growing body of evidence from properly conducted and reported research in favour of the use of low-intensity laser irradiation as a therapeutic modality. Such evidence is derived from results of work spanning cellular, animal and human research, including clinical trials. Based upon this, it is possible to recommend the application of low-intensity laser as an effective therapeutic modality for a range of conditions. While outlined briefly below for the purposes of this introductory chapter, these applications will be fully expanded upon in later chapters.

This then represents one of the primary objectives of the current text:

the provision of critiques of the current literature and the identification of those conditions which appear to be indicated for low-intensity laser treatment. In presenting such reviews together under one cover, the book is very much intended to fill what is perceived as an obvious gap in the literature, and consequently to satisfy the needs of busy clinicians who have limited time and resources to attempt comprehensive library searches.

In a recent survey of the clinical use of low-intensity laser therapy among chartered physiotherapists (Baxter et al 1991), the most common complaint voiced by respondents was a lack of information concerning this relatively new treatment modality. In all, some 94% admitted dissatisfaction with the amount of information and instruction available to them on laser therapy. Apart from a lack of formal courses and lectures on the subject, respondents also identified insufficient detail in manufacturers' literature and a lack of firm guidelines on treatment parameters/dosage etc. as the main causes of such dissatisfaction. However, and most relevant to the current text, almost 70% of all respondents complained of the lack of published articles and textbooks upon which to base clinical practice and application. A number also admitted being confused by the conflicting advice given by different sales representatives and manufacturers; and others by the variable results from the laser research reported in the literature.

While this survey was the first of its kind, these findings were neither novel nor surprising to anyone within the field of low-intensity laser therapy. Confusion exists, not only in the minds of clinicians, but also on the part of researchers and authors. It is therefore hoped that the current text will help to resolve some of the confusion, especially on the part of the clinicians towards whom it is primarily directed. However, it would be surprising if basic and clinical researchers did not find at least some of its contents of use!

THE HISTORICAL PERSPECTIVE

By way of background and introduction to later chapters, it is useful to paint the historical perspective by considering the development of this field. The roots of low-intensity laser therapy are both wide and deep. In a number of important respects, the modality is essentially a relatively recent development of photomedicine, i.e. the use of light for the treatment of disease. In this respect, the growth of laser therapy in the 1970s and 1980s parallels the development of ultra-violet therapy or actinotherapy in the early 1900s, with clinical practice developing and expanding rapidly to exploit the latest technological advances. However, the therapeutic use of low power lasers has also sprung from the field of laser medicine and surgery: early papers by such researchers as Toshio Ohshiro resulted directly from experience in the wider applications of (usually high-power) lasers in medicine. To this end, it is useful to begin this book by considering briefly the history of the use of light in medicine and the development of laser technology.

History of photomedicine

While laser therapy is a relatively new phenomenon, the use of light as a therapeutic modality predates the earliest records. However, as Licht (1983) has indicated, the practice of heliotherapy in ancient times was based largely upon religious beliefs and superstitions. Prehistoric man deified the sun and consequently sunlight, being holy, was thought to be able to drive out the evil spirits which were believed to cause disease (Keele 1957). The ancient Sun gods were thus considered to be gods of health and healing: the Phoenicians and early Hebrews worshipped Baal as god of sun and health, and the Greeks praised Helios as god of light, sun and healing (it is from Helios that the contemporary term 'heliotherapy' is derived). Sun worship was not confined to prehistoric times: it survived as a monotheistic religion for almost four centuries before finally being assimilated into Christian orthodoxy during the rise of the Holy Roman Empire. Licht (1983) identifies the early Christian suppression of sun worship as the reason why no further mention of heliotherapy can be traced in the literature from then until the 18th century.

Although the efficacy of ancient heliotherapy is hard to judge, it was highly regarded and recommended by Greek and Roman physicians such as Celsus and Galen for a range of conditions including epilepsy, arthritis, asthma and obesity. In these cultures, sunbathing was considered healthy and a means of preventative medicine: for instance the importance of sunlight in bone growth had already been recognised by Herodotus in the 6th century BC.

The latter part of the 18th and early 19th centuries saw rediscovery of the beneficial effects of heliotherapy. This was largely as a result of the inevitable illnesses caused by poor housing and dark, sunless streets within rapidly expanding towns where soft coal was in abundant use (Licht 1983). Sun baths were recommended for scurvy, rickets, oedema, dropsy, rheumatic arthritis and depression (Cauvin 1815). This last indication is particularly interesting given the recent recommendations of ultra-violet therapy for seasonal and other affective disorders (Lewy et al 1982, Kripke 1985, Hansen et al 1987, Wehr et al 1988).

While the 19th century saw the increasing use of heliotherapy, it was not, however, regarded as a panacea; the potentially harmful effects of excessive exposure were noted to include ophthalmia. The early 1800s also saw the introduction of various devices to increase the effectiveness of insolation, including lenses to focus the incident sunlight, as well as glass boxes in which patients were to lie during therapy. Interest in the clinical use of sunlight grew and encouraged a number of scientists to investigate the photobiological effects of such radiation. As a consequence, the bactericidal action of sunlight had been shown on a range of bacteria by the end of the 19th century, based upon initial work by Downes & Blunt (1877). These observations led to the use of ultra-violet (UV) radiation for sterilisation, an application which it continues to find today.

Attempts were also made to artificially replicate the UV rays of the sun using various types of lamp. With these early devices, the basis of modern actinotherapy was established and photomedicine became independent of sunlight as a source of radiation. The most successful of these early actinotherapists was Finsen, who used both natural and artificial light to great effect. In what was essentially a development of Ziegelroth's treatment technique using a carbon arc lamp, Finsen designed a lamp incorporating a system of lenses and filters for the treatment of lupus vulgaris (Finsen 1899), his successes leading to the award of a Nobel Prize in 1903. The subsequent popularity of the carbon arc lamp led to a number of improvements in its design over the next two and a half decades, most notably the incorporation of tungsten to enrich the ultra-violet spectra produced.

However these lamps were not the only source of artificial UV radiation to be developed over this period. The use of carbon arc lamps was rivalled by quartz mercury vapour devices, based upon lamps originally designed for street lighting. The original water-cooled Kromayer lamp, which still finds clinical application in some quarters for the treatment of open wounds, was designed in 1904 (Rowbottom & Susskind 1984). The use of light for the treatment of the open wounds found in surgical tuberculosis was first proposed by Bernhard and subsequently developed by Rollier (Bernhard 1926). While Bernhard and Rollier used natural sunlight, the extent of their successes encouraged Reyn (a colleague of Finsen) to use full body irradiation with artificial UV for such patients (Licht 1983).

Apart from tuberculosis and open wounds, the other main indication found for actinotherapy was rickets. Palm had noted the importance of sunlight in the development of the condition in 1890, and had recommended heliotherapy as a preventative measure and therapy of choice (Palm 1890). However it was not until 1919 that the first X-ray evidence was available to support the use of UV in the treatment of rickets. The use of actinotherapy expanded significantly over the following decades so that, by the mid 1930s, Krusen could list literally hundreds of conditions for which success was claimed with actinotherapy, including nephritis, rheumatoid arthritis, haemophilia and herpes zoster (Krusen 1933). One of the most important developments over the period was the recognition of the need for testing of patients to establish skin type, because of variations in response to therapy (Saidman 1930).

In modern clinical practice, many of the conditions for which actinotherapy was the only treatment are now routinely and successfully treated by other means. Furthermore, more enlightened social policy has resulted in improved diet and housing conditions, so making the UV treatment of rickets and tuberculosis redundant. The list of applications and conditions for which actinotherapy is currently recommended is therefore limited but includes the stimulation of wound healing in ulcers, boils and carbuncles (Scott 1983), the treatment of acne vulgaris (Cuncliffe 1973), neonatal jaundice (Ennever 1988) and as a means of inducing counter-irritation for pain relief (Scott 1983, see also Editorial 1989).

However, such use is not universally accepted. This is due in part to the generally poor findings from controlled clinical research (e.g. Mills & Kligman 1978), but particularly in the light of recent reports which have stressed the potentially harmful effects of UV radiation (Prime 1983).

Despite having lost its previously wide appeal, UV radiation does retain an important role in the photochemotherapy treatment of psoriasis and some other dermatoses, especially where topical agents have been tried with little effect, or where sociopsychological factors warrant it (Frain-Bell 1985). In so called PUVA (Psoralen/UVA) therapy, patients are administered a psoralen orally and receive whole-body UVA radiation in conjunction with the drug to produce phototoxic reactions within psoriatic lesions. In common with standard actinotherapy, reservations have been expressed because of the potential carcinogenic side effects of the therapy (Kenicer et al 1981) and there is still some debate over the selection of optimal regimes and dosages for effective treatments (Frain-Bell 1985).

Despite waning popularity, UV therapy continues to form an important but limited part of routine physiotherapy. In summary, the comments of Scott are both succinct and pertinent:

Ultra-violet therapy has been subject to alternating periods of advocacy and denigration and recently there has been a trend towards the latter.
Consequently, some of the more scientific practitioners have tended to use this treatment less. On the other hand there is no doubt that ultra-violet energy is a valuable therapeutic agent when used in certain conditions. However, it is still the case that some of the more 'artful' physicians who regard the practice of medicine as an art as well as a science can still use ultra-violet light to the benefit of their patients. (Scott 1983)

The development of medical lasers

The principles upon which all laser devices are based (see Ch. 2) were developed at the turn of the century by the physicists Planck and Einstein. During this period a certain amount of speculation and discussion had surrounded Maxwell's concept of considering electromagnetic radiation as waves. It was obvious that the theory had a number of shortcomings and failed to explain some commonly observed phenomena. In order to explain these anomalies, Planck proposed quantal theory: the idea that radiation could be considered as discrete quantas or bundles of energy. Building upon Planck's concept of quantal energies, Einstein published a paper in 1917 entitled 'Zur Quantum Theori der Strahlung' which outlined the key principles for the stimulated emission of photons.

However, it was some 40 years before the dream of building such a device to produce stimulated radiation was realised by a group at Columbia University. Working at microwave wavelengths which fall outside the visible part of the electromagnetic spectrum, this device was termed a MASER (Microwave Amplification by Stimulated Emission of Radiation; see Gordon et al 1955). Within three years Schawlow & Townes (1958) proposed the development of what was originally termed an 'optical maser' based upon the maser used at Columbia University. Despite this, it was Dr Theodore Maiman at Hughes Laboratories in Malibu who published in 1960 the first account of the production of laser radiation using a ruby crystal as the basis for his device. This first ruby device produced pulsed laser visible radiation at a fixed wavelength of 694 nm and thus appeared red.

The 1960s saw rapid developments in laser technology, including the use of a wide range of alternative lasing media as the basis for laser devices working at alternative wavelengths to Maiman's original 694 nm (see Ch. 2). Workers at the Bell Telephone laboratories exploited a mixture of the elemental gases helium and neon to produce a helium–neon (commonly abbreviated to He–Ne) laser operating at 632.8 nm, the same laboratories going on to develop the carbon dioxide (CO_2) laser (Patel 1965). The latter laser was something of an innovation, being able to operate continuously at power outputs well above the usual milliwatt range, and was subsequently to prove extremely popular in surgical applications for a number of reasons which are outlined below.

Other lasers developed over this period included the argon, the neodymium–glass and the neodymium–yttrium–aluminium–garnet (Nd:YAG) lasers. All were to find rapid application in medicine and surgery, although some more successfully than others. Interestingly, the world's first medical laser laboratory, which was established at the University of Cincinnati in 1961, was conceived to investigate the *safety* of the new technology. However, shortly afterwards, a laboratory was established at the Children's Hospital of Cincinnati under the direction of Professor Leon Goldman to assess the potential surgical applications of lasers.

Ophthalmologists were the first medical specialty to successfully use laser in surgical applications. Prior to the development of laser technology, pioneering work by Meyer-Swickerath had led to the use of a xenon-arc photocoagulator to produce intense spots of light energy on the retina as a means of treatment for retinal detachment among other things. During such treatments, the intense energy produced by the photocoagulator was used to 'weld' the retina back in place. However this device was unsatisfactory for a number of reasons, chiefly because the power density was too small and thus allowed energy to dissipate (as heat) to surrounding structures during the relatively large treatment times required.

Given the characteristics of the ruby laser developed by Maiman, with its ultrashort pulse width coupled with high peak power, it was not long before it was trialled by a number of ophthalmologists, initially on experimental animals. The generally favourable results of early work on humans reported by, for instance, Flocks & Zweng (1964) represent the first successful application of laser technology in surgery. The pulsed ruby laser thus found wide usage in ophthalmology, as did a number of other lasers based upon alternative lasing media, including the argon, krypton and dye lasers. The continuous wave argon laser first developed by Bridges (1964) proved to be a particularly useful tool in ophthalmology, due to the fact that the blue-green light produced by the gas is preferentially absorbed by the sort of highly vascularised tissues frequently requiring treatment (Zweng 1971).

Oncology was another area that seemed full of early promise, with a number of groups reporting varying success with laser irradiation of malignant tumours (e.g. Goldman et al 1965). This flirtation with the new pulsed laser technology was short lived after a number of groups reported finding viable tumour cells in the explosive debris produced during short-pulse laser irradiation (e.g. Minton et al 1965). Given the very real danger of encouraging the formation of metastases during such laser treatment, pulsed laser treatment of cancers was abruptly curtailed.

Fortuitously for the surgeons, the CO_2 laser proved to be more promising for surgical application, being readily absorbed by biological tissue and capable of operating in the continuous wave (CW) mode. This reduced the explosive nature of the laser–tissue interaction which is common with high-power pulsed machines, and consequently did not give rise to the propagation of viable cancer cells to other parts of the body. The CO_2 laser thus became popular with surgeons during the early part of the 1970s and has since remained the standard laser system for a number of surgical applications including neurosurgery, dermatology, plastic surgery and podiatry.

Laser medicine has developed rapidly since the late 1960s, in parallel with more recent innovations in laser technology. The intervening years have thus seen the introduction of tunable dye lasers, excimer (excited dimer) lasers and metal-gas lasers into clinical practice (see Table 1.1). As far as low-intensity lasers for therapeutic applications are concerned, the most significant developments took place within the field of semiconductor diode technology, culminating in the production in 1979 of the first gallium–arsenide laser diode by Yariv and colleagues at the California Institute of Technology. Together with the He–Ne laser already identified, it is diode lasers based upon this gallium–arsenide prototype that are mainly used in low-intensity laser therapy.

LASERS IN SURGERY AND MEDICINE: CURRENT APPLICATIONS

It would be inconceivable to complete the current text without providing

Table 1.1   Some lasers in common clinical use (after Carruth & McKenzie 1986)

Laser medium	Wavelength (nm)	Colour	Typical applications
Carbon dioxide (CO_2)	10 600	IR[1]	Surgical laser: general, gynaecology and ophthalmology Oncology, bronchoscopy Otolaryngology: laryngeal microsurgery, otology
Argon (Ar)	488	blue	Surgical laser: ophthalmology, dermatology (port wine stains)
	514.5	blue-green	Photodynamic therapy (PDT)[2]
Krypton (Kr)	568	yellow	Ophthalmology
	647	red	
(Krypton violet)	407 413 415	violet	Localisation of HPD-bearing tissue in PDT
Neodymium– yttrium–aluminium– garnet (Nd:YAG)	900 1060 1350	IR	Ophthalmology, bronchoscopy, oncology, cancer therapy
(Tunable) dye	variable		Dermatology: vascular lesions
Copper vapour	510	blue-green	Ophthalmology
	578	yellow	
Excimer	351[3]	UV	Dermatology, ophthalmology

[1] Infra-red
[2] Use of haematoporphyrin derivative (HPD) and laser to cause phototoxic reactions in cancers
[3] Example only, variable output

at least an overview of the applications of lasers and laser technology in medical and surgical practice. However, it must be stressed from the outset that is not possible (nor intended) within this short introductory chapter to cover the area in sufficient depth to do justice to such a wide and diverse field. For those interested in further detail, such texts as Carruth & McKenzie's short book (Carruth & McKenzie 1986) or the American Society for Laser Medicine and Surgery's *Introduction to Laser Biophysics* (ASLMS 1988) each provides an excellent introduction to the physics of high-power medical lasers as well as outlining current clinical applications and practice. Current clinical applications for a range of various types of laser system are summarised in Table 1.1.

Ophthalmology

As already indicated, ophthalmologists were the first medical specialty to use laser, employing the pulsed ruby laser as a treatment for retinal detachment. In addition to retinal detachments, a host of conditions are currently treated by laser ophthalmologists, including retinal tears, diabetic retinopathy, glaucoma and tumours. Several laser systems have found successful application in addition to the ruby laser, including argon and Nd:YAG systems.

Argon lasers were initially used to arrest neovascularisation in diabetic retinopathy where the progressive development of neovascularisation can lead to loss of vision. Such systems later found application in the treatment of glaucoma. Applications for the Nd:YAG laser include the excision of opaque or semi-opaque membranes, particularly in cataract surgery. More recently, excimer ('excited dimer') lasers operating in the near ultra-violet part of the spectrum have been investigated for their potential application in the treatment of a number of conditions including astigmatism and corneal transplantation.

Dermatology and plastic surgery

The main applications for high power lasers in the field of dermatology are for the treatment of angiomas and other vascular lesions, principally port wine stains, and for the coagulation of pigmented lesions such as melanomas. Lasers have been successfully used by dermatologists in the treatment of such vascular lesions as cavernous angiomas, Kaposi's sarcoma and malignant vascular tumours, as well as for certain types of recalcitrant wart and for florid condylomata acuminata. In the removal of tattoos, treatment with high power laser has been found to be partically useful as the pigment within the tattoo readily absorbs the incident radiation and fragments. The resultant phagocytosis produces a good cosmetic result with minimal scarring or epidermal damage.

In the hands of a number of plastic surgeons, lasers have been successfully employed for the excision of massive angiomas, as well as for selected types of head, neck and hand surgery. More recently a number of laser systems have been trialled for microvascular welding of blood vessels and peripheral nerve welding with some encouraging results being reported to date.

For such applications in dermatology and plastic surgery argon, CO_2 and Nd:YAG have remained the most popular laser systems to date, although more recently the xenon–fluoride excimer and heavy metal vapour lasers have been used with some success.

Gynaecology

The CO_2 laser has been the most commonly used laser in gynaecology to date, usually for the treatment of pre-invasive cancer of the vulva, vagina and cervix. For early and inoperable cancers, some types of laser have also been successfully used to administer so-called photodynamic therapy (PDT) or photoreactive therapy (PRT) in gynaecology (see below). Apart from such cancer treatments, laser is also routinely employed in some centres for endometriosis, laparoscopy and to perform tuboplasty as a treatment for infertility.

Diagnostic/non-surgical applications

Apart from the above applications, which are largely dependent upon the thermal effects of laser upon irradiated tissue, a number of the medical applications for laser are based upon the other special characteristics of this type of radiation. Perhaps the best known of these is the He–Ne laser Doppler flowmeter for the in vivo monitoring of bloodflow. More recently, laser spectroscopy has been used in conjunction with magnetic resonance imaging (MRI) scanners to enhance the imagery and it might reasonably be expected that laser holography will soon be routinely available for the provision of three-dimensional images for a range of diagnostic applications.

Photodynamic therapy/photoreactive therapy

One of the most exciting developments in the field of oncology in recent years has been the use of relatively low-power dye lasers in so-called photodynamic or photoreactive therapy (PDT or PRT). Operating at powers of about 1 W, these machines are considered to be of little use in general surgical applications. However when used in conjunction with the haematoporphyrin derivative (HPD) dihaematoporphyrin ether (DHE) such lasers can be selectively applied to produce phototoxic reactions or laser-induced fluorescence specifically in skin and soft tissues. As DHE tends to concentrate predominantly in cancerous lesions, laser irradiation can be used either to induce fluorescence as an effective means of detecting early cancers or alternatively to induce phototoxicity and thus destroy the cancer. While this application is still relatively new, encouraging results have been reported to date from a number of centres. Possible future developments within the field of PDT will be outlined in Chapter 8.

THE DEVELOPMENT OF LOW-INTENSITY LASER THERAPY (LILT)

As can be seen from the above account, the introduction of laser technology into medical and surgical practice was rapid and parallelled its expanding use in other fields. However, most of these applications relied upon the exploitation of photothermal and ablative interactions of laser with tissues at relatively high power and energy densities. Additionally, the biological effects of lasers at lower power and energy densities were initially unclear; in fact low-power He–Ne units were considered to have no biological effects whatsoever and were (and are still) consequently incorporated into higher-power lasers as 'pointers'.

Given that some of the higher-power lasers could only produce laser radiation in very short pulses, the potentially highly destructive nature of their interaction with biological tissue and the fact that these devices frequently operated in the invisible parts of the spectrum, the use of a visible red He–Ne laser operating in the milliwatt range seemed an ideal solution to the problem of targeting the main laser. It was against this background that several groups initiated studies on the possible biological and clinical effects of low-power laser. Most notably these included the late Professor Endre Mester in Budapest and Dr Friedrich Plog in Canada.

In Budapest, Mester initiated a series of studies on isolated cells and experimental animals during the late 1970s in which he attempted to demonstrate what he considered to be the potential carcinogenic effects of low power He–Ne and argon laser. In one of these early experiments, Mester used He–Ne laser to irradiate experimental carcinomas in laboratory mice, expecting to find an acceleration in the growth of carcinomas as a result of irradiation. To his surprise, the experimental carcinomas were unaffected by the He–Ne irradiation. However, and most surprising of all, irradiated animals regrew hair (which had been shaven for the purposes of the experiment) faster than controls.

In an extension of these early experiments in mice, Mester and his group embarked on a series of animal studies, the results of which were published during the next 2 years (Mester et al 1985). All showed a *photobiostimulation* effect on the rate of tissue repair in various experimentally-induced wounds as a result of low power He–Ne laser irradiation. Spurred on by the success of this animal work, Mester's group began some simple clinical trials on small numbers of patients suffering from chronic unhealed wounds and sores of various aetiologies which had previously been found to be unresponsive to other treatments. Similarly encouraging results were found in these patients, who provided the first direct evidence of the photobiostimulative potential of low-energy laser therapy in humans in vivo. As a result of this pioneering work, a laser therapy clinic was quickly established at Budapest to exploit the benefits of the new therapy in patients with chronic intractable wounds. Despite the unfortunate death of Professor Endre Mester in 1987, this important work has continued at Budapest since.

The possible biological effects of low power laser was also of interest to Dr Friedrich Plog in Canada, who, quite independently to Mester, began to investigate He–Ne laser as a potential alternative to metal needles for acupuncture treatments in 1973. Findings from Plog's initial studies suggested that irradiation of acupuncture points with the He–Ne laser was a viable alternative to invasive needling.

Based upon the reported successes of Plog and Professor Mester's group at Budapest, a range of research projects were initiated during the next decade, principally in eastern Europe, China and the Soviet Union. The generally positive findings of this research has resulted in laser therapy subsequently becoming a popular modality in the countries indicated, which is reflected in the relatively large proportion of published papers which originate from these countries. Throughout the latter part of the 1970s and particularly the 1980s, reports emerged of laser's potentially beneficial effects on a range of conditions including postoperative wounds (Burgudjieva et al 1985), angina pectoris (Agov et al 1982) and stomach ulcers (Dotsenko et al 1985). These applications have relied almost exclusively on the use of He–Ne units, often used with fibreoptic delivery devices.

However, for some of the reasons already identified, the acceptance of laser therapy in the West and particularly in the USA has been limited. It was not until the early 1980s that reports began to appear in the West of low-power laser's use in clinical practice (e.g. Calderhead et al 1982, Kleinkort & Foley 1984, Goujon et al 1985, Kamikawa & Kyoto 1985). It is interesting to note that, in contrast to those described above, such publications have tended to be based upon the use of semiconductor lasers and superluminous diodes (see Ch. 2). This reflects the norm in clinical practice in western Europe, where the cheaper and more robust semiconductor-based diode lasers are more popular with clinicians than He–Ne lasers.

The use of, and applications for, low-energy laser therapy have steadily grown in the ensuing years among a number of clinical groups including physiotherapists and dentists. However, while therapeutic laser currently enjoys a degree of acceptance in Europe and Asia, the Food and Drug Administration (FDA) in the USA has yet to approve its use for a single application. In spite of this, as research continues and the potential therapeutic benefits of low-intensity laser therapy become clearer it may reasonably be expected that it will not be long before this modality enjoys similar popularity in America.

A note on terminology

It is common to hear lasers of the type used for therapeutic applications variously described as 'soft', 'cold' or 'low-power' lasers, and consequently their therapeutic use has tended to be labelled accordingly. Thus early papers referred to 'soft laser treatment' and 'cold laser therapy' etc. in an attempt to distinguish the lasers used from the higher-power lasers commonly employed in other medical applications. Such terminology is inappropriate and tends to confuse rather than enlighten, as it is based upon the laser *system* rather than its effects upon the irradiated tissue; relatively powerful machines operating in the 1 W range which could normally produce destructive thermal reactions in irradiated tissue have been successfully used in conjunction with a scanning device to deliver *therapeutic* laser treatment (Goldman et al 1980).

Thus definitions based upon the power output of the laser system are essentially meaningless. Essentially it is the laser–tissue interaction which defines the therapeutic applications which are the subject of the current text. Specifically excluded are thermal effects such as thermal coagulation and vaporisation as well as explosive ablation which are common features of laser–tissue interactions at much higher power and energy densities. During such interactions, focal temperature rises of several hundred degrees can easily be achieved. In contrast, therapeutic laser–tissue interaction is essentially athermic, in that it produces no significant measurable heating of the irradiated tissue. This is not to exclude *photothermal* interactions as one possible mechanism of photon absorption in tissue during therapeutic laser treatments. However, as will become evident in later chapters, the main type of reaction with tissue during laser therapy would appear to be *photochemical*: the absorption of incident photons by irradiated tissue producing chemical rather than thermal energy.

Consequently, a more appropriate term that has been suggested for this relatively new modality *is low (reactive) level laser therapy (LLLT)* (Ohshiro & Calderhead 1988). This terminology is thus framed in terms of the *reaction* between laser and the irradiated biological tissue. Alternatively the term *low-intensity laser therapy (LILT)* is equally accurate as, for a given wavelength of laser light, the energy density is the most important factor in determining the tissue reaction.

However, it should be noted that use of the term *low-energy laser therapy*, although coined by the authors of some reviews, is imprecise and cannot be recommended: while a total incident energy of 4 J of laser radiation may be regarded as 'low', if focussed on to a 0.02 cm^2 area by a lens would result in an energy density of 200 J/cm^2 which could not be regarded as within the therapeutic range. The relationships between energy and power, energy density and power density and their clinical relevance are considered further in subsequent chapters.

Another phrase which is commonly used to describe therapeutic laser and its effects in tissue is *laser photobiostimulation*, which is sometimes shortened to *photobiostimulation* or more simply *biostimulation*. This terminology essentially derives from the early work completed on wound healing, in which acceleration in rates of tissue repair was usually seen (see Chs 5 and 6). However the use of such terminology requires caution. In the first instance, the clinical applications for therapeutic laser extend beyond promotion of wound healing (see below) and thus photobiostimulation does not adequately describe or define current clinical practice. Furthermore, and as will become apparent in later chapters, a number of the therapeutic applications of laser depend upon *bioinhibition* rather than biostimulation. To this end a more useful umbrella term that has been suggested for laser's cellular effects is *laser photobiomodulation*.

CURRENT CLINICAL APPLICATIONS

For the purposes of this introductory chapter, the following briefly outlines current clinical applications for low-intensity laser therapy under four headings: physiotherapy, dentistry, veterinary medicine and laser acupuncture. While these give a good indication of the range and variety of current applications for low-intensity laser, it should be stressed that these are not exhaustive: clinicians from other clinical specialties such as chiropody/podiatry and osteopathy have found that therapeutic laser can form a useful addition to their clinical repertoire. Later chapters will consider specific applications such as wound healing and pain relief in greater depth.

Physiotherapy

While a variety of professional groups currently employ low-intensity laser, such devices remain most popular within physiotherapy, with over 40% of chartered physiotherapists canvassed for the purposes of a recent survey indicating clinical experience of therapeutic lasers (Baxter et al 1991). In terms of comparative efficacy, respondents in this survey rated low-intensity laser highly against other more established electrotherapeutic modalities such as ultrasound, interferential therapy and pulsed electromagnetic energy (PEME) for a number of treatment effects including the relief of pain and reduction of oedema. Indeed, laser achieved premier ranking for both the promotion of wound healing and pain relief. It is therefore perhaps not surprising that laser has, within a relatively short period of time, become an accepted part of routine physiotherapy management for a variety of conditions.

Indications

The main indications for low-intensity laser therapy in physiotherapeutic practice are:

*1. **Wound healing.*** The photobiostimulation of wound healing remains the cardinal indication for therapeutic laser in physiotherapy. In this, laser therapy has come to be recognised by many therapists as superior to a range of other alternative electrotherapeutic modalities, including ultrasound. For this reason, laser therapy is often the physiotherapeutic modality of choice in a variety of conditions including trophic, varicose, diabetic and decubitus ulcers ('pressure sores'), particularly where these have become chronic and/or are unresponsive to other treatment approaches. In addition, cases of necrosis, burns and post operative wounds would also seem to respond favourably to low-intensity laser treatment. In cases of scarring, it has been reported by some therapists that laser therapy may not only accelerate remodelling of the scar tissue, but also give a more cosmetically acceptable result.

*2. **Soft tissue injuries,*** including traumatic, inflammatory and overuse-type injuries. While variable results have been reported for the laser treatment of bursitis and muscle spasm, other common soft tissue injuries such as muscle tears, haematomas and tendinopathies would seem to respond particularly well to therapeutic laser, which has led to its wide use in sports medicine. To the athlete, whether recreational or competitive, such injuries represent an unavoidable lay-off from training with consequent loss of form. For such individuals, the prospect of shorter recovery times as a result of low-level laser therapy is an attractive one, and thus many specifically request laser treatment when attending sports injury clinics. Consequently an increasing number of sports physiotherapists regard low-intensity laser as an essential part of their treatment repertoire.

3. Pain relief, including both acute pain (e.g. postoperative pain) and more chronic pain syndromes such as herpes zoster/post-herpetic neuralgia. This represents the most enigmatic and controversial area of low-intensity laser application (see Ch. 6), not least because of the lack of an obvious mechanism(s) of action and the conflicting findings of clinically based research. However, in the experience of clinicians, therapeutic laser is at least comparable, if not actually superior, to a number of other electrotherapeutic agents including interferential therapy and shortwave diathermy for analgesic effect.

4. Arthritic conditions of various aetiologies, particularly where these have affected the small joints of the hands and/or feet. While variable results have been reported from clinical research in this area, low-intensity laser would still appear to offer substantial therapeutic benefits in the management of a number of painful arthropathies (see Ch. 6).

Dentistry

While not enjoying the same popularity among dentists as it does among physiotherapists, low-intensity laser therapy has been recommended by a number of authors as a useful therapeutic tool in dentistry for a range of applications, used either as an adjunctive to other more traditional treatments or in isolation.

Indications for laser treatment

The main indications for therapeutic laser in odontology (see Zhou Yo Cheng 1988, Christensen 1989) would appear to be:

1. Reduction of oedema and hyperaemia, principally in the pulpae during treatment of dental caries. For this, it is usually recommended that the dentine and gingiva of the tooth are irradiated just before filling to reduce inflammation and thus minimise subsequent pain. In cases of gingivitis, irradiation of the affected gingiva using low-intensity laser can also help reduce bleeding and pain, thus improving patient comfort and allowing for more thorough depuration.

2. Promotion of wound healing. Laser photobiostimulation has been successfully employed by dentists in the treatment of such conditions as necrosis of the pulpae, where low-intensity laser is used as an adjunctive treatment after the root canals have been effectively cleared of necrotic tissue and treated with an antibacterial agent.

3. Relief of pain of various aetiologies, including dentine hyper-aesthesia, acute pulpitis and both perioperative and postoperative pain. It has even been reported by some authors that laser acupuncture can be successfully used for the induction of preoperative anaesthesia prior to minor oral surgery. While most commonly applied directly to the painful area, therapeutic laser may also be used to irradiate myofascial trigger points as an effective means of treating orofacial pains.

4. Treatment of herpes labialis ('cold sores') and herpetic gingival stomatitis. An increasing number of practitioners have come to regard low-intensity laser as the treatment of choice for infection of the lips and mucous membranes with the herpes simplex virus.

Veterinary practice

Therapeutic lasers have been successfully used by a number of veterinary surgeons and physiotherapists for over 10 years. Although they are not yet as widely employed as in human practice, this situation is beginning to change. This is especially true in equine practice, where it is increasingly felt that laser therapy offers significant benefits over traditional treatments, which are typically expensive and time-consuming and, most important of all in the case of racehorses, involve long periods of rest. A typical example would be the condition commonly termed 'bowed tendon' (tendinitis), which can mean resting the animal for a period of a year or more. During such periods the injured horse cannot race, with concomitant loss of revenue, and may require an extensive period of rehabilitation and retraining before returning to competition, giving rise to considerable expense for the owners. It is not surprising that an increasing number of veterinary surgeons and physiotherapists are eager to try therapeutic laser in an attempt to reduce significantly recovery time and thus expense for clients, nor indeed that the papers published in this particular field are almost exclusively concerned with equine practice.

In the United States the FDA has no regulatory authority over the use of therapeutic lasers in animal practice, which may explain why the majority of papers published on this particular application have originated from America.

Indications for laser treatment

The main indications for low-intensity laser therapy in veterinary practice (McKibben 1983, Bromiley 1990) are:

1. Relief of pain, principally musculoskeletal pain syndromes of various aetiologies. These include dorso-lumbar pain, splints, rigbones, plantar desmitis ('curb'), check ligaments tendinopathies ('bowed tendon') and fetlock forsians with oedema.

2. Promotion of wound healing processes through laser photo-biostimulation. Laser therapy has been successfully used, principally in equine practice, to accelerate the healing of postoperative incisions and burns, and to enhance recovery from soft tissue trauma.

3. Treatment of respiratory tract infections in horses. Applied to the sides of the neck and the underside of the throat, low-energy laser has been successfully employed as an adjunctive treatment in the management of pharyngeal lymphoid hyperplasia and other respiratory tract infections.

4. Reversal of neuropraxia, including radial paralysis in the horse and vertebral nerve compressions in small animal practice. While the precise mechanism(s) of action underlying this application is unclear, the positive results reported by a number of clinicians are supported by well documented evidence from controlled laboratory-based research on animals (see Ch. 6).

5. Improvement of the rate of foot growth in horses. Laser irradiation of the coronary band has apparently been successfully used to improve the texture and rate of growth of the hoof wall.

Laser acupuncture

In addition to the other uses and applications already outlined, usually based upon the direct application of laser to the lesion or site of pain etc., some clinicians and authors have also recommended the use of low-intensity laser radiation as an alternative to metal needles in acupuncture treatments, most commonly for the relief of pain (Kroetlinger 1980). This irradiation of acupuncture points with low-intensity laser is commonly known as *laser acupuncture*, and a number of commercially available laser systems are specifically advertised as being suitable for this type of treatment. The appeal of using laser in such treatments is obvious given current fears of infection by viruses such as HIV or hepatitis through the use of invasive procedures. Apart from the decreased risk of infection, some practitioners have also reported that very young or nervous patients may sometimes respond better to laser rather than traditional (needle) acupuncture. Furthermore, laser has also come to be recognised as a practical and effective alternative to needles for auricular acupuncture treatments.

As already indicated above, the pioneering work in this field was carried out during the early 1970s by Dr Friedrich Plog of Canada (see e.g. Plog 1980). Based upon Plog's early work, a number of He–Ne laser systems were subsequently developed specifically for acupuncture treatments, principally in China, Japan and the Soviet Union (e.g. Kamikawa 1983). In these countries, laser acupuncture represents an important field for low-intensity laser application, with trials having been success-fully completed for a range of conditions including exophthalmic hyper-thyroidism, pelvic inflammation and particularly for the relief of a range of painful conditions (Wei 1981, Wu 1983, Qin 1987, Ohshiro & Calderhead 1988, Shiroto et al 1989, Baxter 1989). While laser acupunc-ture does not enjoy the same level of acceptance in the West, its popu-larity and use is increasing, particularly through the use of laser diodes as an alternative to acupuncture needles in the deactivation of painful musculoskeletal trigger points.

SUMMARY OF KEY POINTS

1. LASER is an acronym for Light Amplification by Stimulated Emission of Radiation.
2. The first laser was produced in 1960, based upon a ruby crystal.
3. Lasers operating at relatively high power and energy levels have found application in a range of medical and surgical specialties.
4. In contrast to other medical and surgical applications of laser which usually rely upon photothermal mechanisms of action, low-intensity laser therapy (LILT) is by definition athermic, causing no biologically significant rise in temperature in the tissues so irradiated.
5. LILT has been used successfully in a number of fields, including physiotherapy, veterinary medicine, dentistry and as an alternative to metal needles in acupuncture.

REFERENCES

Agov B S, Devyatkov N D, Zhuk A E et al 1982 Treatment of angina pectoris by helium–neon laser. Klinicheskaia Meditsina 5: 65–67
ASLMS (American Society of Laser Medicine and Surgery) 1988 Introduction to laser biophysics. Rockwell Laser Industries, Longwood, Florida
Basford J R 1986 Low energy laser treatment of pain and wounds: hype, hope or hokum? Mayo Clinic Proceedings 61: 671–675
Basford J R 1989 Low-energy laser therapy: controversies and new research findings. Lasers in Surgery and Medicine 9: 1–5
Baxter G D 1989 Laser acupuncture analgesia: an overview. Acupuncture in Medicine 6: 57–60
Baxter G D, Bell A J, Allen J M et al 1991 Low level laser therapy: current clinical practice in Northern Ireland. Physiotherapy 77: 171–178
Bernhard O 1926 Light treatment in surgery. Edward Arnold, London
Bridges W B 1964 Laser oscillation in singly ionised argon in the visible spectrum. Applied Physics Letters 4: 128–130
Bromiley M W 1991 Physiotherapy in veterinary medicine. Blackwell Scientific, London
Burgudjieva T, Katranushkova N, Blazeva P 1985 Laser therapy of complicated wounds after obstetric and gynecologic operations. Akusherstvo I Ginekologiia 6: 60–69

Calderhead G, Ohshiro T, Itoh E et al 1982 The Nd:YAG and GaAlAs lasers: a comparative analysis in pain therapy. Laser Acupuncture 21: 1–4

Carruth J A S, McKenzie A L 1986 Medical lasers: science and clinical practice. Adam Hilger, Bristol

Cauvin J F 1815 Des bienfaits de l'insolation. Paris

Christensen P 1989 Clinical laser treatment of odontological conditions. In: Kert J, Rose L 1989 Clinical laser therapy: low level laser therapy. Scandinavian Medical Laser Technology, Copenhagen

Cuncliffe W J 1973 Diseases of the skin. Acne vulgaris. British Medical Journal 4: 667–669

Devor M 1990 What's in a beam for pain therapy? Pain 43: 139

Dotsenko A P, Grubnik V V, Melnichenko Yu A M 1985 Use of the helium–neon laser in the complex treatment of duodenal ulcer. Klinicheskaia Khirurgiia 8: 21–23

Downes A, Blunt T P 1877 Researches on the effect of light upon bacteria and other organisms. Proceedings of the Royal Society 26A: 488–500

Editorial 1989 New developments in phototherapy. Lancet 1 (8647): 1116

Ennever J F 1988 Phototherapy for neonatal jaundice. Photochemistry and Photobiology 47: 871–876

Finsen N R 1899 La Phototherapie. Carre et Naud, Paris

Flocks M, Zweng H C 1964 Laser coagulation of ocular tissues. Archives of Opthalmology 72: 604

Frain-Bell W 1985 Cutaneous photobiology. Oxford University Press, Oxford

Goldman L, Wilson R, Hornby P et al 1965 Laser radiation of malignancy in man. Cancer 18: 533–545

Goldman J A, Chiapella J, Casey H et al 1980 Laser therapy of rheumatoid arthritis. Lasers in Surgery and Medicine 1: 93–101

Gordon J P, Zeiger H J, Townes C H 1955 The maser. New type of amplifier, frequency standard and spectrometer. Physics Review 99: 1264–1274

Goujon C, Divol J, Moulin G 1985 Preliminary results of mid laser treatment of chronic ulcerations of the legs. Lasers in Surgery and Medicine 5: 78

Hansen T, Bratlid T, Lingjarde O et al 1987 Midwinter insomnia in the subartic region: evening levels of serum melatonin and cortisol before and after treatment with bright artificial light. Acta Psychiatria Scandinavica 75: 428–430

Kamikawa K 1983 Development of laser acupuncture systems and their clinical applications. In: Atsumi K (ed) 1983 New frontiers in laser medicine and surgery. Excerpta Medica, Amsterdam

Kamikawa K, Kyoto J 1985 Double blind experiences with mid-lasers in Japan. International Congress Laser Medicine Surgery. Monduzzi Editore, Bologna

Keele K D 1957 Anatomies of pain. Charles C Thomas, Springfield, IL

Kenicer K J A, Laksmipathi T, Addo H A et al 1981 An assessment of the effect of photochemotherapy (PUVA) and UVB phototherapy in the treatment of psoriasis. British Journal of Dermatology 105: 629–632

Kleinkort J A, Foley R A 1984 Laser acupuncture: its use in physical therapy. American Journal of Acupuncture 12: 51

Kripke D F 1985 Therapeutic effects of bright light in depressed patients. Annals of the New York Academy of Science 453: 270–281

Kroetlinger M 1980 On the use of laser in acupuncture. International Journal of Acupuncture and Electrotherapeutics Research 5: 297–311

Krusen F H 1933 Light therapy. New York

Lewy A J, Kern H A, Rosenthal N E et al 1982 Bright artificial light treatment of a manic-depressive patient with a seasonal mood disorder. American Journal Psychiatry 139: 1496–1498

Licht S 1983 History of ultra-violet therapy. In: Stillwell G K (ed) 1983 Therapeutic electricity and ultra-violet radiation, 3rd edn. Williams & Wilkins, Baltimore

McKibben L S 1983 An evaluation of the effects of the low-energy laser on soft tissue in horses. In: Atsumi K (ed) 1983 New frontiers in laser medicine and surgery. Excerpta Medica, Amsterdam

Mester E, Mester A E, Mester A 1985 The biomedical effect of laser application. Lasers in Surgery and Medicine 5: 31–39

Mills O H, Kligman A M 1978 Ultraviolet phototherapy and photochemo-therapy of acne vulgaris. Archives of Dermatology 114: 221–223

Minton J P, Carlton D M, Dearman J R et al 1965 An evaluation of the physical response of malignant tumour implants to pulsed laser radiation. Surgery, Gynecology and Obstetrics 121: 538–544

Ohshiro T, Calderhead R G 1988 Low level laser therapy: a practical introduction. Wiley, Chichester

Palm T A 1890 The geographical distribution and aetiology of rickets. Practitioner 14: 270–273

Patel C K N 1965 CW high-power N_2–CO_2 laser. Applied Physics Letters 7: 15–17

Plog F M W 1980 Biophysical application of the laser beam. In: Koebner H K 1980 Lasers in Medicine. Wiley, New York

Prime D 1983 Harmful effects of ultra-violet radiation from sunray lamps. Journal of the Royal Society of Health 103: 161–164

Qin J N 1987 Laser acupuncture anaesthesia and therapy in People's Republic of China. Annals of the Academy of Medicine of Singapore 16: 261–63

Rowbottom M, Susskind C 1984 Electricity and medicine. History of their interaction. San Francisco Press, San Francisco

Saidman J 1930 Introduction à l'actinotherapie rationelle: la sensiometrie cutanée. Doin, Paris

Schawlow A L, Townes C H 1958 Infrared and optical masers. Physics Review 112: 1940–1949

Scott B O 1983 Clinical uses of ultraviolet radiation. In: Stillwell G K (ed) 1983 Therapeutic electricity and ultraviolet radiation, 3rd edn. Williams & Wilkins, Baltimore

Shiroto C, Ono K, Ohshiro T 1989 Retrospective study of diode laser therapy for pain attenuation in 3635 patients: detailed analysis by questionnaire. Laser Therapy 1: 41–48

Wehr T A, Rosenthal N E, Sack D A 1988 Environmental and behavioural influences on affective illness. Acta Psychiatria Scandinavica (Suppl) 341: 44–52

Wei X 1981 Laser treatment of common diseases in surgery and acupuncture in the People's Republic of China: preliminary report. International Journal of Acupuncture and Electrotherapeutics Research 6: 19–31

Wu W 1983 Recent advances in laserpuncture. In: Atsumi K (ed) New frontiers in laser medicine and surgery. Elsevier, Amsterdam

Zhou Yo Cheng 1988 Laser acupuncture anaesthesia. In: Ohshiro T, Calderhead R G 1988 Low level laser therapy: A practical introduction. Wiley, Chichester

Zweng H C 1971 Lasers in opthalmology. In: Wolbarsht M L (ed) 1971 Laser applications in medicine and biology. Plenum Press, New York

2. Laser physics

INTRODUCTION

The primary purpose of this chapter is to present, simply and succinctly, the relevant physical principles underlying the production of laser radiation by therapeutic units and to outline the special characteristics of such radiation. To this end, unnecessary complexity has been avoided as far as is possible. However, some review of the basics of opto-physics is essential in order to provide a basis for the discussions presented in later chapters, particularly Chapters 3 and 4 which the current chapter is intended to complement, and in order to equip the reader for more critical review of the published literature on therapeutic laser.

At the outset of this chapter, it is important to draw the reader's attention to two important points which are covered in more detail below. The first is that while 'Laser' is the acronym for '*Light* Amplification by Stimulated Emission of Radiation', the term is equally applied to devices producing radiation in the infra-red and ultra-violet (and therefore invisible) portions of the electromagnetic spectrum (see Table 1.1). Indeed, the majority of therapeutic devices currently available produce infra-red rather than visible radiation.

Secondly, the term 'laser' is rather loosely applied within the field of LILT, and has been used to refer to devices which technically are not 'pure' lasers. The reason for this is that a certain amount of debate still exists as to the clinical necessity for pure (and therefore relatively expensive) laser systems, with some insisting that some of the characteristics of laser such as coherence and polarisation (which are considered further below) are unnecessary and expensive options on clinical laser therapy devices. Thus some manufacturers have produced and marketed therapeutic systems based upon non-coherent superluminous diodes (commonly abbreviated to SLDs) rather than more expensive laser emitting diodes. While this debate is presented in more detail below, the reader should be aware from the outset that for the moment a definitive answer is not forthcoming from the literature; in common with a lot of aspects of laser therapy, more research is still required.

The electromagnetic spectrum and quantum theory

The term 'electromagnetic radiation' may sound very grandiose (and not a little awesome!), but in fact describes a variety of common phenomena. The electromagnetic spectrum (Fig. 2.1) spans X-rays, radio waves and visible light as well as infra-red and ultra-violet radiation. It therefore encompasses, in addition to the radiation produced by therapeutic lasers, that which forms the basis of other common physiotherapeutic treatment modalities such as short wave (radio frequency) diathermy, pulsed electromagnetic energy, microwave, ultra-violet and infra-red. What these apparently very different types of radiation have in common is that they all comprise alternating electrical and magnetic fields which fluctuate in synchrony and perpendicularly to the direction of propagation (Fig. 2.2). The strength of the electrical field rises first to a positive maximum, then falls through zero to a negative maximum, before rising again to zero and on to complete another cycle. This sinusoidal fluctuation in the electrical field is mirrored (at right angles) by an identical variation in the magnetic field.

It is this combination of fluctuating electrical and magnetic fields that gives such radiation the name 'electromagnetic'. What distinguishes radio waves from X-rays, and microwaves from ultra-violet radiation, is the *frequency* of these fluctuations in their electromagnetic fields over time. Similarly, wavelength also characterises electromagnetic radiation (Fig. 2.2), as higher frequencies are synonymous with shorter wavelengths and vice versa. The precise relationship between frequency and wavelength is summarised in the equation:

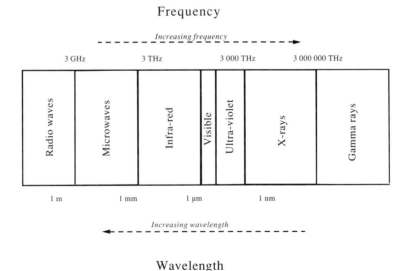

Fig. 2.1 The electromagnetic spectrum.

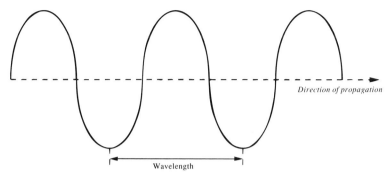

Fig. 2.2   The wave-like nature of light.

$$\lambda = c/f$$

where: λ = wavelength of light in metres
          c = speed of light in metres per second
          f = frequency in hertz ('per second').

The wavelengths in that portion of the spectrum in which therapeutic lasers operate are very small and are usually measured in fractions of a metre, for instance nanometre (abbreviated nm = 1/1 000 000 000 or 10^{-9} metres), or micrometre (abbreviated μm = 1/1 000 000 or 10^{-6} metres). Considering the figure of the electromagnetic spectrum (Fig. 2.1) the term 'laser' as used in LILT embraces a range of electromagnetic radiation of various wavelengths from (approximately) 600–1000 nm, including both visible (red) radiation at the lower end of the visible range and invisible (near infra-red) radiation.

So far, this discussion has concentrated on light (and indeed electro-magnetic energy generally) as if it were composed of waves. This view is commonly referred to as the Maxwell concept and is a valid and useful way of thinking about such radiation, and particularly light. In addition to considering light as a propagated waveform, physicists such as Planck and Einstein proposed at the turn of the century that it was also possible to consider radiation as being composed of quanta (packets) of energy in minute particles called photons. This idea of electromagnetic energy being at once both wavelike and particulate is nothing out of the ordinary for physicists, yet most lay people tend to get confused and ask which is the most appropriate (or 'real') concept. The simple answer is that light is essentially both, for it can be regarded as simultaneously existing as both a waveform and as a beam of particles. The key point is that it is useful (at least theoretically) to consider light as one or the other, depending on the situation. Thus, when accounting for photoelectric effects, physicists find that it is more useful to consider light as photons; in explaining the relationship between frequency and wavelength it is easier and more practical to consider light as a waveform.

It is important to bear in mind that the two concepts are not mutually exclusive. Rather the two are linked, in that there is a fixed relationship between the energy carried by an individual photon of light and its associated wavelength. The photons of a particular wavelength of light all have a discrete, invariable quantal energy, the amount of which can be calculated from the light's inherent frequency by Planck's constant. The formula for this is:

$$E = hf$$

where: E = energy of the photon in joules
h = Planck's constant
f = frequency of the light in hertz.

Given that wavelength and frequency are related as already described on p. 25, a simple substitution into the above equation gives the following:

$$E = \frac{hc}{\lambda}$$

where: E = energy of the photon in joules
h = Planck's constant
c = speed of light in metres per second
λ = wavelength of light in metres.

If the second of these equations is considered, it can be seen that the shorter wavelengths of light are associated with photons carrying higher quantal energies. Conversely, photons from the longest wavelengths of light in the red and infra-red portions of the spectrum carry relatively low quantal energies. Note that the amount of energy carried by a photon is extremely small and is therefore usually expressed in electronvolts. The photon energies that appear to be important for laser photobiomodulation are usually found within the 1–2 electronvolt range.

PRINCIPAL COMPONENTS OF A LASER SYSTEM

In order to produce laser radiation, the laser device ('laser' applying as equally to the means of production as to the resultant radiation) must consist of three essential components: these are presented schematically in Figure 2.3 and are described in detail below.

Lasing medium

A lasing medium is a material which is capable of absorbing the energy produced by an external excitation source through changes in the sub-atomic configuration of its component molecules, atoms or ions, and to subsequently give off this excess energy as photons of light. This is usually achieved through the excitation of electrons to higher energy levels,

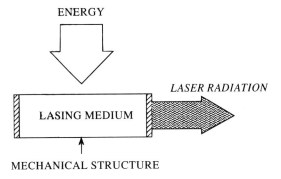

ENERGY

LASER RADIATION

LASING MEDIUM

MECHANICAL STRUCTURE

Fig. 2.3   Laser: principal components.

with photons of light being generated as these electrons drop to lower energy bands (see below). Lasing media can be gaseous, liquid, solid crystal or semiconductor.

While examples of all these types of lasing media can be found in various medical and surgical applications, for the laser systems commonly used in low-intensity laser therapy the medium will either be gaseous (i.e. He–Ne), or semiconductors based upon gallium arsenide (GaAs) or gallium aluminium arsenide (GaAlAs) diodes. This latter type of medium comprises a so called 'p–n junction', which is similar in many respects to the light emitting diodes (LEDs) commonly found in stereos or on the dashboard consoles of cars. Such semiconductors can be thought of as comprising two halves, each containing either positive 'holes' or electrons. Under the influence of an external electrical potential, these charged particles may 'hop' across the junction into the active region of the semiconductor to interact with each other and in so doing give off photons of light (see 'Laser emission: sequence of events' below).

The selection of the lasing medium used in the production of a laser is vitally important as this dictates the wavelength(s) of the machine's output, and hence (for visible radiation) the apparent colour of the radiation produced by a given device. Because of this, the medium is frequently used to describe the laser apparatus used in a particular piece of research or clinical report, rather than specifying the wavelength of the laser's emitted radiation. Thus, for example, sales representatives or published papers may refer to a 'He–Ne laser' or a 'gallium arsenide laser'. It should be noted however that while the wavelengths associated with GaAs or He–Ne laser systems are fixed at 904 nm and 632.8 nm respectively, the same cannot be said of gallium *aluminium* arsenide (GaAlAs) systems. In these the wavelength of the radiation emitted by the device is dependent upon the amount of aluminium used in the manufacture of the unit's laser diode; such semiconductor diodes can be manufactured to produce radiation at various wavelengths ranging from the visible red to the near infra-red parts of the spectrum.

While the lasing media commonly used in commercially available therapeutic laser systems typically produce only a single wavelength of emitted laser light, it is worthy of note that a number of the other media routinely used in medical applications simultaneously generate more than one wavelength of laser radiation (see Table 1.1). A good example of this is the argon laser, which because of the subatomic structure of the active argon ion produces no less than 10 different wavelengths. However, the predominance of output at 488 nm and 514 nm gives the output of these laser devices a blue-green appearance.

Energy source

An energy source is used to excite or 'pump' the lasing medium to the higher energy levels that are necessary for the production of laser radiation (see below). For the types of lasing media commonly found in therapeutic applications, i.e. gaseous or semiconductor, this excitation source is invariably electrical, such systems usually being driven from a local mains power supply. For therapeutic systems which are intended to be more portable (e.g. for use in sports medicine), a rechargeable power unit may also be provided by the manufacturer as the electrical energy source. However with other types of laser media, chemical or optical energy may also be used. The latter is typically employed with tuneable dye lasers (i.e. liquid media), or the types of solid crystal based system (e.g. Nd:YAG) more commonly found in (high-power) medical laser applications.

Mechanical structure

The mechanical structure contains the lasing medium within a central chamber, with two 'mirrors' at either end. These mirrors are normally selectively reflective to the wavelength of light produced by the machine, and are precisely mounted so that they are exactly parallel to one another, with (for coherent sources) the distance between them fixed at a multiple of the laser's wavelength. This arrangement allows for the reflection of photons of light back and forward across the chamber, eventually resulting in the production of an intense photon resonance within the medium. While the reflectance of one of these two mirrors is for all practical purposes 100%, the reflectance of the other is slightly less and consequently this second mirror (sometimes called the output coupler) allows a small percentage of the photons incident upon it to escape as the output of the device.

In the case of semiconductor lasing media, the ends of the diode (p–n junction) can be highly polished to act as mirrors. Additionally, an increasing number of the commercially available diode-based therapeutic units have lenses incorporated into the mechanical structure as an integral part of the unit. Such lenses help to concentrate the output of the therapeutic unit onto a smaller area of target tissue and thus increase the density of photons on the irradiated tissue.

The mechanical structure may also provide the mounting for the energy source and for the control devices (e.g. most He–Ne systems), or provide suitable terminals for connection to a separate control unit. For the type of semiconductor laser system most commonly used in therapeutic laser applications, the mechanical structure containing the lasing media is mounted within a hand-held treatment unit or probe, which is usually connected by flex to a separate control unit.

LASER EMISSION: SEQUENCE OF EVENTS

Precisely how radiation is generated by a particular laser device will vary slightly depending upon the lasing media used in its construction. For the purposes of this text, the following will concentrate upon a description of the sequence of events leading to output of laser radiation in He–Ne and semiconductor-based systems.

Absorption, spontaneous and stimulated emission of radiation

By way of background to the following account, it is first necessary to outline the processes of absorption, spontaneous emission and stimulated emission of radiation at subatomic level. These processes are depicted schematically in Figures 2.4a–d respectively.

Figure 2.4a represents the atomic energy levels within a hypothetical atom of the lasing medium. Under normal circumstances, the vast majority of atoms comprising the lasing medium remain at the lowest energy level (i.e. with their electrons at E_0). This 'resting' energy level is termed the *ground state*. When energy is supplied from an outside energy source, this may be *absorbed* by the atom through excitation of its electrons to a higher energy level (i.e. E_1, E_2 or E_3). This method of energy absorption is depicted in Figure 2.4b. Once in this excited state, atoms are inherently unstable and therefore cannot, and do not, remain at this higher level for very long. Instead, their electrons *spontaneously* return or 'drop' to resting levels and in so doing give off their previously absorbed excess energy as a photon of light. This type of light production is therefore termed spontaneous emission, and represents the means by which most light sources (i.e. incandescent and fluorescent sources) produce their output.

These processes of absorption and spontaneous emission are governed by the laws of subatomic physics. Most notably these state that for energy to be absorbed by the hypothetical atom in Figure 2.4b, the amount of energy delivered must exactly match the difference between ground or resting state (E_0) and one of the other energy levels available within the atom (in this hypothetical example, E_3). Similarly, the quanta ('bundle') of energy released or emitted by the atom when moving from its excited

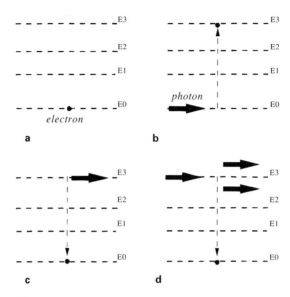

Fig. 2.4 Absorption, spontaneous and stimulated emission. **a.** Hypothetical atom at ground state. **b.** Absorption of incident photon. **c.** Spontaneous emission of photon. **d.** Stimulated emission of radiation.

to its resting state is fixed and precisely equal to the difference in energy levels through which the electron 'falls'. The distance through which the electron falls (i.e. the difference in the respective energy levels E_3–E_0) therefore determines the quantal energy of the emitted photon. Furthermore, as we have already seen, the energy carried by a photon is inversely related to wavelength, thus the difference in energy levels E_3–E_0 in turn dictates the wavelength of the light produced by this atom in returning to its ground state. As the energy difference E_3–E_0 becomes greater, so the wavelength of the light emitted by the atom decreases and vice versa.

In contrast to spontaneous emission, stimulated emission of radiation (Fig. 2.4d) occurs where an atom that has already been excited to a higher energy level is stimulated to emit a photon of light by an incident photon. For stimulated emission of radiation to occur the incident photon must have a quantal energy exactly equal to the amount of energy which will be released when the electron, and thus the atom, returns to its resting state (i.e. E_3–E_0). This condition is vitally important, as without it stimulated emission of radiation will not take place. It is this process of stimulated emission which produces the special characteristics of laser radiation which are described in more detail below. Most importantly, the second, stimulated photon will be identical in all respects to the incident photon which stimulated its production. This results in the production of coherent light (see below), as the photon produced by stimulated emission will be 'in step', in phase, with the incident photon.

Production of laser radiation by He–Ne units

These events are summarised schematically in Figure 2.5. Once the unit is activated, electrical energy is delivered to the lasing medium (Fig. 2.5a) as already described above. Initially this energy will result in excitation of the neon atoms, neon being the active medium within He–Ne units. Within such lasers the helium merely acts as a buffer gas, assisting with excitation of the neon atoms and cooling processes. Spontaneous emission of radiation from the neon atoms occurs readily as the excited state is inherently unstable.

However, the rate of supply of energy to the neon atoms within the medium is far greater than that dissipated through the process of spontaneous emission by these atoms. Consequently, after a short period of time the majority of the neon atoms will be in the higher energy states. This condition is known as *population inversion*: instead of the majority of neon atoms being at resting states and relatively few at higher energy levels, as is normally the case, the reverse situation occurs.

The majority of photons produced by the neon atoms during this initial stage of (predominantly) spontaneous emission, depicted in Figure 2.5b as photons P1, P2 and P3, are lost. However any photons which strike the reflecting surfaces (the 'mirrors') will be reflected according to basic physical principles, so that the angle of reflection equals the angle of incidence (e.g. photons P4, P5 and P6). Consequently any photons incident upon the mirrors at right angles to its plane will be reflected back along their incident path and will traverse the length of the laser's resonating

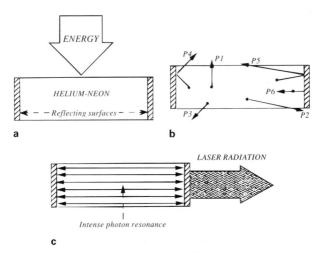

Fig. 2.5 Emission from He–Ne laser: sequence of events. **a.** Initial activation of unit supplies energy to medium. **b.** Spontaneous emission of photons by medium. **c.** Stimulated emission leads to intense photon resonance.

cavity, subsequently being reflected back and forth between the parallel mirrors (P6).

Over a period of time, photons parallel to that depicted as P6 will encounter, on their successive travels back and forth between the mirrors, atoms already in their excited state. When such a collision occurs, stimulated emission results: the photon's impaction causing the excited electron to fall to its resting state and give off a photon of exactly the same energy, due to the fact that the excited atom is identical in terms of subatomic structure to the one that produced the original photon.

After a further period, the number of parallel photons moving back and forth between the mirrors grows dramatically, as an intense photon resonance builds up. At this point some of the intense light produced within the chamber leaks out through the partially transmissive optical coupler. Thus the device emits laser light as shown in Figure 2.5c.

Production of laser radiation by semiconductor systems

As indicated above, for semiconductor-based systems both the structure of the laser and the means of laser production differ somewhat to that already described for He–Ne-based systems. The structure of a typical semiconductor laser is represented schematically in Figure 2.6. Under the influence of an externally applied electrical field, positively charged 'holes' are injected from the p-type gallium aluminium arsenide layer downwards into a so-called *active layer* of gallium arsenide. Simultaneously, electrons are driven upwards into the active layer from the *n*-type layer of gallium aluminium arsenide. As the excess populations of holes and electrons interact within the active layer the energy produced by the combination of electron and hole is released as a photon of light, the precise quantal energy and thus the wavelength of which is determined by the amount of aluminium present within the gallium aluminium arsenide layers.

In a similar manner to that already described above for He–Ne lasers, photons which strike the highly polished ends of the semiconductor at

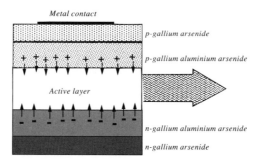

Fig. 2.6 Semiconductor laser: gross structure.

right angles are reflected back and forward within the active gallium arsenide layer, eventually causing an intense photon resonance within this layer. 'Leakage' through one of the polished ends of the semiconductor diode allows a percentage of the photons to escape, and thus the device emits laser light.

CHARACTERISTICS OF LASER LIGHT AND BASIC TERMINOLOGY

Laser devices produce very intense beams of light which differ from the type of light produced by other, non-laser, sources in a number of important respects. Most notably, laser light differs from ordinary light by being *monochromatic*, highly *directional* and *coherent*.

Unfortunately the terms used to describe these differences and, perhaps more importantly, their relevance to the clinical application of lasers in low-intensity laser therapy are poorly understood. Consequently the following will, in the first instance, provide working definitions of the majority of the terms commonly used when discussing the physics of therapeutic lasers, and outline briefly the possible clinical significance of each of the special properties which serve to characterise laser light.

Monochromaticity and wavelength

As far as biological and clinical effects are concerned, monochromaticity is considered perhaps the most important attribute of laser light, and distinguishes the radiation produced by such devices from that produced by other commonly used light sources. Consider Figure 2.7a. This represents in diagrammatic form the output in terms of wavelength (i.e. *spectral emission*) produced by an average domestic light bulb or fluorescent tube. It can be appreciated immediately from this figure that a range

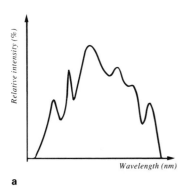
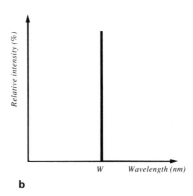

a   b

Fig. 2.7 Monochromaticity and wavelength. **a.** Typical spectral emission from non-laser source. **b.** Spectral emission from laser source.

of wavelengths is produced by such light sources. As each of the wavelengths within the visible range corresponds to a colour, the radiation produced by such sources produces a sensation of the colour white when it is focussed onto the retina. In contrast, Figure 2.7b represents the emission spectra of a typical laser, which can be seen to be clustered around a single, central value of W nm, with very little spread of wavelengths (or *bandwidth*) about this value. As this wavelength W nm corresponds to a single colour, the light produced by a laser source is consequently said to be highly *mono-* (single) *chromatic* (coloured).

It should be stressed at this point that even the infra-red and ultra-violet lamps which still commonly find application in clinical practice produce a selection of wavelengths within a certain limited range, so that while the name used to describe the radiation produced by these devices might suggest that they are monochromatic, this is in fact incorrect. It should be apparent from Figure 2.1 that the terms ultra-violet and infra-red are used to describe a wide range of wavelengths within the electromagnetic spectrum. Thus, even if it were possible to provide equal dosages of each modality, irradiation of tissue with an infra-red laser would not be directly comparable to an equivalent dosage of radiation delivered by an infra-red treatment lamp.

Absorption and wavelength specificity

As already outlined, wavelength and photon energy are linked by Planck's constant, so that for a given laser all the photons produced by that particular system have exactly the same quantal energy. For absorption of light to occur by an atom, the quantal energy carried by each of the laser's photons must exactly equal the energy required by one of the atom's electrons to move from its lower (ground) energy state to a higher energy state. In Figure 2.4b, this photon absorption was represented by the transition of the electron from ground state (E_0) to the highest available energy level (E_3). In other words, given the formula presented on p. 26, the following condition applied:

$$E_3 - E_0 = hf$$

where: E = electron's energy at a given orbit/valence band
h = Planck's constant
f = frequency of the incident laser radiation.

As has already been stated above, the electron cannot be raised to some 'intermediate' energy level, it can only absorb that precise amount or quanta of energy that represents the difference in energies between the two states. Photon absorption is thus dependent upon subatomic structure, being dictated by the differences in energy between the various valence levels within the atom. These energy levels vary from molecule to molecule, atom to atom, and ion to ion. For the case depicted in Figure 2.4, the quantal energies which this hypothetical atom is capable of absorbing would be: $E_3–E_0$, $E_2–E_0$, and $E_1–E_0$ respectively. Thus, as a photon's quantal energy dictates its wavelength and vice versa, this atom can only absorb three *specific* wavelengths of incident radiation. These three wavelengths are collectively known as the *absorption spectra* of the atom and are specific to it. Thus, absorption for a given atom is sometimes said to be *wavelength specific*.

In moving from the hypothetical to the conditions applying within biological tissue, the main difference is that atoms such as the hypothetical example considered here are rarely found in isolation in tissue, but are usually encountered only as small components within the much larger, complex molecules found in tissue. However the conditions described above apply equally to such biological molecules (or *biomolecules*). Consequently the various biomolecules contained within a volume of tissue irradiated during an LILT treatment will differ from one another in their absorption spectra and thus the wavelengths of radiation which they are capable of absorbing. The wavelength specificity of absorption is one of the single most important concepts in laser photobiomodulation and represents the reason why clinical or research results obtained with a laser unit operating at one wavelength cannot necessarily be expected after irradiation with an alternative unit operating at another wavelength. Absorption is considered further in Chapter 4.

Collimation and divergence

Non-laser light sources typically radiate uniformly in all directions. Attempts to produce parallel beams of light with such sources, e.g. through the use of lenses, are at best only partially successful. In contrast, the output from a laser is highly *collimated*. Collimation simply refers to the degree of 'parallelity' of the emitted light beam, consequently describing lasers as being highly collimated means that the emitted light is highly parallel. However, there is usually no specification of collimation given with commercial laser treatment systems, instead *divergence* is more usually quoted in manufacturers' literature. This is essentially the opposite of collimation and is the angle of 'spread' of the emitted beam. (Fig. 2.8). The value of divergence is usually quite small and is in the range of 3–10° for an average diode-based system. This angle varies greatly between treatment units. He–Ne systems are the most highly collimated systems in routine clinical use in therapeutic applications, however it should be stressed that the divergence of such systems is increased by several factors when a fibreoptic applicator is used in conjunction with these lasers, as the small aperture at the end of the applicator serves to increase the divergence.

The clinical significance of collimation/divergence is twofold. Firstly,

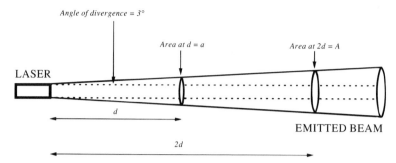

Fig. 2.8 Divergence. *NB*: Doubling the distance between the source and the target tissue squares the area of irradiation (i.e. $A = a^2$). The intensity of radiation is therefore proportionately decreased (inverse square law).

highly collimated beams maintain a small spot size over a relatively large distance. Therefore higher collimation equates with a potentially greater ocular hazard (see Ch. 3). Secondly, the specified power output of therapeutic laser devices is usually as measured at the point of emission of the laser light: the output coupler at the end of the treatment head or fibreoptic tube. If such treatment units are used out of contact with the irradiated/target tissue, for example when treating an open wound, those treatment units with relatively greater divergence will produce relatively larger spot sizes on the surface of the irradiated tissue (Fig. 2.8).

As the total radiant power output of the unit is essentially fixed, such increases in irradiated area equate to relatively smaller power densities on the irradiated site (Fig. 2.8). Consequently when recording such *non-contact* treatments for research papers, the divergence of the unit used and the distance between the treatment head and the target tissue should be specified. In clinical applications, the distance between the treatment head and the treated tissue should be kept as small as possible as the intensity of the laser irradiation is so drastically reduced by increases in distance. The precise relationship between distance and relative intensity of irradiation over the treatment site is given by the so called 'inverse square law' (Fig. 2.8).

Coherence

Coherence refers to the inherent 'synchronicity' of the radiation produced by lasers. Consider Figure 2.9a, which represents in diagrammatic form the radiation produced by a normal everyday light source (e.g. a fluorescent light tube). The main means by which such light is produced is spontaneous emission of radiation, which has already been described above (see Fig. 2.4c). With a true laser, the emitted light is coherent (Fig. 2.9b). This implies two things simultaneously. In the first instance laser light is temporally coherent, the photons being in phase or 'in step', with the crests and troughs of the individual waves of light matching each other

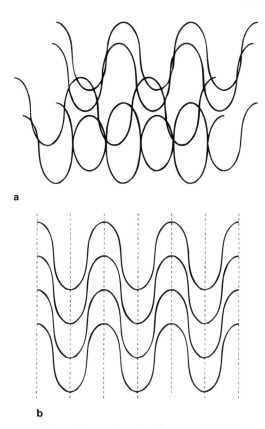

Fig. 2.9 Coherence. **a.** Non-coherent (non-laser) source. **b.** Coherent source.

precisely. Furthermore the light emitted from laser devices possesses spatial coherence, meaning that the photons are essentially unidirectional and stay in phase over very long distances, with relatively little beam spread.

The biological and clinical significance of coherence is not at all clear. Indeed, Karu (1987), based upon her findings in bacterial and cell cultures, has insisted that coherence is not an important factor in photobiological reactions. This is supported by the findings of Dyson's group at Guy's Hospital in London, whose work on macrophage- and fibroblast-like cell lines has demonstrated significant photobiostimulative effects using non-coherent light sources (e.g. Young et al 1989). Findings from the cellular research completed to date in this area are reviewed and considered further in Chapter 5.

A note on superluminous diodes

Findings at the cellular level would imply that the property of coherence is largely unnecessary for the *clinical* effects of low-intensity laser therapy.

Such a contention would appear to be supported by the fact that the temporal coherence of a laser beam is largely lost by the time the incident beam has passed through the first millimetre of irradiated tissue. Consequently, as already indicated at the start of this chapter, despite use of the terms 'laser' therapy, 'laser' biomodulation etc., a growing number of manufacturers do not provide coherent (laser) diodes with their apparatus, but instead use non-coherent and thus relatively cheaper superluminous diodes or SLDs. These diodes produce light or infra-red radiation which is both highly monochromatic and collimated but is non-coherent. This means that the units are easier (i.e. cheaper) to manufacture. Consequently the multiwavelength/multidiode arrays or so called 'cluster' heads which are commonly used in laser treatments usually combine no more than a couple of laser diodes, the remainder being SLDs. Such units would be prohibitively expensive if they were based solely upon laser-emitting diodes. While these cluster units have been in wide clinical usage for some time now, with no obvious difference in efficacy in comparison to true lasers (Baxter et al 1991), many sources still maintain the requirement for coherent sources in clinical applications (e.g. Moore & Calderhead 1991).

Polarisation

The term polarisation is familiar to most people through commercially available 'polarised' sunglasses, which help limit glare by allowing only light polarised within a single plane to pass through their lenses. In polarised light, the waves of light are all orientated within the one plane, so that the fluctuations or vibrations in their electrical fields occur in a single direction, rather than the random orientation typically found in the light produced by non-laser sources. A polarised output beam can be obtained from a randomly polarized laser beam by the use of suitable polarising materials in the construction of the unit. However it must be stressed that in doing so, a significant reduction in power output occurs. It is further possible with some types of polarised lasers to alter the direction or plane of polarisation to produce more complex forms of polarisation such as circular and elliptical polarisation. However, such complex forms of polarisation are beyond the scope of the current text and are therefore not considered further here.

As with coherence, the clinical significance of polarisation is not clear. This has not, however, prevented a number of manufacturers from providing polarisation as an option on some of their more expensive machines. It is certainly theoretically possible that significant biological effects of polarisation might yet be found at the subcellular or cellular level, as the associated electrical and magnetic fields generated by polarised light are uniplanar, which serves to intensify these fields for a given optical radiant power. This may possibly have subtle effects upon key biological structures such as cellular membranes or mitochondria and thus represents one possible area for future cellular research.

Power (*radiant power*) and power density (*irradiance*)

Apart from the special characteristics of laser radiation which have already been considered above, lasers also differ from other light sources in producing extremely brilliant radiation, which has been described for some laser systems as being 'point for point' brighter than the sun. This extreme brilliance is in the first instance essentially a product of the high degree of collimation found in laser light. Despite producing only a fraction of the output of a light bulb, a therapeutic He–Ne laser system has all its output 'bundled' into a small parallel beam, with a diameter well under 1 cm, and hence the ocular hazard associated with the use of such devices. Furthermore, it must also be remembered that while the output from a light bulb is spread across a range of wavelengths, that from the laser is highly monochromatic, in this example being clustered around a value of 632.8 nm (see Fig. 2.7). The net result of this is that the laser will produce a greater number of photons *at 632.8 nm* than the light bulb.

In radiometric terms, the output (or more correctly the *radiant power*) of lasers (and indeed other sources such as light bulbs) is measured and specified in watts (W). As the He–Ne and semiconductor lasers routinely used in therapeutic applications operate well below 1 W, the milliwatt (mW = 0.001 W) is more commonly used to specify radiant power for such systems. While some manufacturers have produced and promoted units with power outputs as low as 0.1 mW, some of which have been used as the basis for published papers showing positive effects, the market and clinical trend has been towards units with higher radiant power. Thus treatment probes incorporating single laser diodes producing 100 mW of radiant power are currently commercially available, as well as units containing arrays or 'clusters' of photodiodes with total radiant powers of over 600 mW.

While radiant power is a useful measurement in the comparison of therapeutic laser units, it is only a starting point. When assessing and comparing the potential biological and clinical effects of such devices, the area of irradiation and distribution of the incident photons across this area are important considerations. Where treatment units are used directly in contact with the target tissue, the area of irradiation is for all practical purposes the same as that of the output coupler found at the end of the treatment probe, or the cross sectional area of the fibreoptic applicator. However, as will become apparent in later chapters, laser therapists and researchers frequently use therapeutic lasers out of contact with the target tissue. In these situations, and despite the minimal divergence of such units, the area of irradiation will be larger than it would have been had the unit been used in contact (see Fig. 2.8).

As has already been indicated above, as the area of irradiation increases, there will be a relatively smaller number of photons *per unit area* for the same radiant power. In other words the optical 'power density' or *irradiance* will decrease with increasing distance between the treatment unit and the target tissue. Irradiance or power density is defined by the equation:

$$\text{Irradiance (mW/cm}^2) = \frac{\text{Incident power (mW)}}{\text{Area of irradiation (cm}^2)\star}$$

It should be stressed that the above formula only calculates average irradiance, as in the first instance the distribution of the incident optical power, and thus the incident photons, is not uniform across the laser beam. A typical distribution of the optical power within a laser beam is represented schematically in Figure 2.10a. From this it can be seen that the beam is most intense (or strongest) near its central axis, with intensity decreasing towards the edges of the beam. For a stationary incident beam, the actual pattern of irradiance on the irradiated target tissue (Fig. 2.10b) will therefore not be uniform, but rather will reflect the distribution of optical radiant power found within the incident laser beam.

The calculation of optical power and energy densities are important criteria in comparing dissimilar laser treatment protocols. While the clinical importance of these is considered further in subsequent chapters, guidelines on calculations are presented in Chapter 4.

MODE OF EMISSION

Whether assessing radiant power output, calculating irradiance, or indeed comparing research or clinical reports, it should always be borne in mind

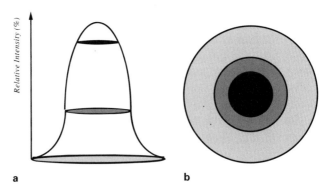

Fig. 2.10 Beam profile. **a.** Distribution of power/photons across beam. **b.** Beam imprint on target tissue.

★Note:
1. Incident power usually equals radiant power of the treatment unit used
2. If incident power is specified in mW, irradiance will be in mW/cm².

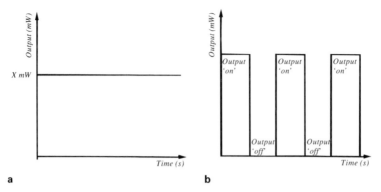

Fig. 2.11   Mode of emission. **a.** Continuous wave output. **b.** Pulsed output.

that the mode of radiation emission (in other words the pattern of emission over time) may vary greatly between different therapeutic units. The simplest form of output is represented in Figure 2.11a. As can be seen from this figure, this particular type of laser system produces a relatively constant, unvarying radiant power output of X mW over the period of time for which the unit is activated by the operator or therapist. Such units are therefore termed *continuous output* or more commonly *continuous wave* (abbreviated *CW*) lasers, with their outputs being labelled accordingly.

As will become apparent in later chapters, continuous wave lasers based upon various lasing media (e.g. He–Ne, GaAs and GaAlAs) have been successfully employed within a wide range of clinical applications for many years. Furthermore, a substantial proportion of the research papers published on therapeutic laser have been based upon the use of such units. However, many manufacturers now market therapeutic lasers which provide or allow *pulsing* as an alternative to CW output on their units. Pulsed output is represented in Figure 2.11b.

From this it can be seen that the output of the machine alternates over time between 'off' and 'on' periods. The reason for manufacturers providing such an option is because it is felt by some that, under certain conditions, pulsing the emitted radiation may be an important factor in enhancing the photobiomodulative effects, and thus the clinical efficacy, of the laser treatment unit. In much the same way as only specific wavelengths of radiation are absorbed by biomolecules within irradiated tissue, biomolecules will further preferentially absorb only certain sized packets (or pulses) of radiation, pulsed at certain frequencies or repetition rates. At a given wavelength, how much energy a given biomolecule will absorb during irradiation will depend upon:

1. The 'size' or more precisely the amount of energy contained within each pulse, which is in turn dependent upon the height or amplitude of the pulse and its duration.
2. The inter-pulse interval.

These parameters are represented diagrammatically in Figure 2.12. Taken together, these parameters will dictate the total cycle time and thus the 'pulsing frequency' or more precisely the *pulsing* (or *pulse*) *repetition rate* of the machine: the number of pulses produced by the unit per second. It should be noted that while some authors and manufacturers will often use the term *pulsing frequency*, this can cause some confusion as the emitted radiation possesses an inherent frequency (see p. 25). It is therefore recommended that this nomenclature is avoided as far as possible.

Although the theoretical basis of frequency-specific absorption might be well established, the biological and clinical significance of such beam pulsing is less clear. While the evidence in support of significant frequency-specific effects from the published literature is reviewed in later chapters where appropriate, it is useful to note two examples here.

In the first instance, research in healthy human volunteers completed by Martin and colleagues at the University of Ulster (Martin et al 1991) would suggest that photobiological effects upon lower limb blood flow may, at least under certain circumstances, be frequency-specific. Furthermore, research on experimental animals would indicate that the latency and duration of the pain relief produced by laser irradiation (laser-mediated hypoalgesia) is dependent upon the pulse repetition rate used in the treatment (Ponnudurai et al 1987). As such, pulse repetition rate represents an important treatment parameter which must be considered and fully accounted for when comparing research reports based upon dissimilar treatment protocols, or when planning or progressing treatment regimes.

While a substantial proportion of the commercially available laser units may produce some form of pulsed output or provide a selection for the same, the means by which such output is achieved can vary

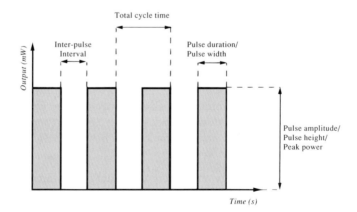

Fig. 2.12 Pulsed output: chief pulsing parameters/characteristics.

enormously between machines. In the first instance, on some machines the various characteristics of the pulsing regime (i.e. pulse width or duration, amplitude, repetition rate) are fixed, either because the diode used in the construction of the unit is inherently pulsed with these characteristics, or because of the specifications of the control systems incorporated into the machine's manufacture. Alternatively, and more commonly, machines allow for some alteration of the pulsing characteristics within predefined limits. Of the various range of options provided by manufacturers, three main type of pulsing option can be identified for the purposes of the current text: *fixed pulsed, chopped output* and *modulated output* units. These are each considered in more detail below.

Fixed pulse systems

In these units, the control system allows for the production of a well defined, 'fixed' pulse, with constant pulse width and amplitude. With such systems, the consistency of the emitted pulse will depend upon the quality of the diode used in the unit's manufacture and the sophistication of the printed circuit boards incorporated within the unit's control systems.

Where such systems are used, alteration of pulse repetition rate will change the number of these fixed pulses produced by the apparatus over a unitary time period. At 5 Hz, five such pulses will be emitted per second; at 5000 Hz (or 5 kHz) 5000 pulses will be emitted per second. This has a profound effect upon the radiant power output of these machines. The net effect is illustrated in Figure 2.13: increasing pulse repetition rate in these units also increases the *average* radiant power output and in turn, for a stationary treatment head, the irradiance upon

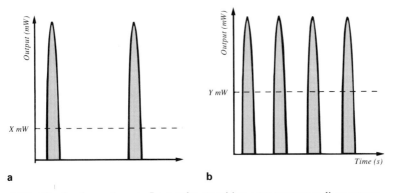

Fig. 2.13   Fixed pulse system. **a.** Low pulse repetition rate: average radiant power output $= X$ mW. **b.** High pulse repetition rate: average radiant power output $= Y$ mW ($> X$ mW).

target tissue. This is due to the fact that, as each pulse contains a fixed amount or bundle of light energy (i.e. a fixed number of photons), by having a greater number of pulses within a defined period, the average radiant power delivered over that period is correspondingly greater. The higher the pulse repetition rate, the greater the average radiant power emitted by this type of device.

Chopped output unit

In contrast to the fixed pulse type units outlined above, another popular means of pulsing the output of therapeutic laser relies upon 'chopping' the output either electrically or mechanically. Such units are based upon a continuous wave diode or He–Ne base unit which can be chopped to give a pseudo-pulsing effect. This is depicted schematically in Figure 2.14. It is important to note that, with its output chopped in this way, the unit's average radiant power output drops dramatically. Where such units allow for *alteration* of the pulse repetition rate, two important characteristics of the emitted output will change with changes in the pulse repetition rate:

1. The pulse width or duration varies, usually decreasing with increasing pulse repetition rate
2. The average radiant power output falls as the pulse repetition rate is increased. This is summarised in Figure 2.14b.

The latter represents perhaps the most important distinction between the fixed pulse and the chopped output type units, and obviously must be borne in mind when planning treatment protocols or comparing research reports.

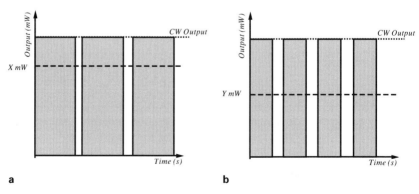

Fig. 2.14 Chopped output system. **a.** Low pulse repetition rate: average radiant power output = X mW. **b.** High pulse repetition rate: average radiant power output = Y mW ($< X$ mW).

Modulated output units

As already indicated above, for both fixed pulse and chopped output type units, average radiant power output varies enormously for alterations in pulse repetition rate. This is synonymous with variation in duty factor or unit cycle (see below). In an effort to overcome this variation in duty factor, at least one manufacturer has provided apparatus with so-called *modulated output* to provide a fixed average radiant power or constant duty factor across all pulse repetition rate settings. How this is achieved is represented diagrammatically in Figure 2.15.

At low pulse repetition rates, the pulse width is relatively greater than at higher pulse repetition rates. At various (preset) pulsing repetition rates, the control system in such units modulates the pulse parameters/characteristics to maintain the duty factor and thus the average radiant power output. It should be noted that the pulse amplitude or peak power remains constant, being essentially fixed for a given diode. It should be stressed that in checking the specification of a therapeutic unit, while the power output specified by the manufacturer is most usually the peak power, it is obviously also important to check or preferably measure the average radiant power output of the unit (see Ch. 3).

Duty factor/unit cycle

Duty factor, sometimes also known as unit cycle, is an important specification for pulsed laser systems. It is the proportion of the unit's maximum radiant power or peak power that the unit will emit on average over an extended period of time. Duty factor can thus be expressed as:

$$\text{Duty factor (\%)} = \frac{\text{Average radiant power output (mW)}}{\text{Peak radiant power output (mW)}}$$

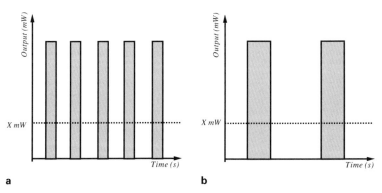

Fig. 2.15 Modulated output system. **a.** Low pulse repetition rate: average radiant power output = X mW. **b.** High pulse repetition rate: average radiant power output = X mW.

As shown in this equation, duty factor is usually expressed as a percentage. As already indicated, in many instances the radiant power output as detailed in the manufacturer's specifications or on the side of the laser treatment unit is the peak radiant power. This can be misleading, as a laser diode rated by the manufacturer at 30 mW may in fact only deliver an average radiant power of 15 mW when used in pulsing mode. In this case the duty factor would be 50%. It should also be stressed here that the duty factor or unit cycle will usually vary on therapeutic devices when the pulse repetition rate setting is changed, in some cases ranging from less than 10% to well over 80% of the rated or specified radiant power of the unit. Where this is the case, either the average radiant power or the duty factor should be specified *for each pulsing repetition rate* by the manufacturer.

A number of sources will refer to the duty factor as the percentage ratio of laser 'on' time (i.e. pulse width or duration) to the total cycle time (i.e. pulse width plus inter-pulse interval). This simplification of the above formula is certainly correct for laser units producing and emitting so called 'square wave' pulses, such as the typical chopped output units already considered above (Fig. 2.14). It is the essentially rectangular profile of the resulting pulse produced by these and similar units that gives rise to the description of 'square wave'. However, it is important to realise that where the emitted pulses are not square wave (e.g. Fig. 2.13), this simplified relationship does not hold true.

SUMMARY OF KEY POINTS

1. Laser is no more than a special form of electromagnetic energy, comprising electrical and magnetic fields which fluctuate perpendicularly to the direction of propagation.
2. The units commonly used in LILT include devices operating in the visible as well the near infra-red (and thus invisible) portions of the electromagnetic spectrum.
3. Laser devices comprise three essential components: a lasing medium, an energy source and a mechanical structure.
4. Lasers are highly monochromatic, essentially producing only a single wavelength of light. This is an important characteristic of laser as absorption of light is wavelength-specific.
5. Lasers produce highly collimated output, which has very little divergence.
6. Laser radiation is coherent, the individual waves of radiation moving in synchrony.
7. Output from superluminous diodes or SLDs possess all the attributes of laser radiation except coherence. They are less expensive than true laser emitting diodes and, since coherence is thought by

some to be unnecessary for LILT applications, are becoming more popular.

8. Although typical radiant power levels are in the milliwatt range, lasers produce highly brilliant radiation, which in turn produces high levels of irradiance (power density) on the target tissue.

9. Therapeutic units may produce continuous wave or pulsed output. Where pulsing units are used, it is important to check or measure the average radiant power output as this can vary enormously as the pulse repetition rate is altered.

REFERENCES

Baxter G D, Bell A J, Allen J M et al 1991 Low level laser therapy: current clinical practice in Northern Ireland. Physiotherapy 77: 171–178

Karu T I 1987 Photobiological fundamentals of low power laser therapy. IEEE Journal Quantum Electronics QE-23, 10: 1703–1717

Martin D M, Baxter G D, Allen J M et al 1991 Effect of laser pulse repetition rate upon peripheral blood flow in human volunteers. Lasers Surgery Medicine Suppl. 3: 83

Moore K C, Calderhead R G 1991 The clinical application of low incident power density 830 nm GaAlAs diode laser radiation in the therapy of chronic intractable pain: a historical and optoelectronic rationale and clinical review. International Journal Optoelectronics 6: 503–520

Ponnudurai R N, Zbuzek V K, Wu W 1987 Hypoalgesic effect of laser photobiostimulation shown by rat tail flick test. Acupuncture Electrotherapeutics Research International Journal 12: 93–100

Young S, Bolton P, Dyson M et al 1989 Macrophage responsiveness to light therapy. Lasers Surgery Medicine 9: 497–505

3. Safety and good treatment practice

INTRODUCTION

This chapter outlines the key principles of safety and good treatment practice as these apply to low-intensity laser therapy, beginning with an overview of the various types of therapeutic laser system currently on the market. In this, the chapter represents a logical and practical extension of the previous chapter. As a result, an understanding of the physical principles of laser devices and laser emission, as outlined in Chapter 2, is required before completing this chapter.

COMPARISON OF TYPES OF LASER DEVICE

An appreciation of the variety of therapeutic laser devices currently available for clinical applications, and consequently an understanding of their relative advantages and deficiencies, is important for the laser therapist. Hence the reason for this overview of the types of laser systems and devices currently employed in therapeutic applications. The following section is complemented by Appendix I, which presents specific examples of treatment units currently available from manufacturers and suppliers.

He–Ne lasers and fibreoptic applicators

The He–Ne laser was the first laser system to be used in clinical and research applications, principally in eastern Europe and China, commencing in the mid to late 1970s. It should be remembered that laser-emitting diodes were not available until the early 1980s. Even since then, He–Ne lasers have continued to be the standard unit for therapeutic applications in these countries, as laser diode technology has largely been unavailable to clinicians and researchers based there. In contrast, while He–Ne systems have certainly been used in the British Isles and in Europe, the trend has been towards diode-based systems.

This may be attributed to at least three factors. In the first place, therapeutic He–Ne lasers are relatively expensive compared to similar diode-based units. Secondly, He–Ne systems pose a greater ocular hazard as their output is highly collimated. For this reason, a greater degree of care is required when using such systems to minimise the attendant danger of accidental *intrabeam* viewing (see below). Finally, compared to the relatively portable and robust treatment probes used with diode-based systems, He–Ne systems are cumbersome and relatively easily damaged.

In an attempt to overcome these problems, He–Ne units have traditionally been mounted on a movable arm which can be manipulated by the therapist to irradiate the desired target tissue (see e.g. Zhou Yo Cheng 1988). Alternatively, fibreoptic applicators are sometimes provided with such units to enable the operator to direct the output onto the target area more easily. It is important to stress, however, that where such devices are used the divergence at the end of the fibreoptic applicator is several times greater than that found on diode-based systems. With this type of treatment unit, the use of so-called *contact technique* (i.e. with the applicator kept firmly in contact with the target tissues) wherever possible is critically important to maximise the optical power density (irradiance), and thus the therapeutic effect, upon the treated tissue (see Ch. 2).

Semiconductor diode systems

Semiconductor diode lasers based upon the gallium arsenide (GaAs) or gallium aluminium arsenide (GaAlAs) diode are by the far the most popular units in routine clinical use in therapeutic applications in the British Isles and in Europe. In such units the laser or superluminous diode is normally mounted into a hand-held 'probe' for ease of application by the therapist. This treatment probe (alternatively sometimes called the treatment 'head') is usually connected by flex to a separate control unit containing an electrical transformer which provides an appropriate source of energy from a mains supply, and a control panel via which the irradiation parameters can be alternatively controlled, programmed or at least monitored by the laser operator. More recently, at least one manufacturer has introduced a 'no leads' treatment system in which a mains-powered base unit is used to charge the treatment head which can then be slipped into a pocket or sports bag for ease of transport (see Appendix I).

Semiconductor diode lasers can be divided into two main types: continuous wave (CW) and pulsed systems. Whereas CW lasers have been the most popular treatment units in continental Europe and particularly in Japan, pulsed systems of various types (see Ch. 2) have tended to be more commonly used in the British Isles (Baxter et al 1991a).

A variety of cases and boxes have been provided by manufacturers for the transport of their therapeutic laser systems, including adapted photographers' cases. With a number of these devices, the design of the case is such that accidental closure of the lid can 'nip' the mains power supply lead (and/or the flex connecting the treatment probe to the control unit) between the lid and the main body of the case. Over a period of time, repeated episodes of such accidental nipping will result in damaged or unserviceable cables, and in the case of the power supply cable, a potentially dangerous piece of equipment. With such units, it is imperative that care is exercised to minimise the risk of damage, especially to the power cable, which should be routinely examined at regular intervals to assess possible damage.

Scanners

Scanning devices (or more simply 'scanners') have been offered as an optional extra by several manufacturers (see Appendix I). These are usually fitted over the end of the output coupler and, by a system of slowly moving optical reflectors/mirrors, scan the laser's output across a predefined area. The primary purpose of such devices is to simplify the application of therapeutic laser where relatively large areas of tissue are to be treated. Thus rather than using a single treatment probe or fibreoptic applicator to treat a 'grid' of individual points (see Ch. 7) across the target tissue, the scanner allows the laser therapist a relatively simple means of applying a uniform dosage across the *whole* area in a carefully controlled and prescribed manner.

While scanners have apparently been successfully employed in the treatment of a variety of conditions including sports injuries, osteoarthritis and musculoskeletal pain of various aetiologies (Mayordomo et al 1985, Morselli et al 1985a, b), and are usually promoted as being the device of choice for the treatment of extensive areas of burn injury or surgical scarring, such devices have never enjoyed the same degree of popularity as semiconductor lasers. This may be attributed to three main factors.

In the first place, the units are relatively costly and have typically been used in conjunction either with high-powered systems such as the CO_2 laser to carefully control and limit the dosage delivered during treatments, or with He–Ne systems to provide a practical, 'no hands', means of delivering laser therapy without recourse to fibreoptic applicators. Furthermore, the movement or scanning of the laser's radiant output across the target tissue makes calculation of therapeutic dosages difficult and may compromise the effectiveness of laser treatment, especially through the reduction of irradiance levels on the target tissue. The latter may be a particular problem where the scanning unit defocusses the output of the laser to produce a straight line or an ellipsoid beam imprint. Finally, the use of a scanner significantly increases the optical hazards associated with laser therapy treatments, which makes the strict observance of safety measures even more important.

These factors notwithstanding, the use of a scanner to accelerate the healing of burns or large wounds while minimising the associated pain and risk of hypertrophic scarring would seem an attractive option and consequently strongly indicates the desirability of a controlled clinical trial in this area to assess the efficacy of scanning laser treatments.

Multidiode arrays or 'cluster' units

As has already been indicated in the previous two chapters, treatment units based upon various arrays of diodes have been successfully used in the laser therapy of a range of conditions (e.g. Mester & Mester 1987). Such units vary enormously in design, from custom-built devices incorporating only laser-emitting diodes all operating at a single wavelength (McKibben 1991), to commercially available units based upon both superluminous and laser-emitting diodes (i.e. non-coherent and coherent sources) producing radiation at a range of wavelengths in both the visible and near infra-red parts of the spectrum (see Appendix 1). Although extremely popular in clinical practice if not necessarily with researchers (Baxter et al 1991a), such units present a number of practical problems in their use.

Firstly, the specification of dosage with such units is not straightforward: while measurement and calculation of the radiant power and irradiance for individual diodes contained within the array is relatively easy, problems arise in trying to express the pattern of irradiation upon the target tissue. While in routine clinical practice, treatment may be commonly recorded as *Laser: 2 min/5000 Hz/'cluster' head*, this is not sufficient to allow attempts to replicate this treatment by therapists using alternative laser apparatus. Indeed, some cluster units vary so enormously in emission spectra and design of array that any attempt at replication with alternative systems is pointless.

In spite of these practical difficulties, the point to be stressed is that although the treatment record as specified here may be adequate in defining the treatment given with the particular treatment unit used and allow other therapists working within the same department or with the same unit to repeat the treatment, it does not adequately define the irradiation parameters used for those unfamiliar with the apparatus. In such circumstances, the calculation of total radiant power output represents the very minimum with respect to correct recording of treatment parameters with cluster treatment units. For this the radiant power of each of the diodes comprising the array should be totalled. Thus for a hypothetical diode array containing the following diodes:

1. 1×50 mW
2. 10×30 mW
3. 10×15 mW

the total radiant power would be: $(50 + 300 + 150) = 500$ mW.

This figure might seem unusually high, but it must be remembered that this output is dispersed over a comparatively large incident area; 2 min of 'in contact' irradiation with such a unit would thus in no way be comparable to 2 min 'in contact' irradiation with a (single) 500 mW probe. In the latter case, the irradiance (power density) would be significantly higher than for the hypothetical multisource array with its 21 diodes spread across the face of the cluster unit and consequently the target tissue.

The calculation of irradiance for any cluster is therefore not as simple as for treatment with single diode or indeed He–Ne units. At best, only an average irradiance over the target tissue can be calculated, usually achieved by dividing the total radiant power output of the cluster unit by the surface area of the unit. If, for the hypothetical unit described above, the surface area of the array was 12.5 cm², the average irradiance across the area of target tissue immediately under the cluster head, where the unit is used in contact, would be:

Average irradiance $= 500$ mW/12.5 cm² $= 40$ mW/cm².

The accuracy of this as a measure of the irradiance over the target tissue will depend upon a number of factors, including:

1. The actual pattern or *configuration* of the diodes across the face of the cluster array. Where these are evenly distributed across the unit, the average irradiance figure will be a more accurate and thus more useful estimate of the actual irradiance at any given point on the surface of the irradiated tissue.

2. The variation in radiant power outputs between individual diodes comprising the array. In the hypothetical example given above, the actual irradiance directly under the 50 mW diode will obviously be significantly and commensurately higher than that directly under one of the 30 mW or 15 mW diodes. Thus in such cases, the average irradiance is less accurate than where all diodes emit the same radiant power.

3. The convention adopted for (and accuracy of) measurement of the area of irradiation on the target tissue. Some sources, given the divergence of the diodes and the distribution of light within the first few mm of irradiated tissue insist that the total area of the face of the array is accurate enough for the purposes of such calculations.

Quite apart from these problems relating to radiant power output and irradiance, cluster units will frequently incorporate a mixture of diodes, some emitting visible and others near infra-red radiation at various wavelengths as determined by the manufacturer. Consequently for the purposes of recording of laser treatments and for research reports, the wavelengths emitted by the unit used should be listed, together with the associated radiant power output and numbers of each different type of diode, e.g.:

1. 5 × 660 nm/15 mW
2. 10 × 820 nm/30 mW
3. 5 × 880 nm/30 mW
4. 1 × 904 nm/15 mW *(coherent)*.

Note that in this hypothetical example, the single laser-emitting diode has been identified to distinguish it from the other superluminous diodes comprising the array.

It should be obvious from the above that multiwavelength cluster arrays produce a complex pattern of irradiation, the precise biological and clinical significance of which are not yet clear. While good clinical research using multiwavelength multisource arrays is lacking, positive results from recently completed laboratory-based research on cellular effects and experimental pain would at least support the continued clinical application of such devices pending the provision of objective data from future research in the clinical setting (Baxter et al 1991b, El Sayed 1992).

INTERNATIONAL STANDARDS AND REGULATIONS

Lasers are classified into four groups according to an internationally agreed system. The basis of this classification is the potential danger posed to the exposed skin and to the unaccommodated eye.

Class 1

This includes low-power laser devices operating in both the visible and invisible portions of the electromagnetic spectrum. Lasers in this group pose no immediate danger to the eye or skin, even with extended periods of viewing directly into the path of the beam (*intrabeam viewing*). They are typically enclosed systems which do not emit hazardous levels of radiation. The commonly used laser lecture beam pointer is an example of a class 1 laser device. Some He–Ne and semiconductor diode laser units satisfy the requirements for inclusion in this class. However the exceptionally low radiant power output of these units (< 0.5 mW) means that they are generally considered unsuitable for therapeutic applications.

Class 2

This classification is limited to low-power lasers *in the visible range* which are considered safe for accidental momentary viewing. Such lasers are further considered safe for extended periods of irradiation on the unprotected skin. Whereas an extended period of intrabeam viewing is not advisable, the brilliance of the visible lasers within this group will invoke the blink reflex and thus preclude such extended intrabeam viewing. While none of the GaAs or GaAlAs diode lasers operating within the near infra-red fall within this category (regardless of power output), He–Ne lasers with radiant power outputs of up to 1 mW are class 2 lasers. Although some class 2 He–Ne systems have been used as therapeutic devices, their relatively low output severely limits the usefulness of these devices for routine clinical application.

Class 3

This class includes both visible and invisible mid-powered lasers which are considered to pose a potential hazard to the eye, but relatively little to exposed skin. The vast majority of commercially available therapeutic laser systems fall within this category and therefore pose a significant ocular hazard. For this reason, procedural controls are normally required and protective goggles should normally be worn where these lasers are used. The range in radiant power output of the lasers in this class is extremely wide, extending from under 1 mW to 500 mW (or 0.5 W), although few therapeutic devices other than research prototypes produce more than 200 mW. It is important to realise that, although posing a relatively lesser hazard than that of a laser operating at the same wavelength and radiant power, non-coherent superluminous diodes operating above 1 mW should also be treated as class 3 lasers.

Class 4

Class 4 lasers are much more hazardous than those included in class 3, posing a significant hazard to unprotected skin and the eye, even after diffuse reflection. In use they also represent a significant fire hazard. Although the units falling within this category are unsuitable for routine clinical use as a therapeutic laser, a number of investigators have assessed the photobiomodulative effects of relatively low doses from such systems (e.g. Goldman et al 1980). High-powered lasers such as the argon, Nd:YAG and CO_2 lasers, which are the standard units for surgical applications, are class 4 lasers.

DHSS regulations (see DHSS 1984)

In the UK, the Department of Health and Social Security (DHSS) has provided for the appointment of laser safety officers within the National Health Service with much the same powers and remit as radiological safety officers; indeed in many cases the role is carried out by the same individual. While the primary concern of the laser safety officer will be with the safe operation of high-power lasers, these individuals can be a useful source of advice on safety matters pertaining to the use of therapeutic laser for therapists within the health service, and should be consulted when drawing up local rules for the safe use of a particular unit.

Interestingly, it should be noted that, for health practitioners using therapeutic laser in private clinics, strict interpretation of current regulations would require both registration and licensing of the privately used laser unit with the attendant expenses associated with each. This would appear rather excessive given the relatively minor dangers associated with therapeutic compared to higher-power class 4 units. As a result, to date the majority of private practitioners have not registered the laser therapy units used in their clinics.

Current Food and Drug Administration position

In the USA, the Food and Drug Administration (FDA) has yet to approve the use of low-intensity laser therapy for a single application. Despite this prohibition, various health professionals in the US circumvent the ban by offering laser therapy to patients at privately run centres and clinics located close to the American border in Mexico and Canada, where the use of therapeutic laser is not so restricted.

Considerable debate and controversy surrounds the ban on therapeutic laser devices in America, and recently there has been some apparent softening of the FDA's position. In this respect, Goldman (1991) has recently provided a succinct outline of current thinking on Laser bio-stimulation (sic) in America, and how in the future the FDA might co-operate in the design and implementation of well designed and controlled research (both basic and clinical) to definitively establish or refute the putative efficacy of low-intensity laser therapy.

POTENTIAL DANGERS ASSOCIATED WITH LILT

Electrical safety

Therapeutic laser equipment is electrically powered and should therefore be operated with care. Complacency in the operation of any electrical equipment is dangerous and potentially fatal. For this reason, attention should be paid to the routine care and maintenance of the laser equipment (see below), which should be serviced at least once per year and repaired by a competent person when a fault is suspected. As already indicated above, because of the risk of damage to the power supply cable in certain units where the cable can become nipped between carrying case and lid, cursory inspections of the power cable by operators should be part of routine care and maintenance.

Ocular hazards

The potential for ocular damage during treatments through accidental intrabeam viewing represents the most obvious and significant danger associated with the use of therapeutic laser devices. This is essentially due to the high degree of collimation of lasers, even operating at the relatively low radiant powers routinely used in therapeutic applications. When the lens within the anterior compartment of the eye is completely relaxed, objects at infinity are focussed onto the retina, light incident from such sources being essentially parallel. The almost parallel rays from a laser unit will likewise be focussed, only in this case onto a tiny spot on the retina. In doing so, the magnification provided by the visual apparatus is in the region of $\times 10^5$. It should be noted that this will also apply to output from lasers operating in the near infra-red, as radiation within this portion of the spectrum is equally well focussed by the eye. Thus, although invisible to the naked eye, the output from such lasers still poses a potential hazard for the unprotected eye. For this reason it is a now a requirement that such systems incorporate a second diode to provide a visible aiming beam (usually operating $\leqslant 1$ mW) within the treatment probe which is simultaneously operated with the main infra-red treatment diode.

A note on laser goggles

The use of laser-protective goggles by therapist and patient is so widely recommended and well established that most manufacturers now include two pairs of goggles in the cost of their unit. However some older units (especially where these are purchased second-hand) may not come supplied with *suitable* goggles. In these circumstances, the acquisition of appropriate eye protection must be considered essential.

It is important to stress a number of points in the assessment and selection of goggles for use with a particular treatment unit. The first is that not all goggles are equally effective in protecting the eyes from a given wavelength of laser radiation. Goggles are usually designed to be selective filters and thus will only protect wearers against ocular damage from a certain range of wavelengths of visible, infra-red or indeed ultra-violet radiation. This is a critical factor in assessing goggles for use with a given system as they must be designed to filter the wavelength(s) emitted by that particular apparatus. If not, unwitting but inappropriate use of the goggles by operators and patients may be more dangerous than their non-use, as they may provide a false sense of security.

Although the filtered wavelength band should be specified by the manufacturer or supplier and clearly marked on the sidepiece of the goggles, where this is not the case the goggles can be relatively easily checked. The simplest method of testing the adequacy of a particular pair of protective eyewear is by using the output meter provided with the apparatus to measure the output of the therapeutic unit through the goggles. This will provide a rough but useful estimate of the suitability of the goggles for use with the machine. Where a more accurate assessment is required, or where the unit is not provided with a power meter, most hospital physics departments and many technical laboratories can relatively easily measure the transmission of the eyewear's filters. Finally, the local laser safety officer (see above) will be able to have the suitability of the goggles tested.

It should be noted that goggles can vary enormously in price, in some instances by a factor of more than 10. In general, the relatively cheaper units are less selective filters, whereas more expensive goggles filter only the narrow band of wavelengths necessary to provide compatibility with a particular machine. The relevance of this for the clinical user is that cheaper goggles tend to make equipment operation and treatment more difficult as they can significantly affect vision, making control panels and the treatment area harder to see. In contrast, more expensive goggles allow for relatively easy vision and yet afford maximum protection. For this reason, at least two manufacturers who supply protective eyewear with their apparatus provide one of each type of goggles: a more selective (and thus relatively more expensive) set of filters for use by the operator and wide-band filters for the patient. In these circumstances, both operator and patient are equally well protected, and yet the overall cost is kept low without compromising the operator's ability to perform treatment. This therefore represents a useful and cost-effective strategy where goggles have not been provided with the machine.

However, the inappropriate designs of some the cheaper goggles available may represent more of a safety hazard than intrabeam viewing. In the only reported case of eye injury during therapeutic laser treatment, a chartered physiotherapist using a treatment unit on loan from a supplier suffered 60% corneal abrasions from the protective 'wings' on the side of the goggles provided with the apparatus (Chartered Society of Physiotherapy 1988). It would seem that the goggles in question were poorly designed in that the folding wings, provided to minimise the risk of oblique viewing of the laser beam 'out of the side of the eye', were not permanently attached to the sidepieces. Because of this, the physiotherapist, in attempting to put the goggles on, scratched her cornea on one of the wings which was only half open.

Thus, in assessing protective eyewear for routine use in clinical practice and/or for purchase, the safety aspects of the design of the goggles need careful consideration as the risk of eye injury from this source represents a real danger to both therapist and patient. In this current litigation-conscious climate, it is hardly sufficient for the therapist to claim that he/she was 'only using the goggles supplied with the apparatus' in an attempt to avoid charges of professional negligence after a patient has suffered eye injuries as a result of being supplied with badly designed protective eyewear!

Contraindications

As with any electrotherapeutic modality, the specification of contraindications to low-intensity laser therapy is based more upon prudence rather than hard experimental or clinical data. Only as research becomes the norm rather than the exception will definitive pronouncements on contraindications be possible. Having stressed this caveat, the following should, for the time being at least be regarded as *absolute* contra-indications (CSP Safety of Electrotherapy Equipment Working Group 1991):

1. Direct treatment of the eye for whatever reason

While a number of high-power laser systems are routinely used by laser ophthalmologists (see Ch. 1); even the relatively low-power units used in therapeutic applications pose a significant ocular hazard through accidental intrabeam viewing and thus their use to treat the eye is contraindicated other than by suitably trained ophthalmologists.

2. Irradiation of the fetus or treatment over the pregnant uterus

This represents a standard contraindication for all electrotherapeutic modalities and requires no further explanation.

3. Irradiation in the presence of active neoplasm

While *direct irradiation over the site of neoplastic tissue* is commonly regarded as an absolute contraindication, recent research at the University of Ulster would suggest that laser treatment at any site should be contraindicated in those patients in whom active neoplasms are suspected (Shields et al 1992). This study, which is considered further in Chapter 5, was completed in circulating mononuclear leukocytes obtained from healthy human volunteers; its results would suggest that irradiation of these cells at therapeutic doses (660 nm; 0.6–3.6 J/cm^2; pulsed at 5 kHz) mediates the release of certain *growth factors* (see Ch. 5). In vivo, it is likely that laser irradiation would mediate similar release and thus that these growth factors would be available to act upon a range of cell types including neoplastic cells at sites distant from that actually irradiated. Thus prudence would dictate that, at least for the present, LILT should be regarded as contraindicated at any site in those patients with active neoplasms.

4. Areas of haemorrhage

This is regarded as an absolute contraindication to laser treatment because of the possibility of laser-mediated vasodilation exacerbating the loss of circulating fluids. However, it should be noted that Martin's findings using a multisource, multiwavelength array would suggest the possibility of laser-mediated decreases in blood flow in the lower limb in vivo at certain pulsing repetition rates (Martin et al 1991a, b). While this evidence from work in healthy human volunteers is not sufficient to justify reassessing areas of haemorrhage as an absolute contraindication, it would indicate the necessity for further work in this area.

Apart from these absolute contraindications, caution is further recommended in the following cases (CSP Safety of Electrotherapy Equipment Working Group 1991):

1. Areas of hypoaesthesia, particularly decreased sensitivity to heat and/or pain

While routine skin testing should be the norm before application of any electrotherapeutic modality, the presence of hypoaesthesia cannot be regarded as an absolute contraindication for therapeutic laser treatment for two main reasons. In the first instance, LILT is by definition an athermic modality and thus the danger of producing a burn in the presence of decreased thermosensitivity, common to modalities such as ultrasound or infra-red, is negligible. Secondly, work carried out by Rochkind's group in Israel upon experimental lesions in the peripheral and central nervous systems of animals has demonstrated significant photobiostimulative effects following low-energy-density laser irradiation (e.g. Rochkind et al 1990a, b). Based upon this, it would appear that laser may be an effective therapeutic modality in the treatment of peripheral nerve lesions. However further work is required before any definitive pronouncements can be made in this respect.

2. Infected tissue such as infective dermatitis or infected open wounds

Specification of the presence of infection as a contraindication for laser therapy is based upon the assumption that, in addition to photobiostimulating the wound healing process, laser may also stimulate the bacteria usually responsible for wound infection. This view is supported by the findings of workers such as Karu (e.g. Karu 1987), who have used bacteria such as *Escherichia coli* as the basis for a large proportion of their work on laser photobiomodulation. Given that *E. coli* is very similar to the types of bacterium commonly found in infected wounds, the fact that photobiostimulative effects are so readily demonstrated in this bacteria would reinforce the contraindication of laser therapy for infected wounds. However, this ignores the potential of low-intensity laser irradiation to stimulate the *host response* and thus the ability of the patient's immune system to combat the infection.

Interestingly, in a recent survey of current clinical practice in laser therapy among chartered physiotherapists (Baxter et al 1991a), while some respondents specified the presence of infection as an absolute contraindication, others regarded such infection as an indication for laser treatment. It would thus seem, given the clinical experience of this latter group, that laser may represent a useful modality in the treatment of such wounds. While further research is required before LILT could be recommended for the management of infected wounds, it is useful to note here that laser can be successfully used in combination with ultra-violet treatment to utilise the photobiostimulative effects of the former and the bactericidal action of the latter (see Ch. 7).

3. Treatment over epiphyseal lines in children

Although extreme care should always be exercised in such cases, regard-less of the electrotherapeutic modality concerned, it should be stressed that recent research completed at the Tissue Repair Research Unit at Guy's Hospital in London would suggest that the risks to the healthy growth plate are minimal (Cheetham et al 1991).

4. Treatment over the sympathetic ganglia, the vagus nerves and the cardiac region of the thorax in patients with heart disease

Given the large volume of papers which have demonstrated the poten-tial of low-energy-density laser irradiation to significantly alter neural function (see Ch. 6), the rationale for the inclusion of this contraindication is obvious and requires no further explanation.

5. Irradiation of the gonads

Care should always be exercised in the application of any therapeutic modality over the site of, or directly to, the gonads. However it should be stressed that therapeutic laser, applied directly to the testes at a dose of 1.3 J/cm^2, has been successfully used in Indonesia as a treatment for infertility (Hasan et al 1989), an application that would seem to be supported by research at the cellular level, which has demonstrated the potential of low-intensity laser irradiation to increase sperm motility (Sato et al 1984). Additionally, it is also relevant that laser acupuncture has apparently enjoyed similar success in the treatment of prostatitis in at least one centre in the People's Republic of China (Shirui Li et al 1989). Finally, low-intensity lasers are routinely used at a number of centres in eastern Europe for the treatment of postoperative wounds following gynaecological surgery (e.g. Burgudjieva et al 1985). Such apparent success with these types of applications, with no reported side effects or complications, would suggest that the dangers associated with low-intensity irradiation of or near the gonads are minimal.

6. Patients with obtunded reflexes

While this case is commonly cited for most electrotherapy modalities, its relevance in the case of low-intensity laser irradiation would seem to be limited.

7. Treatment over areas of photosensitive/sensitised skin or tissue

Although such cases are rare in routine clinical practice, patients should be screened for any previous history of adverse reactions to sunlight or current use of photosensitising drugs (e.g. a psoralen in patients also receiving PUVA treatment) or chemicals (e.g. coal tar soap). In such cases, skin testing should initially be carried out to assess the potential tissue reaction, and dosages should be kept low and progressed only gradually. To date only one report of such adverse patient reaction to laser treatment has appeared in the professional or scientific literature (Wigmore-Welsh 1991).

8. Patients with cognitive difficulties

Where it is the opinion of the therapist that the patient has difficulties in comprehending the significance of verbal warnings, and thus the dangers associated with laser treatment, care should be exercised to minimise the risk to such patients of accidental intrabeam viewing.

Long-term effects: the need for further research

In spite of over 20 years' clinical application of low-intensity lasers, there have been no reports to date of any serious unpredicted iatrogenic effects as a result of such treatment. However, it must be stressed that further research is still necessary to establish the probable long-term effects of low-intensity laser exposure. To this end, it is interesting to note that preliminary work by McKelvey at the University of Ulster has provided some evidence of DNA damage in Friend mouse erythroleukaemia cells as a result of relatively low doses ($1.2-7.2$ J/cm^2) of 660 nm laser irradiation (McKelvey et al 1991). While the results of this study might seem damning, it should be stressed that the production of DNA damage in this study (assessed here by a so-called Comet assay) does not necessarily imply a mutagenic potential with low-intensity laser. Rather, the mutagenic potential of the particular lesions found in this study require further investigation (McKelvey et al 1991).

ADDITIONAL RECOMMENDATIONS FOR CLINICAL PRACTICE

Verbal warning

In order to minimise the risk of ocular damage, the patient should be briefed on the attendant hazards of intrabeam viewing and, where it is deemed necessary, other staff should be advised that a laser is in use. The audible alarm provided on treatment units should, however, be sufficient to warn staff of the laser's operation.

Safety of the laser environment

As has already been indicated above, the laser safety adviser should be consulted in the drawing up of local rules for the safe use of a therapeutic unit. These should include the designation of a controlled area, with restricted access and suitably marked with warning symbols, for the provision of laser treatments. Depending upon the type of unit used, the dangers associated with reflected rays from mirrors and other reflective surfaces may also have to be considered. Within the designated laser area, routine safety and ergonomic considerations also apply: e.g. the treatment unit should ideally be mounted on a treatment trolley of suitable height, close to the electrical supply and adjacent to the treatment plinth. In addition, the safety features provided by the laser manufacturer should be exploited. While this is normally limited to the controlled distribution and issue of the unit's safety keys to prevent unauthorised or dangerous misuse, a relatively recent development in the design of therapeutic units has been the provision of a deadlock-type control on some machines. Where such controls are provided, their feasibility might need careful consideration in conjunction with the local laser safety adviser.

Care and maintenance of therapeutic units

In the first instance it is imperative, as with any electrotherapeutic device, that the unit is kept clean, dry and dust-free. Water ingress or accumulation of dust and dirt around such key components as switches and electrical connections can seriously impair the operation of the unit and may be potentially dangerous. Most importantly, the output coupler/treatment head must be routinely inspected and cleaned to ensure the effective operation of the unit. To this end, some manufacturers provide swabs and cleaning fluid to be used with their particular unit. Where these are not provided by the manufacturer or supplier, satisfactory results can be obtained with cotton-wool sticks (e.g. Q-Tips or Cotton Buds) and alcohol.

How often the treatment head or probe is cleaned will vary depending upon usage and the type of clinical conditions typically treated. Even in a busy outpatient department where the laser unit is in almost continual use throughout the clinic opening times, routine cleaning could well only be required twice a day. This however relies upon irradiated skin being well prepared with surgical spirit or cleansing swabs before 'in contact' treatment, to remove surface lipids. Where open wounds and/or infected skin is treated, the treatment head should ideally be cleaned immediately before and after irradiation. This in the first instance helps prevent the introduction of infection where broken skin or open wounds are treated, and secondly minimises the risk of cross-infection from infected lesions.

Furthermore, a number of therapists have used transparent plastic barriers such as clingfilm in an apparently successful effort to prevent contact between treatment heads and infected wounds. It must be stressed however that, even though positive results might be achieved with such treatment techniques, the transmission of laser through this type of material has not been systematically assessed and thus requires further investigation before such practices could be endorsed for routine clinical application.

As a part of the routine inspection procedures, the radiant output of the unit should be assessed on a regular basis. European legislation will make the provision of an output meter or photometer an essential requirement for all new therapeutic laser units. Indeed, many manufacturers already provide such meters with their apparatus, usually built into the casing of the control unit. In contrast, others provide or sell hand-held meters to be used with their apparatus. Two points need to be stressed concerning the use of such meters. In the first instance, they are *wavelength-specific* and thus a meter designed for use with a diode unit operating at 830 nm will not be capable of accurately measuring the 632.8 nm output of a He–Ne laser. Secondly, where the output is pulsed, the reliability of the meter cannot be guaranteed and thus under these circumstances the measurement of radiant output is best left to technical services. It can therefore be seen that power meters frequently cannot be used to measure anything other than the output of the unit for which it is designed.

While a number of units incorporate a digital LED unit in the construction of their control unit that ostensibly provides a continuous reading of output, it must be stressed that such readings cannot be guaranteed to provide an accurate measure of the radiant output of the unit under all conditions. At best they can provide only a rough estimate of the output of the treatment head.

SUMMARY OF KEY POINTS

1. Therapeutic lasers are usually based either upon a semiconductor diode or a He–Ne source; however, scanners and multidiode arrays or cluster units are also available for routine clinical application.
2. An internationally agreed system classifies lasers into four groups according to relative hazard to the eye and exposed skin. The devices routinely used in the therapeutic applications are class 3 lasers and thus pose a potential hazard to the unprotected eye.
3. The associated ocular hazard means that therapeutic lasers should normally be used with protective goggles.
4. Absolute contraindications to laser treatment include direct treatment to the eye, irradiation of the fetus, any treatment in

the presence of active neoplasm or irradiation over areas of haemorrhage. Caution is also recommended in a number of other circumstances (see pp. 60–62).

5. While there are no reports of serious side effects as a result of low-intensity laser treatment, further research is required to exclude the possibility of iatrogenic effects in the longer term.

6. Patients should be verbally warned of the dangers associated with laser treatment.

7. Therapeutic laser units should be routinely cleaned, inspected and serviced by a competent person.

8. Laser therapy treatments should be provided in a designated area marked with warning symbols and restricted access. Safety devices provided on the apparatus should be utilised to the full.

REFERENCES

Baxter G D, Bell A J, Allen J M et al 1991a Low level laser therapy: current clinical practice in Northern Ireland. Physiotherapy 77: 171–178

Baxter G D, Mokhtar B, Allen J M et al 1991b Effect of laser irradiation of ipsilateral Erb's point upon tourniquet-induced ischaemic pain. Lasers in Surgery and Medicine (Suppl) 3: 11

Burgudjieva T, Katranushkova N, Blazeva P 1985 Laser therapy of complicated wounds after obstetric and gynecologic operations. Akusherstvo I Ginekologiia 6: 60–69

Chartered Society of Physiotherapy (CSP) 1988 Hazard warning: laser safety goggles. CSP Safety News, August 1988

Cheetham M, Young S, Dyson M 1991 820 nm irradiation of the healthy growth plate. Lasers in Surgery and Medicine (Suppl) 3: 12

CSP Safety of Electrotherapy Equipment Working Group 1991 Guide lines for the safe use of lasers in physiotherapy. Physiotherapy 77: 169–170

Department of Health and Social Security (DHSS) 1984 Guidance on the safe use of lasers in medical practice. Her Majesty's Stationery Office, London

El Sayed S 1992 PhD Thesis, United Medical and Dental Schools Guy's and St Thomas'

Goldman J A 1991 Laser biostimulation. In: Goldman L (ed) Laser non-surgical medicine. Technomic, Lancaster, PA

Goldman J A, Chiapella J, Casey H et al 1980 Laser therapy of rheumatoid arthritis. Lasers in Surgery and Medicine 1: 93–101

Hasan P, Rijadi S A, Purnomo S et al 1989 The possible application of Low reactive level laser therapy (LLLT) in the treatment of male infertility. Laser Therapy 1: 49–50

Karu T I 1987 Photobiological fundamentals of low power laser therapy. IEEE Journal of Quantum Electronics QE-23, 10: 1703–1717

McKelvey V J, Keegan A L, Allen J M 1991 Induction of DNA damage by low level laser irradiation in friend mouse erythroleukaemia cells. Abstracts, EEMS Meeting Prague 1991

McKibben L 1991 Personal communication

Martin D M, Baxter G D, Allen J M et al 1991a Effect of laser pulse repetition rate upon peripheral blood flow in human volunteers. Lasers in Surgery and Medicine Suppl. 3: 83

Martin D M, Ravey J, McCoy P et al 1991b The effect of laser pulse repetition rate in low level laser therapy on human peripheral blood flow. Proceedings, 11th International Congress World Confederation Physical Therapy Book II: 1093–1095

Mayordomo M M, Failde J M G, Cabrero M V et al 1985 Laser in painful processes of locomotor system: our experience. Proceedings International Congress on Laser in Medicine and Surgery. Monduzzi Editore, Bologna

Mester A F, Mester A R 1987 Biotherapy 3 and argon ion, He–Ne, ruby lasers. Comparative study of their biostimulative effects. Abstracts, Fifth Annual Congress, 28-30 January 1987. British Medical Laser Association

Morselli M, Soragni O, Anselmi C et al 1985a Very low energy-density treatments by CO_2 laser in sports medicine. Lasers in Surgery and Medicine 5: 150

Morselli M, Soragni O, Lupia B P et al 1985b Effects of very low energy-density treatment of joint pain by CO_2 laser. Lasers in Surgery and Medicine 5: 149

Rochkind S, Lubart R, Wollman Y et al 1990a Central nervous system transplantation benefitted by low-level laser irradiation. In: Joffe S N, Atsomi K (eds) Laser surgery: Advanced characterisation, therapeutics and systems II. Progress in biomedical optics, SPIE Volume 1200, International Society for optical engineering

Rochkind S, Vogler I, Barr-Nea L 1990b Spinal cord response to laser treatment of injured peripheral nerve. Spine 15: 6–10

Sato H, Landthaler M, Haina D et al 1984 The effects of laser light on sperm motility and velocity in vitro. Andrologia 16: 23

Shields T D, O'Kane S, Gilmore W S et al 1992 The effect of laser irradiation upon human mononuclear leukocytes. Lasers in Surgery and Medicine Suppl 4: 11

Shirui Li, Shizeng You, Shilin Zang 1989 A new approach in the application of the Helium Neon laser in acupuncture therapy for prostatitis: a clinical study involving 114 cases. Laser Therapy 1: 37–40

Wigmore-Welsh J 1991 Drugs and laser [letter] Physiotherapy 77: 682

Zhou Yo Cheng 1988 Laser acupuncture anaesthesia. In: Ohshiro T, Calderhead R G 1988 Low level laser therapy: a practical introduction. Wiley, Chichester

4. Bioenergetics and tissue optics

INTRODUCTION

This chapter concentrates on the bioenergetics of laser light and the optical properties of tissue. It therefore describes the photophysical events which underlie the type of biological responses commonly observed in clinical laser therapy practice. While bioenergetics and tissue optics may seem to be of only academic importance to the average clinician, they require some consideration as they underpin the clinical use of low-intensity laser, particularly as regards determination of treatment dosage. In order to administer optimal and effective laser treatment, it is important that the clinician should have at least a basic understanding of the principles underlying light propagation in tissues and the different possible modes of laser-tissue interaction; it is furthermore *essential* that he or she should be competent in the calculation of dosage. The chapter is (unavoidably) one of the most technical in the book, and for that reason readers with little or no understanding of physics are recommended to familiarise themselves with the material in Chapter 2 on the physical principles of lasers before proceeding further.

The chapter starts with a brief description of the mechanisms of absorption and scattering of light in tissue, which are the most important modes of light–tissue interaction within those wavelength bands commonly used in low-level laser therapy (630–1300 nm). Given the disparate claims for the amount of penetration achieved when irradiating tissue with laser, the methods most commonly used for determination of penetration depth and light distribution in tissue are then overviewed; because of the technical difficulties in measuring light irradiance within tissue in vivo, this is accomplished for practical purposes by the use of mathematical equations that describe the propagation of light in tissues.

In an extension of the material presented in Chapter 2 on radiant optical power and irradiance etc., some principles of dosimetry are described next, focussing on the definitions of those terms in common use in laser therapy for the specification of treatment dosage (i.e. energy and energy density) and the importance of these and other parameters such as pulsing repetition rate in clinical practice. Some practical examples of dosage calculations are also presented: these are included within this chapter as tables for ease of reference. The chapter ends with some notes and considerations on the extrapolation of dosages from cellular or animal studies for human treatment.

LASER–TISSUE INTERACTION

Introduction: the two modes of interaction

Therapeutic laser devices are designed to be used in contact with tissue; where so-called non-contact treatment is used a percentage of the incident light is reflected from the tissue surface, which reduces the energy delivered to the tissues and in turn the potential efficacy of treatment. The two most important modes of light interaction with tissue during laser 'in contact' treatment procedures are *absorption* and *scattering*. Absorption results in the transformation of light energy into some other form of energy, while scattering may be defined simply as a change in the direction of propagation of the light. The relative degree of absorption and scattering that occurs in a particular situation is dependent upon the type of tissue through which the light is passing, as well as the wavelength of the incident light. The following analysis will therefore present an overview of the mechanisms of light–tissue interaction for different wavelength bands and for different tissues.

The interaction between light and tissue may be considered at three levels; firstly the atomic, secondly the molecular and finally the macromolecular level. The atomic level of interaction is predominant in the X- and gamma-ray bands of the electromagnetic spectrum and is not considered any further here since the bands of interest in practical medical laser applications are the far and near ultra-violet, the visible spectrum and the near, mid and far infra-red. The approximate wavelengths for these various bands are shown in Figure 2.1 on p. 24.

The second level of light–tissue interaction is the molecular level. Light absorption predominantly occurs at this level of interaction. This can be described in simple terms as:

1. the excitation of the electron bonds within biomolecules

and/or

2. the excitation of atoms to higher modes of oscillation relative to each other

as well as

3. rotation of the whole biomolecule, or parts of the whole biomolecule by the external electromagnetic field created by the incident light.

These are summarised diagrammatically in Figure 4.1.

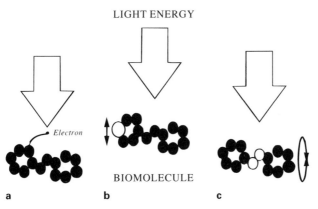

LIGHT ENERGY

BIOMOLECULE

a   b   c

Fig. 4.1 The three possible methods of light absorption by biomolecules. **a.** Excitation of electron bonds. **b.** Excitation of atoms to higher modes of oscillation. **c.** Rotational changes within the biomolecule.

In the case of organic molecules, the excitation of the electron bonds can result in the breakage of some relatively larger molecules, or even changes within the carbon chain. It should be noted that such changes may be reversible or irreversible depending upon the intensity of irradiation, with higher intensities of radiation tending in general to produce irreversible changes. Excitation of atoms to higher modes of oscillation or rotational stages within biomolecules may be seen macroscopically as temperature elevation. While of only limited relevance to low-intensity laser therapy applications, these processes are of primary importance for those applications relying upon or involving heat production (i.e. photothermal reactions), as well as for photochemistry (photodynamic therapy).

Failure to observe significant temperature increases during irradiation with low-intensity laser has led to its classification as an athermic modality. However the possibility of temperature elevation at the microscopic level cannot be discounted. Thus, while perceptible temperature increases are not observed at whole body level, such increases may and in all likelihood do occur at cellular or subcellular level.

Finally, the third level of interaction is at the macromolecular and microstructural level. These interactions result in scattering (changes in direction) of light as it propagates in tissues. Scattering is considered in more detail below.

Absorption

The basis of absorption has already been presented above. The following outlines the different absorption mechanisms for the various therapeutic wavelength bands and for different types of tissue. It is useful to remember from the outset that the principal constituent of biological tissue is water. In adult humans the average water content is about 70%, this figure decreasing slightly with age, the remaining 30% consisting mainly of organic molecules. Therefore any consideration of light–tissue interaction is best regarded in terms of light interaction with either water and/or organic molecules.

Light absorption by water predominates in light–tissue interaction in the infra-red spectrum for wavelengths longer than 1200 nm, and in the ultra-violet spectrum for wavelengths shorter than 200 nm. For these wavelengths, optical properties of tissue can be assumed to be similar to the optical properties of water. In contrast, within the visible and near ultra-violet spectrum, water can be considered transparent for all practical applications of laser–tissue interaction. In this portion of the spectrum, absorption is dominated by the absorption characteristics of organic molecules. Within the therapeutically important near infra-red range of the spectrum, absorption properties vary between these two extremes. Water absorption curves are shown schematically in Figure 4.2, together with the optical absorption properties of melanin, oxygenated and reduced haemoglobin.

The organic molecules responsible for light absorption can be divided into two groups. The first of these contains the amino acids and nucleic acid bases, and the other group the so-called *chromophores*.

In the former group, the amino acids and nucleic acid bases form the building blocks of DNA as well as the proteins in cells. The amino acids have significant absorption in the mid and far ultra-violet, through

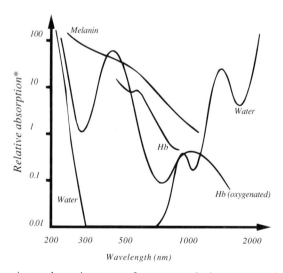

Fig. 4.2 Approximate absorption curves for water, melanin, oxygenated and reduced haemoglobin.
*Molar extinction coefficient $(10^{-3}.M^{-1}.cm^{-1})$; a H_2O (cm^{-1})
Hb = haemoglobin

the process of electronic excitation (see Fig. 4.1a). Their ability to absorb radiation within this part of the spectrum is due to the presence of sulphur in the *aromatic residues* of these molecules. These aromatic residues of amino acids link together to form proteins and polypeptides. All of the naturally occurring proteins are formed from the so-called 'canonical' amino acid residues. Of these, three contain sulphur. In contrast to their absorbency characteristics within the ultra-violet, amino acids show no significant absorption in the near ultra-violet or visible spectrum, because of their molecular structure.

In the visible, near and middle infra-red parts of the spectrum, amino acids can be excited by external radiation fields. However, excitation in this case is not electronic. Instead the radiation changes atoms from resting into higher modes of excitation relative to each other, and whole molecules or parts of molecules into different rotational stages (Figs 4.1b, c). With sufficient energy, this will be seen macroscopically as heating of the biological tissue, as with treatment using infra-red or radiant heat lamps. However, the transition energies required to produce these changes are much lower than the energies required for the electronic excitation produced by the ultra-violet radiation discussed above. Hence relatively small energy densities in the visible, near and middle infra-red parts of the spectrum can produce non-electronic excitation. As already outlined earlier, such changes may occur without discernible increase in temperature.

Smaller organic molecules exhibit similar behaviour at the infra-red wavelengths. Nucleic acid bases show similar absorption characteristics in the mid and far ultra-violet as well as the infra-red bands; however they show little absorption in the near ultra-violet and visible parts of the spectrum.

Where amino acids are linked together with peptide bonds to form proteins, the optical behaviour of the resultant protein within the ultra-violet spectrum is dominated by the properties of the individual amino acids. At a macromolecular level, the helical structure of the protein does not absorb ultra-violet radiation, but is excited to higher vibrational stages by incident infra-red radiation. At higher energy densities, the resulting macroscopic temperature rise can easily result in the breakage of atomic bonds. The same is valid for DNA and RNA, where optical properties in the ultra-violet spectrum are dominated by those of the nucleic acid bases, and their absorption in the infra-red by the bonds of the helix. While the above is true in general, it must be stressed that in some circumstances, there may be some minimal response to near ultra-violet and visible light, due to the precise spatial alignment of the structural elements. In this region, response is dominated by the chromophores.

The biomolecules which absorb light in the visible region are those proteins which have an added functional group containing a chromophore. Chromophores may be defined as molecular structures which absorb light in the visible spectrum. The most commonly occurring chromophores are those derived from the porphyrin groups. Porphyrins are highly complicated bio-organic molecules which are common in most species. In mammals, for example, haemoglobin, the biomolecule which transports oxygen to the tissues, is the result of binding the haem group with the globin protein. The former group is largely formed from iron porphyrins.

Depending on whether the haemoglobin biomolecule is in its oxygenated or its reduced state, it shows two slightly different but characteristic absorption curves (see Fig. 4.2). Oxygenated haemoglobin has absorption peaks at 577 nm and 420 nm, while reduced haemoglobin has an absorption peak at 560 nm. These haemoglobin absorption characteristics in the visible spectrum can be very useful for laser treatment procedures, particularly in the visible red range. Equally, absorption of incident radiation by haemoglobin results in fewer photons being available within the tissue at the site of irradiation to produce more localised treatment effects. The practical problems resulting from absorption of incident laser radiation by blood is considered further in Chapter 7.

The other important chromophore is melanin. Melanin is the dark brown pigment found in the skin as well as in the pigment epithelium of the retinal fundus. The biosynthesis of melanin is triggered by near ultraviolet radiation, resulting in the tanning effect produced in human skin by irradiation at these wavelengths. The biosynthesis of melanin starts with the amino acid thyrosine, which is converted through several biochemical steps into the indolylquinone ring. Indolylquinone then polymerises within the cell and forms melanin. Absorption characteristics of melanin are given in Figure 4.2. The absorption characteristics of melanin within the therapeutically important near infra-red should particularly be noted.

Both haemoglobin and melanin play an important role in converting incident laser radiation energy into heat. They thus mediate *photothermal* effects of laser irradiation. They do not exhibit any photochemical reaction, as opposed to other chromophores (such as rhodopsin in the eye or chlorophyll in plants) which convert optical energy into chemical energy.

Summary

In summary, the absorption properties of tissue are determined by amino acids in the mid and far ultra-violet spectrum, chromophores in the visible and the near ultra-violet, and water within the infra-red spectrum. In addition, vibrational changes induced in biomolecules also play a role in the absorption properties of tissue within the infra-red part of the spectrum.

Scattering

The other important parameter for determination of light propagation in tissue is scattering. Put most simply, scattering is due to the differing *relative* refractive indices of the various cellular substrates and molecules *with respect to water*, which is the main ingredient of tissues.

As already indicated, scattering in tissues may be defined as the change in the direction of light propagation and is due to the complex geometry of biomolecules, as well as to the precise configuration of the interfaces between water and cell, or water and organelle membranes. Subcellular structures thus act as scattering particles for the incident light.

In physics, two different types of scattering are recognised. These are termed Mie and Rayleigh scattering. The most important factor in determining the type of scattering caused by the type of relatively small particles found in cells is the ratio of the size of the particle to the wavelength of the incident light. In addition the optical properties of the particle material is also important. Mie scattering theory applies where the particle size is comparable to the incident wavelength (Kerker 1969, van der Hulst 1980). Rayleigh scattering theory is essentially a simpler formulation of the equations used to describe Mie scattering and applies where particle size is relatively small compared to incident wavelength. For a given concentration of biological particles to mediate scattering, the degree of Rayleigh scattering is generally smaller than the degree of Mie scattering. Thus the latter is more important for an understanding of the interaction of laser light with biological tissue.

Scattering of electromagnetic radiation can be determined theoretically for simple geometrical shapes where the absorption and refractive properties of the scattering particles are known. However, in biological tissues, it is impractical (and indeed unnecessary) to formulate scattering equations using Mie scattering theory, as tissue is a random non-homogeneous medium with extremely complex geometry. If the problem of defining scattering and thus light distribution in tissue is approached in this way, the solution becomes extremely complex. However, there are some assumptions that can simplify the formulation and solution of this problem. Simple light distribution theories that incorporate scattering can apply to tissue under certain assumptions: these are considered further in the following sections.

As already outlined above, the type and degree of scattering in tissues varies with wavelength; for the band of wavelengths commonly used in laser therapy, in general, the degree of scattering in tissues decreases with wavelength. Furthermore, as the ratio of tissue particle size to wavelength changes, the relative proportion of Mie and Rayleigh scattering changes, so that Rayleigh scattering becomes more prevalent at the longer wavelengths.

In the commonly cited 'therapeutic window' of 660–1300 nm, scattering is composed of a forward-directed scattering component and an additional random or *isotropic* component. It has been found that scattering in certain tissues is not wholly or even largely isotropic, but instead has a predominantly forward component in common with the predictions of Mie scattering theory. This means that the probability of a photon being scattered through a narrow angle is much higher than the probability of it being scattered through a wider angle. Measurements in human skin irradiated with a He–Ne laser (632.8 nm) have shown that the forward scattering portion is about 90% of the total scattering, while isotropic (random) scattering is only about 10% (Jacques et al 1987). In other words, 90% of the He–Ne radiation is scattered parallel to the incident beam and only 10% is scattered 'sideways'.

The relative degree of isotropic scattering (i.e. compared to total scattering) is indicated by the *anisotropy coefficient*. This anisotropy co-efficient is an important measure, as its value dictates the degree of broadening which the incident beam will undergo as it travels through the tissues; this in turn therefore helps determine the depth of penetration. The anisotropy coefficient takes values between −1 and 1. In cases where scattering has a predominantly forward component, anisotropy values will be close to 1, while totally isotropic or random scattering will have an anisotropy value of 0. When the incident beam is totally scattered in a backward direction, the factor is −1. In tissues, for wavelengths between 400 nm and 1400 nm, the anisotropy coefficient increases with wave-length and has a value of approximately 0.80 for the lower wavelengths and between 0.90 and 0.95 for the higher wavelengths. Blood, because of the red blood cells which function as scattering particles, has anisotropy coefficients ranging between 0.95 and 0.99 for the above wavelengths.

Additionally, heating of tissues in conjunction with photo-irradiation not only gives rise to bloodflow and associated changes at a physiological level, but also in turn causes a significant change in the scattering pro-perties of the tissue. This alteration in the optical properties of the heated tissue needs to be borne in mind where laser treatment is used in conjunction with thermal modalities, either in routine clinical practice or for the purposes of research trials. At its most extreme, sufficient tem-perature elevation causes coagulation, which forms globular structures as the protein chains shrink and molecular structures become attached together. The resulting shrinkage increases tissue density. Macroscopically the coagulated tissue whitens because of the increased reflectance due to the light-scattering properties of these globular structures (Jacques 1989). This has important clinical implications for the laser treatment of scar tissue, as increased reflectance at the surface scar calls for use of com-mensurably increased dosages when treating such tissue.

Absorption versus scattering: attenuation of light in tissues

Perhaps the most important consideration in predicting laser–tissue interaction and thus the distribution of light within irradiated tissue is the overall *attenuation* (essentially loss of power) of the beam as it travels through the tissue. This in turn depends upon the ratio of absorption to scattering. This ratio will in the first instance depend upon the type of tissue irradiated: for example the ratio of scattering to absorption is greatest in the dermis. This ratio also varies with wavelength of the incident radiation. In the region of the spectrum where light absorption by tissue is low (600–1200 nm), scattering predominates. In the rest of the visible spectrum there is a wider range of suitable chromophores and therefore absorption plays a more significant role.

LIGHT DISTRIBUTION DURING LASER IRRADIATION OF TISSUE

As already indicated, the prediction of the exact light distribution when tissue is irradiated with a laser is an extremely complicated problem, mainly because of complex structure and geometry of tissue and the variability of its optical properties. In fact, deduction of the actual light distribution in tissues may be impossible. However, a number of different (mathematical) methods, essentially models, can be used to provide a working approximation of the actual distribution.

Beer's law

The most popularly used model is (perhaps not surprisingly) one of the simplest to use. An approximate estimation of light distribution in tissue can be provided using Beer's law (based upon diffusion theory), which assumes that the incident light has exponential attenuation (see Fig. 4.4). The equation that describes this is:

$$I_z = I_{inc}.\exp(-gama.z)$$

(gama = a + s)

where: I_z = the irradiance (W/cm^2) at a given depth
   z = depth in the tissue (cm)
   gama = total attenuation coefficient (cm^{-1})
   a = absorption coefficient (cm^{-1})
   s = scattering coefficient (cm^{-1})
   I_{inc} = incident irradiance (W/cm^2) at the surface of the tissue.

The problem with the use of this equation in low-intensity laser therapy applications is that it gives good results for wavelengths where absorption is dominant (i.e. the ultra-violet and far infra-red), but fails to give an accurate description where scattering has a substantial or greater value compared to absorption, as is the case in the visible and near infra-red parts of the spectrum. The inaccuracy occurs because the scattered photons add to the total amount of light energy within a given volume of tissue or, more correctly, the light *flux* within the tissue (see below). Another problem with the equation is that it works in one dimension only and does not adequately account for those scattered photons incident from different directions.

Radiative transfer theory

A more accurate approach to the problem of describing light distribution in tissue, which accounts for both absorption *and* scattering, is radiative transfer theory. This theory is essentially a development of Mie theory, which itself has a number of limitations. Most important of these is that Mie scattering theory only applies to scattering from a single particle isolated in space with no other particles present. In practice, light is scattered from one particle, impinges upon another particle and is thus rescattered. This process is repeated continuously, resulting in a complex pattern of scattering and rescattering.

The precise formulation of radiative transfer theory and its analytical solutions are beyond the scope of this book; however it is useful to note here that it is derived from calculations of light distribution based on numerical models (Chandralsekhar 1960). These are outlined below. Put simply, the theory describes a unidimensional 'film' of medium, through which the light passes, as comprising a dense array of channels. These channels have various angular orientations, from the perpendicular to the horizontal, so that they cover the entire film of medium. For any incident beam, it is possible to calculate the light that passes into any one channel. For this channel, it is further possible to calculate the amount of light absorbed and, from Mie theory, the amount of light scattered from one channel to another (Joseph et al 1976).

An inherent problem with the equations derived from radiative transfer theory is that they are only capable of providing unidimensional solutions. In order to derive an equation which can provide solutions in two or three dimensions, it is necessary to restrict the angular distribution of the scattered light (i.e. it is necessary to ignore the most extreme angular deviations). There have been some proposed solutions of light distribution problems in three dimensions; however these are beyond the scope of the current text (Ishimaru 1978, Yoon et al 1988).

Monte Carlo models

Despite its limitations, radiative transfer theory can usefully be extended to provide approximations of light distributions in two or three dimensions, using the so-called Monte Carlo method (Keijzer et al 1989). This method computes a random 'walk' for each photon and follows the photon until it is absorbed. Light distribution is then estimated from the distribution of absorbed photons. This distribution, in turn, gives the fluence rate within the tissue.

Fluence may be considered in many respects to be similar to irradiance or power density (see Ch. 2). However, the definition of fluence assumes that the photoacceptor is a small sphere located within the tissue, with its surface irradiated from all directions by photons impinging upon it. In turn, fluence rate may usefully be thought of as absorption of light power per unit volume. The units of fluence rate are therefore W/cm^3 (cf. irradiance and *energy density* – which is defined below – neither of which takes account of absorption, only incident light power and energy respectively). The implications of fluence rate in terms of heat production in tissues are outlined below.

The Monte Carlo method has been used as the basis of a computer program by Keijzer and colleagues which allows prediction of light distribution in tissue (Prahl et al 1989). This program follows the photons on their individual walks. The individual walks are created by a random number generator, using the absorption and scattering coefficients as weighting probabilities in the drawing of the random path. The path is drawn on a grid with cylindrical co-ordinates. Each cell of the grid can have different optical properties to match different layers and types of tissue. The program also takes account of refraction and internal reflections due to mismatch of indices of refraction at the surfaces separating different layers of the grid. The photon source is considered to be an impulse beam co-linear with the axis of the cylindrical grid, light entering the grid through a single point. This implementation of the transfer equation is a state-of-the-art solution to the problem of defining light distribution in tissues, giving a very good estimation of the distribution where tissue is irradiated with a laser source.

A note on heat production and diffusion during irradiation

The absorption of laser light in irradiated tissues produces heat. This absorption of incident energy results in temperature elevation, which may be observed at a whole body level if the energy density is sufficiently high. As already described above, the rate of energy absorption at any point within the tissue is known as the *fluence rate*, which can be calculated as the product of the *fluence* and the tissue's *absorption coefficient*:

$$\text{Fluence rate} = a.\phi$$

where: a = coefficient of absorption of the relevant tissue in cm^{-1}
ϕ = fluence in W/cm^2.

The amount of heat produced at any point in the tissue is directly proportional to the fluence rate, and thus in turn the absorption coefficient at that point. Conversely, the fluence rate can also be calculated for any point in the tissue where the amount of heat at that point and the local absorption coefficient are both known. Depending on the irradiation time, the light distribution and the thermal properties of the irradiated tissue, the amount of heat deposition within the tissues can therefore be modelled. This is usually achieved with the so-called *bioheat transfer equation.*

That the amount of heat deposited in tissue should vary with irradiation time is an important concept, particularly as regards pulsing of laser sources. During irradiation using relatively short, high-energy pulses and high repetition rates, energy is deposited at the target site before a significant amount of heat is diffused to adjacent tissues. Biophysical effects should therefore be more localised and intense with such modes of irradiation (Karu et al 1990). Under these conditions, local temperature rises in a stepwise fashion as represented in Figure 4.3a, corresponding to the pulsing of the incident light. In contrast, for longer pulse durations as well as for continuous wave irradiation, diffusion of energy occurs before a significant amount of heating occurs. Thus with this type of irradiation, steady temperature states (as described in the steady-state bioheat transfer equation) are achieved before the laser is turned off (Fig. 4.3b). Effects should therefore be more diffuse when these modes are used.

For longer irradiation times, the absorbed light is the heat source term of the steady-state bioheat transfer equation (see above). While some have produced analytical solutions using such heat transfer equations, it must be stressed that these equations rely on certain assumptions which are not necessarily valid in all clinical applications; principal among these is that blood flow remains constant.

BEAM PROFILES AND DEPTH OF PENETRATION

The gaussian distribution

In calculating parameters such as irradiance/power density (see Ch. 2)

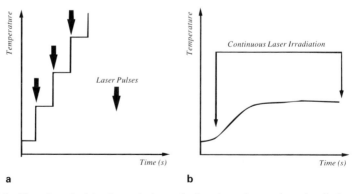

Fig. 4.3 Heat deposited in tissue during pulsed and continuous laser irradiation. **a.** Pulsed irradiation produces step-wise increase in temperature. **b.** Continuous wave laser irradiation causes 'steady-state' temperature rise.

and radiant exposure/energy density (see below), the formulae as they are commonly presented assume that the laser beams in question are uniform or *homogenous*. This implies that the beam delivers the same intensity of radiation across the total area which it irradiates and that outside this well defined beam imprint area there are no photons from the beam. As already indicated in Chapter 2 (p. 40), this is not strictly true, as in most cases the beam imprint does not have abrupt edges, but instead has a bell-shaped profile which approximates to what is known as a gaussian distribution (see Fig. 2.10a). Consequently, the equations as presented in Chapter 2 and below give the average power or energy density over the area of irradiation. It should be noted that, in practical applications, while the beams are not exactly gaussian it is a fair and valid approximation to assume them to be so. While the gaussian profile does not have clearly defined edges, certain assumptions can be employed in order to assist with calculations.

Where a gaussian beam is incident on the surface of an area of target tissue, the edges are assumed to be at the points where the intensity of the beam falls to 12.9% of the intensity at the centre of the beam. The value of 12.9% is $1/e^2$ (i.e. 1 over the square of e) where e is the base of the natural logarithm 2.78. The area defined by these edges includes more than 90% of the total power of the beam. This area is typically used for the calculations of power densities.

Depth of penetration

Gaussian distribution is also assumed for the purposes of calculation of depth of penetration. Where absorption is dominant, there will be exponential attenuation of the beam in the treated tissue (Fig. 4.4). The

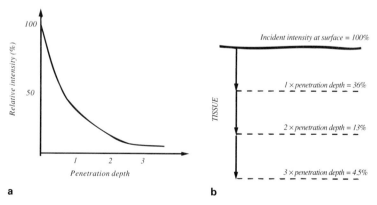

a   b

Fig. 4.4 Exponential attenuation of laser radiation intensity within irradiated tissue. **a.** Approximate graph of relative intensity (%) versus penetration depth. **b.** Approximate percentage values of incident intensity at various penetration depths.

depth at which the intensity of the beam is 36% of the original incident intensity on the surface is called the *depth of penetration* and is typically given in centimetres, millimetres or micrometres. This value of 36% is equal to 1/e. The penetration depth is also the point where the product of the attenuation coefficient (*gama*; see p. 75) and depth is 1. Thus, where absorption is dominant, the depth of penetration is given by the reciprocal of the attenuation coefficient, or 1/*gama*. With calculations it can be further shown that the intensity at a distance of two penetration depths within the tissue is about 13% of the incident intensity on the surface and about 4.5% at three penetration depths (Fig. 4.4).

Even in cases where absorption is not dominant (as is the usual case in laser irradiation of tissue), the depth of penetration term is still used to describe the depth where the intensity is 36% of the incident value on the surface. This is done in order to ease calculations and comparisons. A more accurate distribution can be measured or calculated using, for example, the Monte Carlo method already described earlier and then extrapolating the depth at which the light intensity is equal to 36% of the incident intensity on the surface.

Wavelength and depth of penetration (Table 4.1)

As depth of penetration depends upon scattering and more importantly upon absorption, its value is wavelength-dependent. For practical purposes in biostimulation treatment the spectrum can be divided into the categories described in Table 4.1. Corresponding depths of penetration in the skin are given in this table, assuming normal resting blood circulation and caucasian subjects with a low melanin content.

It should be noted that precise values cannot be given for the depth of penetration because optical properties vary so greatly from individual to individual, depending on such factors as condition of the skin, age, hydration of the skin, blood and fat content etc. However, this variation is not usually more than 20–30% of the values given in Table 4.1.

Table 4.1 Wavelength and approximate penetration depth in tissues

Wavelength in nm		Depth of penetration in mm
Ultra-violet	150–380	< 0.1 mm
Violet to deep blue	390–470	approx. 0.3 mm
Blue to green	475–545	approx. 0.3–0.5 mm
Yellow to orange	545–600	approx. 0.5–1 mm
Red	600–650	approx. 1–2 mm
Deep red to near infra-red	650–1000	2–3 mm
Near to mid infra-red	1000–1350	3–5 mm
Infra-red	1350–12000	< 0.1 mm

Difference between incident and absorbed light

It is important to distinguish between incident light and absorbed light. Incident light at a surface consists of all the photons that impinge upon that surface. The total power associated with a given number of photons *crossing* a surface is called light flux (see above) and has units of power (watts) per surface area (W/cm^2). In situations where the light is diffuse, photons will cross the surface in two directions and the total flux is the sum of the two fluxes. The incident light cannot be absorbed by the surface alone: in order to have absorption, a finite absorbing volume is also required. The light absorbed by this volume will be the sum of the photons entering the surface that defines this volume, minus the sum of the photons that leaves the volume, i.e. the net influx of photons (Fig. 4.5). This absorbed light can be described in terms of volumetric absorption. The volumetric absorption is described in energy units per volume (J/cm^3). The following describes some practical methods for calculating volumetric absorption.

The parameters of incident light such as power, energy, power density (irradiance) and energy density (radiant exposure) are described below and in Chapter 2 (see pp. 39–40). Light distribution charts can give the predicted values of these properties at certain depths within the tissue, where the incident property on the surface is known. If the value of one of the incident properties, for example power density/irradiance, is I_{inc} then the value of the power density at 1 penetration depth will be $0.36\,I_{inc}$. At 2 penetration depths, it will be $0.129\,I_{inc}$, and at 3 penetration depths the power density will be $0.045\,I_{inc}$ etc.

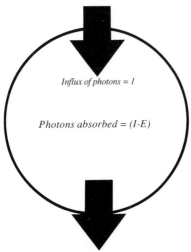

Influx of photons = I

Photons absorbed = (I-E)

Photons exiting volume = E

Fig. 4.5 Absorption of light by a given volume of tissue.

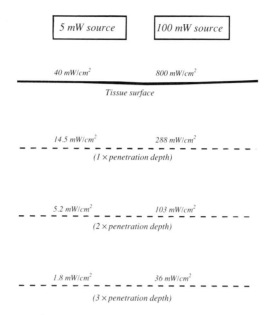

Fig. 4.6 Penetration of two hypothetical 820 nm laser treatment diodes. Reflectance is ignored for this comparison; treatment is 'in contact'; area of irradiation at surface is assumed to be 0.125 cm².

If two hypothetical laser treatment 820 nm wavelength probes are compared using these equations (see Fig. 4.6), with one probe having an average power output of 5 mW and the other an output of 100 mW, the importance of power output to successful treatment becomes clear. From Figure 4.6 it can be seen that in clinical practice, incident power density (usually the power output of the treatment unit divided by the spot size of its beam on the tissue surface) is critically important, especially where the lesion to be treated is relatively deeply located within the tissues. Furthermore, it is also important to stress that volumetric absorption is greater when multisource irradiation is present, as is the case when 'cluster' units are used; in such circumstances the cross-interference from neighbouring diodes in three dimensions increases the fluence below the dermis.

However, it is the absorption of the incident energy that produces the therapeutic effects during (and subsequent to) irradiation. The approximate absorbed energy within a thin layer of tissue is given by:

$$E_{abs} = I_{inc}.d.\gamma.t$$

where: E_{abs} = energy absorbed in J/cm²
I_{inc} = incident irradiance in W/cm²
d = tissue thickness in centimetres
γ = absorption coefficient of the tissue
t = time of irradiation in seconds.

If the layer of interest is to be found at a substantial depth within the irradiated tissue, the above formula is not very accurate and a more precise result will be given by:

$$E_{abs} = (I_{inc} - I_{base}).t$$

where: I_{base} = irradiance at the base of the layer in W/cm^2.

Where the target is a small cell or organelle within the tissue, then it is most appropriate to assume the particle of interest to be a small disc and calculate the absorbed light as:

$$E_{abs} = I_{inc}.d.\gamma.a.t$$

where: a = surface area of the particle in cm^2.

Note: γ for the particle may be different from that of the rest of the tissue.

BASICS ON DOSIMETRY

When it comes to use of laser devices for treatments in clinical practice the above theoretical considerations have to be translated into dosage units, so that treatment may be planned and recorded. This section therefore gives the basic units used in laser treatment. The reader should be conversant with the physical principles of lasers, as outlined in Chapter 2, before reading further.

Energy

As already outlined in Chapter 2, the power unit used for laser equipment is the watt, abbreviated W. Because of the low power outputs typically employed in laser therapy, the unit milliwatt (one thousandth of a watt; abbreviated mW) is more commonly used. A single watt of power applied for a period of 1 second (s) gives an energy of 1 joule (J). Similarly, 1 mJ is one thousandth of a joule and 1 µJ one hundred thousandth of a joule; these are typically the energy parameters per pulse for the millisecond and microsecond pulses emitted by therapeutic laser devices.

In low-intensity laser therapy, the output of a laser is always described in watts or milliwatts, and the energy delivered to a region of target tissue over a period of time is always described in joules or millijoules. Time should always be specified or recorded in seconds. The relationship between power, energy and time is given by the following equation:

   Energy (J) = *power* (W).*time* (s)

Consequently, if a specific energy is required for a treatment and the power of the laser is known, the time needed for treatment can be calculated by dividing the dosage energy by the power of the laser, the result

Table 4.2 Sample energy calculations

Radiant power output (mW)	Irradiation time (s)	Energy (J)
5	10	0.05
5	30	0.15
5	60	0.30
5	120	0.60
15	10	0.15
15	30	0.45
15	60	0.90
15	120	1.80
30	10	0.30
30	30	0.90
30	60	1.80
30	120	3.60
50	10	0.50
50	30	1.50
50	60	3.00
50	120	6.00

being the irradiation time required in seconds. A number of examples of energy calculations are shown in Table 4.2.

Pulsed output systems

With a laser which produces pulsed output, the usual terms used to define the pulses produced by the apparatus are the *pulse energy* and *peak power* (see Fig. 2.12). Pulse energy and *pulse duration* may be specified, from which peak power can be calculated, as peak power is equal to the pulse energy divided by the pulse duration, assuming that the pulse has a rectangular shape. In contrast if the shape of the pulse is triangular, then the peak power is usually assumed to be twice the pulse energy divided by the pulse duration.

As already indicated in Chapter 2, the *average power* of a pulsed laser is always less than the peak power specified for the unit and it is the former value which should be used in calculating the energy delivered during laser treatments. Apart from calculating average power from peak power and duty cycle as already outlined in Chapter 2 (p. 45), it may also be obtained by multiplying the pulse energy by the number of pulses per second (i.e. the pulse repetition rate), as power may be defined in terms of work done *per second*. Under these circumstances, the above formula becomes:

Energy (J) = *pulse energy* (J).*repetition rate* (Hz).*time* (s)

Energy density (radiant exposure)

While some authors insist that calculation of energy delivered during laser therapy is sufficient to define treatment dosage (Kert & Rose 1989), this is more usually specified in terms of *energy density* or *radiant exposure* on the target tissue. Power density or irradiance, as already explained in Chapter 2, is the total incident power divided by the area of the irradiated surface. Similarly, radiant exposure or energy density is obtained by dividing the total incident energy by the irradiated area, and is usually given in joules per square centimetre (J/cm²). It can also be obtained by multiplying the power density or irradiance (in W/cm²) by the total time of irradiation in seconds. For all practical purposes in routine clinical practice, the power output of the laser treatment device will be known, and the spot size of the beam can be calculated, so that the equation most frequently used will be:

$$\textit{Energy density (J/cm}^2) = \frac{\textit{power (W).time (s)}}{\text{area (cm}^2)}$$

Note:
1. Power of a therapeutic unit will usually be specified in milliwatts (e.g. '50 mW'), and therefore must be multiplied by 0.001 before inclusion in the above equation (i.e. 50 mW = 0.05 W)
2. While the unit most commonly used for specifying the surface area in laser treatment is the square centimetre (cm²), the square metre has also been used in some publications (1 m² = 10 000 cm²).

A number of examples using the above equation are presented in Table 4.3.

Table 4.3 Sample energy density (radiant exposure) calculations

Radiant power output (mW)	Irradiation time (s)	Area of irradiation (cm²)	Energy density (J/cm²)
5	10	0.16	0.30
5	120	0.16	3.75
5	10	1.0	0.05
5	120	1.0	0.60
15	10	0.16	0.94
15	120	0.16	11.28
15	10	1.0	0.15
15	120	1.0	1.80
30	10	0.16	1.88
30	120	0.16	22.50
30	10	1.0	0.30
30	120	1.0	3.60
50	10	0.16	3.13
50	120	0.16	37.50
50	10	1.0	0.50
50	120	1.0	6.00

Note: Irradiated areas used for the purposes of the above calculations are based upon 'in contact' (0.16 cm²) and no contact (1.0 cm²) irradiation at a distance of approximately 1.5 cm, in each case using an average diode-based treatment unit.

EXTRAPOLATION OF DOSAGES

One of the problems faced by clinicians within this field is the realisation in their human patients of therapeutic effects documented either in other species, in vitro or indeed in cell lines. Given a hypothetical report that laser irradiation of experimentally induced wounds in rats, using a He–Ne source (632.8 nm) at an energy density of 1 J/cm^2, causes photobiostimulation of the repair process, it should not necessarily be expected to achieve similarly positive results using the same treatment parameters in other species. The problem of lack of specification of irradiation parameters by a sizable proportion of authors has already been noted; however even with full disclosure, the difficulty in extrapolating to humans or between species remains. Unfortunately, little work has been done to date in this area so that, for the time being at least, direct conversions cannot be made between species. However the following few points can be made to help clinicians and investigators in consideration of the problem.

In the first instance, the relative size (or more precisely, volume), of the species should be considered. An energy dose of 4 J represents relatively more irradiation per unit volume of body tissue for a mouse than for a human. While for the mouse and human the number of photons incident per unit area under the same treatment head are exactly the same, the relative size of the irradiated areas is vastly different, by a factor of thousands. The same would hold true for extrapolating the dosage for the treatment of (say), racehorses. While it is not suggested for the examples illustrated here that energy densities be multiplied by several thousands in order to obtain equivalent doses, increases in the order of several factors at least would seem prudent. Indeed, while animal studies commonly cite irradiation with radiant exposures of up to but usually no more than 4 J/cm^2, physiotherapists and clinicians treating humans may employ energy densities of up to 30 J/cm^2.

However, species differences extend to more than sheer size. In particular, skin composition and structure vary enormously between species, so that optical properties are vastly different. The consequently greater penetration of laser light in such loose-skinned animals as mice and other small rodents may account for the superior results obtained in research using these species (Basford 1986). In general, therefore, treatment dosages have to be increased when extrapolating from loose-skinned animals such as rodents to species with a more intact tegumen, e.g. humans. However, two points need to be made in this respect. In the first instance, where open wounds are being compared, species differences should matter rather less as the laser is irradiating the wound bed with minimal (if indeed any) attenuation. Furthermore, the *relative* differences in the two species must also be considered: the differences in skin structure between a mouse and a human are obviously more profound than between a pig and a human.

For this reason, porcine wound healing is usually considered superior to murine wound healing as an experimental model of the process in humans.

SUMMARY OF KEY POINTS

1. The two most important modes of light interaction with tissue during therapeutic laser treatment procedures are absorption and scattering.
2. The interaction between light and tissue may be considered at three levels: atomic, molecular and macromolecular levels. Laser–tissue interaction at the wavelengths commonly used in LILT applications is predominantly at the molecular and macromolecular levels.
3. Absorption may be defined as the conversion of light to some other form of energy. The absorption properties of tissue are determined by amino acids in the mid and far ultra-violet spectrum, chromophores in the visible and near ultra-violet and water within the infra-red spectrum.
4. Scattering in tissues may be defined as a change in direction of light propagation and is due to the complex geometry of bio-molecules, as well as to the precise configuration of the interfaces between water and cell, or water and organelle membranes.
5. Light may be scattered in a forward, rearward or random (isotrophic) fashion. Measurements in human tissue would suggest that approximately 90% of the scattering that occurs at therapeutic wavelengths is in a forward direction.
6. The prediction of the precise light distribution when tissue is irradiated with therapeutic laser is extremely complex, mainly because of the complex structure and geometry of tissue and the wide variation in optical properties. Despite this, a number of different mathematical models have been used to provide working approximations of light distribution in tissues. These include Beer's law, radiative transfer theory and Monte Carlo modelling.
7. While it is usually assumed that laser beams are homogenous, the actual irradiance across the beam varies, with greatest values being found in the centre of the beam.
8. Depth of penetration varies with tissue type and wavelength. As absorption is predominant in tissue, there will be exponential attenuation of the laser beam as it passes through treated tissues. The depth at which the intensity of the beam is 36% of the original incident intensity on the tissue surface is called the penetration depth.

9. Energy is equal to the radiant power output of the unit in watts (or mW) multiplied by the irradiation time in seconds. It is expressed in joules (J) or millijoules (mJ). For pulsed output units, this figure can also be calculated by multiplying pulse energy by pulse repetition rate, then by the time of irradiation in seconds.

10. Energy density is expressed in joules per centimetre squared (J/cm^2) or per metre squared (J/m^2) and is given by dividing the energy delivered to the target tissue by the area of irradiation.

11. Extrapolating dosages between animals and humans remains a problem. Apart from such species differences as skin structure etc., the sheer variation in volume between some experimental animals and humans confounds the realisation in human practice of positive results obtained in animals.

REFERENCES

Basford J R 1986 Low-energy laser treatment of pain and wounds: hype, hope or hokum? Mayo Clinic Proceedings 61: 671–675

Chandralsekhar S 1960 Radiative transfer. Dover Press, New York

Hulst van der H G 1980 Multiple light scattering, vol. II. vvv, New York

Ishimaru A 1978 Wave propagation and scattering in random media. Academic Press, New York

Jacques S 1989 Time resolved reflectance spectroscopy in turbid tissue. IEEE Transactions Engineering Medicine Biology 36: 1155–1161

Jacques S L, Aeter C A, Prake S A 1987 Angular dependence of He–Ne laser light scattering by human dermis. Lasers in the Life Science 1: 309–333

Joseph J H, Winscombe W J, Weinman J A 1976 The delta-Eddington approximation for relative flux transfer. Journal of Atmospheric Science 33: 2452–2459

Karu T, Tiphlova O, Samokhina H et al 1990 Effects of near-infrared laser and superluminous diode irradiation on Escherichia coli division rate. IEEE Journal Quantum Electronics 26: 2162–2165

Keijzer M, Jacques S L, Prahl S A et al 1989 Light distributions in artery tissue: Monte Carlo simulations for finite-diameter laser beams. Lasers in Surgery and Medicine 9: 148–154

Kerker M 1969 The scattering of light. Academic Press, New York

Kert J, Rose L 1989 Clinical laser therapy: low level laser therapy. Scandinavian Medical Laser Technology, Copenhagen

Prahl S A, Keijzer M, Jacques S L et al 1989 A Monte Carlo model of light propagation in tissue. SPIE Institute, series 5

Yoon G, Welch A J, Montamedi M, van Gemet M C J 1988 Development and application of three dimensional light distribution model for laser irradiated tissue. IEEE Journal of Quantum Electronics 23: 1721–1733

5. Laser photobiomodulation of wound healing

INTRODUCTION

Wound healing is a complicated, interactive, integrative process involving cellular and chemotactic activity, the release of chemical mediators and associated vascular responses. During the past 20 years there have been numerous reports indicating the potential of low-energy laser irradiation in the facilitation of the wound healing process. Physiotherapists have identified a variety of wounds as responding well to low-intensity laser treatment and indeed have ranked the efficacy of laser above that of other commonly used electrotherapeutic modalities such as interferential, shortwave and, most notably, ultrasound (Baxter et al 1991). Consequently the treatment of wounds represents the primary indication for laser therapy in the minds of most clinicians.

This has prompted the publication of a multiplicity of research papers in this area, encompassing both in vivo and in vitro studies. The purpose of this chapter is to present an overview of the wound healing process and to provide the reader with an up to date review of current research in this area.

THE TRIPHASIC MODEL OF WOUND REPAIR

As already indicated above, wound healing is a complex physiological process involving many different reactions. It begins, essentially, with tissue injury and encompasses the body's innate reactions to such damage. Both the immune and blood clotting systems are alerted and an interrelated sequence of events ensues, modulated by a mixture of chemical and cellular factors.

The sequence of events culminating in total wound closure and repair can be divided into three overlapping phases (Clark 1985, 1988):

1. Inflammation
2. Re-epithelialisation and contraction
3. Matrix remodelling.

A brief description of each stage of repair is essential to the understanding of the types of biological mechanism that may be affected when

89

using low-intensity laser therapy. Consequently the purpose of the first part of this chapter is to give a brief, concise overview of the mechanisms involved in wound repair.

INFLAMMATION AND ACTIVATION OF THE IMMUNE RESPONSE

The basic acute inflammatory reaction to any kind of trauma is ubiquitous regardless of the inciting cause, whether surgical, bacterial or accidental physical injury. The major series of events immediately following tissue wounding are a result of blood and lymph vessel disruption, consequential extravasation (leaking) of blood constituents, platelet aggregation and degranulation, and ultimately blood coagulation. The purpose of these events is to provide a cleansing service in the area, in the form of phagocytic cells which engulf bacteria and other cellular debris. Once this is performed the sequential repair mechanisms can proceed normally. Occasionally, the latter process is not totally efficient and a state known as chronic inflammation ensues.

The acute inflammatory stage usually lasts only 1–3 days and overlaps with the next phase, granulation tissue formation. Figure 5.1 shows a schematic graph of the various processes involved and the time-scale each normally employs.

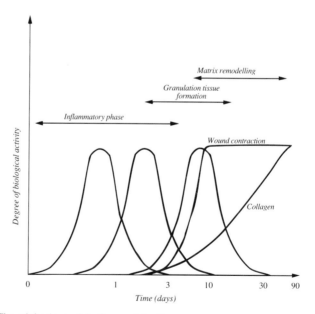

Fig. 5.1   The triphasic model of wound healing.

The vascular response

Vascular reactivity is rapid and results in an immediate, short-lived vaso-constriction mediated by noradrenaline. This partially controls the tendency to haemorrhage, as partial occlusion of small vessels occurs due to contraction of endothelial linings which become sticky (Peacock 1984, Kloth et al 1990). Vasodilation follows after a few minutes and is manifested as the erythema seen at an injured site. The pain felt on tissue injury is due to a combination of stretching of the local nerves, distention of tissue spaces, as well as chemical irritation of nociceptors.

Almost immediately, an influx of white blood cells, primarily neutrophils, begins. The stickiness of the endothelium results in adherence of these leukocytes to it, and within 30 minutes to 1 hour after the beginning of the inflammatory period, the entire surface of the vessels may be covered with neutrophils (Peacock 1984). Platelets and erythrocytes also adhere, but to a much lesser extent, the red cells forming tentative capillary plugs.

Oedema formation

Along with vascular dilation, leakage of fluid from vessels occurs and produces swelling (oedema) in the surrounding tissues. Plasma leakage is due to changes in vascular permeability, initially brought about by histamine. Histamine is released almost immediately by damaged cells, the majority of it emanating from degranulating mast cells, which also release other active mediators: for example prostaglandins, serotonin and heparin. Basophils may also contribute histamine, although this leukocyte appears in very low numbers. Histamine acts on the endothelial cells lining blood vessels, not on the vessels themselves, causing them to swell and contract leaving gaps between cells. Its action is quite short-lived, lasting not longer than 30 minutes. It is clear, therefore, that other factors must be involved at later stages to alter permeability, and a biphasic capillary reaction has been described (Peacock 1984).

Figure 5.2 shows the vascular changes which lead to oedema formation. Normally there is an equilibrium in the capillary with the flow of fluid and cellular material out of the vessel balancing the influx of fluid and waste products. Upon vessel disruption, the net outflow increases as dictated by chemical mediators of permeability. The endothelial cells become 'leaky', resulting in oedema transudate collecting in the tissue spaces. Initially this transudate appears as a clear, serous liquid; however, as the inflammatory reaction continues, effete leukocytes and other cellular particles (e.g. low molecular weight proteins like albumin) diffuse out with the fluid and the oedema exudate assumes an opaque, viscous consistency (Kloth et al 1990) which is known as *sterile pus*.

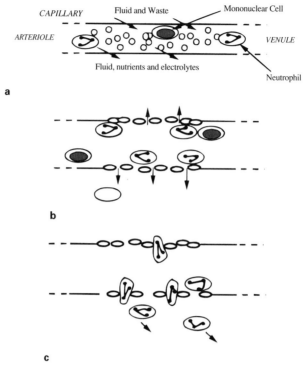

Fig. 5.2 Overview of oedema formation. **a.** Normal situation: balanced flow of fluids and nutrients. **b.** Permeability increased; endothelial cells move apart. Neutrophils marginate. More fluid fills tissue spaces; oedema transudate formed. **c.** Neurophils migrate to tissue spaces along with fluid; oedema exudate increases.

Cellular events and reactions

Neutrophils

Neutrophils are the first cells to arrive in large numbers at the wound site. Once in the area they adhere to the endothelium, a process known as *margination*. Monocytes appear to migrate at the same time (Turk et al 1976), both cells being attracted to the site by a variety of chemotactic factors (Table 5.1). The major function of neutrophils during the early stages of inflammation is to rid the area of bacterial contaminants and other debris by engulfing and then solubilising particles with intracellular enzymes, a process known as *phagocytosis*. Subsequent lysosomal (e.g. proteolytic, collagenolytic and fibrinolytic) enzyme release at low pH (Kanzler et al 1986), and oxygen radical formation associated with neutrophils also help in wound debridement.

Although neutrophils are quite prompt at arriving and efficient in their functions at the wound site, it has been demonstrated experimentally in both neutropenic animals and by injection of antineutrophilic serum that

Table 5.1 Chemotactic factors involved in wound repair (from Clark 1988)

Factor	Chemoattractant for:
C5a and C3a	Neutrophils, monocytes, macrophages
Prostaglandin I_2	Neutrophils
Neutrophil chemotactic factor (NCF)	Neutrophils
Collagen fragments	Macrophages
Bacterial endotoxins	Macrophages
Lymphokines, including:	
Macrophage activating factor (MAF)	Macrophages
Migration inhibition factor (MIF)	Macrophages
Chemotactic factor (CF)	Macrophages
Histamine	Macrophages, monocytes, neutrophils
Leukotriene B_4	Neutrophils, eosinophils, basophils, monocytes
Fibronectin	Fibroblasts
T-cell factors	Lymphocytes, eosinophils, basophils
Platelet-derived growth factor	Fibroblasts, smooth muscle cells
Thromboxane A_2	Platelets
Adenosine diphosphate (ADP)	Platelets
Interleukin 8 (IL-8)	Neutrophils, monocytes

they are not necessary for normal wound healing to proceed (Simpson & Ross 1972, Peacock 1984, Kloth et al 1990).

Following margination, the neutrophils must contact the inflamed extravascular tissue to have any effect. They do this by squeezing between endothelial cells (*diapedesis*) and on to the inflamed site. Recent research in this area has concentrated on elucidating the mechanisms of neutrophilic adherence, diapedesis and attraction towards the target site. There appear to be four basic movements involved (Fig. 5.3). Initially, chemoattractants (Table 5.1) cause the neutrophil to stick to the endothelium and flatten. The mechanism of granulocyte trapping in vessels has been investigated, as it was not known whether the chemoattractant acted on the cell itself or on specialised receptors on the vessel surface. There appears to be a receptor on the neutrophil for the chemotactic substances (Nourshargh & Williams 1990). These mediators also potentiate leakage, thus encouraging neutrophil emigration to the extravascular spaces. The neutrophil positions itself between endothelial cells, then moves further out and is held in a 'sandwich-like' manner between the endothelium and the perivascular membrane. Finally, the cells infiltrate the perivascular barrier, by some mechanism which is still unclear, and move along a concentration gradient of chemoattractant towards the injured site.

The complement component C_{5a} and the chemical mediator prostaglandin I_2 are quite important in chemoattraction and as oedema-inducing agents. It has been demonstrated that peak production of both these mediators occurs approximately 2 hours after injury; however, after

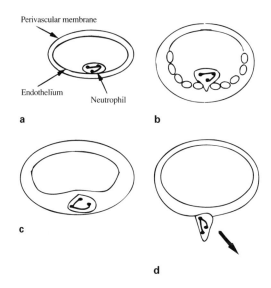

Fig. 5.3 Neutrophilic movement. **a.** Pavementing – neutrophil sticks to endothelium and flattens. **b.** Diapedesis – neutrophil moves between endothelial cells. **c.** Neutrophil 'sandwiched' between endothelial cells and perivascular membrane. **d.** Neutrophil moves along chemoattractant gradient to site of injury.

approximately 6 hours, there is another peak of increased activation. It is therefore assumed that there must be a second mediator released which maintains the state of hyperpermeability and causes further attraction of neutrophils. A process known as amino acid n-terminal sequencing of this second mediator has proposed a substance called interleukin-8 (Collins et al 1991).

Neutrophil infiltration will cease after the first few days and effete cells are phagocytosed by tissue macrophages which essentially take over the role of neutrophils, the latter having a relatively short life-span.

A note on chronic inflammation

Occasionally, the numbers of neutrophils present do not decrease as expected. Bacterial or other contamination may result in a continuation of acute inflammation which would ultimately result in interference with the next stage of healing. Persistence of the inflammatory state is known as chronic inflammation and, although neutrophilic cell levels are elevated, the predominate cells are mononuclear, since neutrophils are mostly destroyed or die after phagocytosing offensive material. The monocytes modulate into phagocytically active macrophages upon migration from capillaries into the tissue spaces. Some of them combine to form multinucleate giant cells. This high level of macrophages may persist for many years, and cellular proliferation is usual in this situation. The mononuclear cells occasionally develop into histiocytes or into epithelioid cells and are often observed in the wound lesion. Granulomas are usually the end result of chronic inflammation. A granuloma is a benign mass of multi-nucleate cells encapsulated by epithelial cells and fibrous tissue which frequently requires surgical removal.

Macrophages

Under normal circumstances, the macrophage population increases significantly from the early inflammatory stage onwards. Macrophages are considered to be pivotal in the wound healing process (Clark 1985) and, unlike neutrophils, are essential if repair is to continue (Liebovich & Ross 1975, Olsen 1984). They are an important source of various active substances which are vital in attracting and activating additional cells as well as substances necessary for the initiation and propagation of granulatory tissue in the next stage. Thus the macrophage plays a crucial role in the continuation of the whole process (Roitt et al 1985, Kanzler et al 1986).

Macrophages appear generally within the first 5 days of inflammation (see Fig. 5.1), and compared to neutrophils have a relatively long lifespan. Mononuclear cell migration may be stimulated by various factors (Table 5.1); for example collagen fragments, plasma, bacterial endotoxins and complement components (Postlethwaite & Kang 1976). Similarly, activation of macrophages in the wound area can also be initiated by an array of substances such as lymphokines, complement component C_{3b}, and fibronectin (a glycoprotein in the tissue matrix).

Macrophages provide the same cleansing functions as neutrophils by producing collagenases (Wahl et al 1974), proteoglycan degrading enzymes (Laub et al 1982) and elastases, and also respond to soluble and phagocytic stimuli by the production of a family of reactive oxygen species (ROS; Clark 1985, 1988). There is a contradiction here in that ROS appear to be toxic to a variety of cells, including endothelial cells, fibroblasts (Simon et al 1981) and epithelial cells (Martin et al 1981). Thus the role of ROS, apart from bactericidal effects, remains unclear. Optimal macrophage activity occurs in well oxygenated tissues (Silver 1984), although their presence in chronic inflammation and at the leading edge of wounds indicates an ability to tolerate severe hypoxia.

Macrophages release a wide variety of biologically active substances such as vasoactive mediators (Humes et al 1977, Ronzer et al 1982), and chemotactic and growth factors (Sporn & Roberts 1986). Chemotactic factors, for example fibronectin, are important in attracting fibroblasts to the area (Tsukamoto et al 1981) and in their adhesion to fibrin in the later stages of fibroplasia. In the absence of macrophages it has been demonstrated that the appearance of fibroblasts in the wound area is delayed and the amount of collagen laid down is therefore decreased (Peacock 1984).

Angiogenesis (or neovascularisation) also benefits from macrophage presence (Polverini et al 1977, Knighton et al 1981). Premature addition of macrophages to a wound results in new vessel ingrowth earlier than expected, and it has been demonstrated that a macrophage-derived growth factor can induce angiogenesis in an avascular area. Optimal release of this factor seems to occur in hypoxic conditions and indeed, if the oxygen tension is altered and macrophages removed from the area, angiogenesis and wound debridement may be temporarily halted (Banda et al 1985).

Lymphocytes, eosinophils and basophils

Other white blood cells present during the inflammatory period include lymphocytes and, to a lesser extent, eosinophils and basophils. Eosinophils have collagenolytic activity and thus may be more important in establishing an equilibrium between collagen formation and lysis during the remodelling stage (Bassett et al 1977). These cells, which comprise only 2–5% of blood leukocytes, are attracted to the area by products released by T-lymphocytes, mast cells and basophils. One of these mediators is called ECF-A (eosinophil chemotactic factor of anaphylaxis). Eosinophils contain multiple granules and can be stimulated to release the enzymes histaminase and aryl sulphatase which inactivate histamine and the so-called slow-reacting substance of anaphylaxis (SRS-A) respectively from mast cells. These reactions help to reduce the acute inflammatory response and reduce neutrophil migration to the wound site (Roitt et al 1985).

Basophils and closely associated mast cells are also characterised by deeply staining granules. Basophils account for less than 2% of circulating white cells and mast cells are found mostly associated with mucosal epithelial cells or connective tissue. Granular contents are basically the same in both cell types, consisting of histamine, heparin (an anticoagulant), SRS-A and ECF-A. The signal for degranulation is usually an allergen molecule associated with immunoglobulin E, a type of antibody (Roitt et al 1985). Histamine is important immediately after injury to establish the body's response and heparin is useful in preventing clotting of excess tissue fluids and blood components.

Lymphocytes are another type of leukocyte which appear at injury sites, although they are not necessary in the furtherance of repair (Peacock 1984). Maximal infiltration can be observed at the sixth day (Fig. 5.1). Lymphoid cells make up approximately 20% of the total white cell population, and can be subdivided into two groups called T cells (65–80%) and B cells (5–15%). Antigen-activated T cells release a group of mediators called lymphokines (Table 5.2) which can also activate macrophages and regulate their functions. The growth factors GM-CSF (granulocyte–

Table 5.2   Platelet-derived mediators of inflammation (from Clark 1988)

Mediator	Actions
Thromboxane A_2, B_2	vasoconstrictor, proaggregant
Prostaglandins D_2, E_2, F_2	vasoactive, modulate haemostasis and leukocyte function
Leukotriene synthesis	inhibitors, stimulate leukocytes
Serotonin	vasoconstrictor, increases vascular permeability, fibrogenic
Thrombospondin	platelet lectin, inhibits fibrinolysis
Growth factors:	
PDGF	connective tissue mitogen, cell transforming factor, chemotactic
Platelet factor 4	proaggregant, chemotactic, inhibits neutral proteases, induces basophil and histamine release
TGF α	
EGF	
TGF β	regulation of various processes
Elastase	protease
Collagenase	protease
α_1-antitrypsin	protease inhibitor
α_2-macroglobulin	
α_2-antiplasmin	plasmin inhibitor

macrophage colony stimulating factor) and G-CSF (granulocyte colony stimulating factor) are both important in attracting macrophages to the wound site and retaining them there. Lymphocytes also release a variety of chemotactic factors and other mediators which are not as important in wound healing, for example interleukins 2 and 3.

Platelets and the coagulation system

Platelets are another myeloid-derived cell type. In addition to their role in blood clotting, platelets are important regulatory cells in tissue repair and, as they respond directly to perturbations of vascular integrity, are therefore involved from an early stage. Platelet aggregation and activation are crucial in the initial stages of inflammation. When collagen is exposed in damaged tissue, platelets adhere to this and other subendothelial connective tissues (Hoffbrand & Pettit 1984). Platelets contain many granules, and adhesion or alternatively exposure to thrombin results in degranulation. An array of mediators are released including ADP (adenosine diphosphate), serotonin, fibrinogen, fibronectin, and lysosomal enzymes. Table 5.2 shows platelet-derived mediators of inflammation.

Thromboxane A_2 and ADP have a positive feedback effect on platelet adhesion by enlisting more platelets to adhere to the injury site. ADP also causes platelets to swell and encourages neighbouring platelet membranes to adhere, which at the same time causes further degranulation, liberating more proaggregants. This aggregation results in the formation of a platelet mass which can temporarily occlude bleeding vessels. Following degranulation and aggregation the exposed surface, consisting of substances called phospholipids, forms an ideal template for the essential concentration and orientation of specific coagulation proenzymes (inactive enzymes). The temporary microenvironment provided by the wound allows activation of these proenzymes which would normally be quenched in the circulation by plasma protease inhibitors.

The basic function of the cascade system is to amplify the effect of a few initiation substances by sequential activation of pro-enzymes, resulting in the generation of thrombin which converts plasma fibrinogen to fibrin, which in turn reinforces the unstable primary platelet plug. Platelet-derived ADP also facilitates the cascade, producing more thrombin, and platelet granular fibrinogen gets converted to fibrin which reinforces the final clot.

The coagulation cascade can be activated by either the extrinsic or the intrinsic system. The former occurs when tissue procoagulant factors in the interstitium and from damaged cells activate factor VII which directly activates factor X (Fig. 5.4). The intrinsic system is initiated when

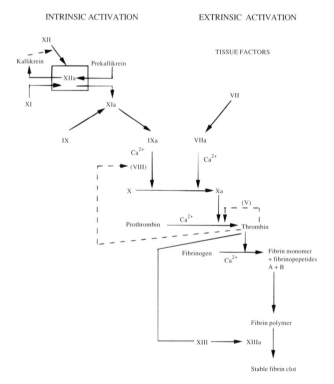

Fig. 5.4 The coagulation cascade.

a proenzyme called Hageman factor (factor XII) is activated on contact with collagen or other negatively-charged components of subendothelial connective tissue. Hageman factor in turn activates factor XI while also converting a substance called prekallikrein to kallikrein. Factor XI and kallikrein are bound to a cofactor, high molecular weight kininogen (HMWK), and the whole arrangement is often referred to as the kinin system.

Kallikrein cleaves a molecule called bradykinin from HMWK. This is a 9 amino acid vasoactive peptide which also appears to induce pain. Kallikrein has a positive feedback effect on Factor XII, and also activates the proenzyme plasminogen of the fibrinolytic system to produce plasmin. This substance is important in splitting the end product of coagulation, fibrin, to produce chemotactic fibrinopeptides, thereby controlling the extent of clotting. In the absence of such regulation, vessel occlusion would occur through unlimited coagulation. Plasmin also has the ability to activate the classical complement cascade, generating different components, for example the anaphylatoxins C_{3a} and C_{5a} which, together with bradykinin, are important in triggering mast cell release of histamine, permeability changes in capillaries and chemokinesis (Roitt et al 1985). They also stimulate release of other vasoactive mediators like leukotrienes C_4 and D_4 from mast cells (Hugli & Muller-Eberhard 1978, Stimler et al 1981), and attract neutrophils and monocytes to the wound site (Fernandez et al 1978), at the same time encouraging them to produce biologically active substances.

Platelet degranulation yields copious amounts of growth factors into the wound area (Table 5.2), notably platelet-derived growth factor (PDGF) which has been demonstrated to be chemotactic and mitogenic for fibroblasts and smooth muscle cells in vitro (Grotendorst et al 1981). Further evidence indicates it is also functional in attracting macrophages (Michaeli et al 1984), monocytes and neutrophils (Deuel et al 1982), and that thrombin-activated platelets have angiogenic activity (Knighton et al 1982). Platelets, like macrophages, have a crucial regulatory function in the whole process of tissue repair.

It is therefore apparent that the clotting, immune, kinin and fibrinolytic systems interact substantially to mediate inflammation and resolve tissue damage, and to maintain vascular integrity and limit the spread of tissue damage whether by physical or infectious causes (Roitt et al 1985). Figure 5.5 shows a simplistic scheme of how this interaction takes place.

Biochemical mediators

Table 5.3 lists the main biochemical mediators involved during the inflammatory period. The actions of cytokines, histamine, bradykinin and the complement components have been described in previous sections.

Serotonin, or 5-hydroxytryptamine (5-HT), is a potent vasoconstrictor

BELMONT UNIVERSITY LIBRARY

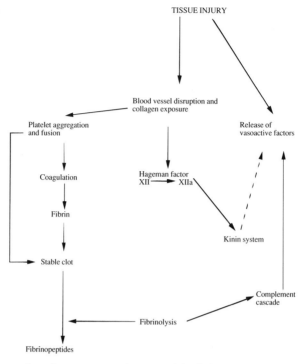

Fig. 5.5 Interaction of systems central to wound healing.

Table 5.3 Biochemical mediators of inflammation

Mediator	Function
Cytokines	Regulation of whole process
Histamine	Initial increase in vascular permeability
Serotonin	Vasoconstrictor. Related to fibroblast proliferation and crosslinking of collagen
Kinins	e.g. bradykinin, potent inflammatory agent, causes increase in vascular permeability
Prostaglandins	PGE_1 – increases vascular permeability
	PGE_2 – chemoattractant for leukocytes, proinflammatory, enhances effects of bradykinin. Sensitises pain receptors

released from platelets and other cells and, in humans, appears to be involved in the latter stages of healing. It potentiates fibroblast proliferation and crosslinking of collagen molecules (Peacock 1984) and promotes DNA synthesis in granuloma cells during chronic inflammation.

Prostaglandins (PG) are the only other major group of chemical mediators with a central role in repair. These are produced by nearly all body cells when the cell membrane is disrupted. Phospholipid is broken down by phospholipase A_2 to form arachidonic acid, which is subsequently converted to leukotrienes by the action of one enzyme (lipoxygenase) or to prostaglandin precursors by another (cyclooxygenase). Two of the leukotrienes, LTC_4 and LTD_4 combine to form SRS-A which alters capillary permeability during inflammation (Roitt et al 1985).

A family of chemically related compounds called thromboxanes are also formed, with some antagonistic functions to those of the prostaglandins; for example whereas PGI_2 and PGF_2 are mostly vasodilatory and encourage antiaggregation of platelets, thromboxane A_2 is a potent vasoconstrictor which also causes platelet aggregation. Some prostaglandins are proinflammatory and enhance the effects of other substances. They are also partly responsible for the hyperalgesic state associated with inflammation by sensitising nociceptors and thus lowering the pain threshold (Wilkerson 1985). Prostaglandins have a contributory effect on successive stages of healing too, in this case by contributing to the synthesis of mucopolysaccharides.

RE-EPITHELIALISATION AND CONTRACTION

This is the proliferative stage of wound healing which evolves over the next 10–14 days and results in regeneration of the epidermis, neoangiogenesis and fibroplasia leading to collagen synthesis. The tissue formed at this stage is often referred to as *granulation tissue* because of its rough granular appearance, which is due to multiple newly formed blood vessels (Clark 1985).

The predominant cells at this stage are fibroblasts and macrophages (see Fig. 5.1) and there is extensive evidence to suggest that macrophages are vital to dermal repair, since they release fibroblast and endothelial cell chemotactic factors and secrete lactate which stimulates collagen synthesis by fibroblasts (Silver 1974). Macrophages also encourage fibroplasia and angiogenesis by releasing growth factors at the wound site. Electron micrographs show intercellular contacts between both types of cell, suggesting interdependence. Fibroblasts respond to the various stimuli by proliferating, migrating into the area, depositing a matrix of extracellular material (collagen, elastin, proteoglycans) and are responsible for wound contraction. The matrix provides a medium through which cells can move, and support for new blood vessels, which in turn supply nutrients and oxygen for the growth of new tissue. This phase, like the others, relies on the interaction of a number of cells for successful completion and progression to the next stage of development.

The formation of granulation tissue and its re-epithelialisation is brought about by various signals including chemotactic and growth factors, changes in structural molecules and loss of nearest neighbour cells (Clark 1985, 1988, Kloth et al 1990). Platelet degranulation in the earlier stages of wound healing results in the release of a plethora of growth factors (Table 5.2), including epidermal and fibroblast growth factors (Sporn & Roberts 1986), while macrophage activation also leads to accumulation of PDGF and other cytokines (Shimokado et al 1985, Sporn & Roberts 1986). As a result, the situation arises in which there is an almost continuous synthesis and release of growth factors.

Re-epithelialisation

Re-epithelialisation begins within the first 24 hours after injury, actually several days before granulation tissue formation, in an attempt to re-establish the protective barrier of the skin. The first noticeable change in epidermal cells (keratinocytes in cutaneous wounds) adjacent to the wound is that they become flattened and develop pseudopod-like extensions of the cytoplasm (Kanzler et al 1986). Intercellular attachments (desmosomes) are lost, as are the structural appendages of the cell (tonafilaments), and actin (a component of muscle) filaments form at the edge. The loss of structural rigidity and formation of actin pseudopodia on the wound side (i.e. basolateral side) of the epidermal cells allows movement.

Movement occurs over viable tissue within 24 hours and is highest in hyperbaric conditions. The rate at which cells move is approximately 12–21 μm/h (Kanzler et al 1986), the epithelial cells being guided by the scaffolding provided by the fibrin clot and the presence of collagen. The orientation of the substrate is vital to epithelial migration and this directing of cellular movement is called contact guidance. The surface glycoprotein fibronectin also provides a matrix over which cells may migrate, although it appears more important in the movement of fibroblasts. The intracellular contractile (actin) filaments of the migrating cells interact with fibronectin filaments that protrude from the surface of the fibrin clot and other fibroblasts, and the cells actively pull themselves over the matrix. The actin filaments disappear from the epithelial cells after healing and are not found in normal epidermis.

Movement can take place by two possible mechanisms. Firstly, it has been demonstrated that an epithelial cell migrates only a short distance and then slides or rolls over other epithelial cells which are already implanted (Winter 1972). The cell then remains in this position and other cells continue to 'leapfrog' over it until a layer of four to six cells advances far enough to close the defect (Kloth et al 1990). The second method proposed is that a single line of cells migrates across a wound with a 'train' of cells behind it, stopping when it comes into contact with other epithelial cells (contact inhibition) or on completion of the re-epithelialisation.

The stimulus for movement is not yet clearly described. It may be due to chemotactic factors, active contact guidance or the loss of neighbouring cells (Clark 1985). A group of tissue-specific substances called *chalones* are thought to be involved in control of cellular events in normal circumstances by inhibition of such processes. In the case of disrupted or injured tissue, chalones would not be produced and thus adjacent normal tissue could proliferate until such time as it was healed and began to secrete chalones once again to control proliferation (Bullough & Lawrence 1961).

Many of the growth factors released by degranulating platelets may be important in epidermal proliferation. Epidermal growth factor (EGF) is known to play a major role in re-epithelialisation (Cohen 1965, Brown et al 1986). Platelet-derived growth factor (PDGF), transforming growth factor (TGF-α), and fibroblast growth factor (FGF)-like peptides are also released from platelets; later macrophages are also involved in the release of such growth factors. The rate of mitosis in the epidermal cells is greatest at 48 hours post-wounding, in some cases reaching 17 times its normal rate; it also loses its normal diurnal rhythm. Once the cells are contact inhibited and basement membranes reformed, resumption of normal cellular phenotype occurs and mitosis falls to three to four times the normal rate (Kanzler et al 1986).

Reformation of the basement membrane occurs soon after cell migration. The first part of the basement membranes to regenerate is an antigen found between the basal plasma membrane of epidermal cells and the temporary matrix, which is called bullous pemphigoid antigen. The two most prominent components, laminin and type IV collagen, are laid down following cessation of cellular migration (Clark et al 1982a). Basement membrane deposition begins at the periphery and advances to the centre of the wound. The resumption of normal epidermal cell phenotype takes place once re-epithelialisation is complete and basement membrane synthesis is nearing completion. Hemidesmosomes reform rapidly (Gipson et al 1983) and anchor the epidermal cells. Healthy re-epithelialisation will take place in a well hydrated wound, although the formation of a scab may well impede the process. It is therefore vital to keep the wound area moistened to prevent scab formation.

Fibroplasia

Fibroblast proliferation (fibroplasia) and migration into the wound site are instigated by numerous interrelated factors including fibroblast growth factors (Zetter et al 1976, Sporn et al 1986) and chemoattractants (Postlethwaite et al 1976, 1987, Seppa et al 1982). During granulation tissue formation, fibroblasts acquire ultrastructural, functional, immunological and chemical characteristics which distinguish them from normal tissue fibroblasts. Such transformed fibroblasts are termed *myofibroblasts* (Montandon et al 1977, Gabbiani et al 1978, Majno 1979).

Morphologically, they retract their Golgi body and endoplasmic reticula to areas surrounding the nucleus and develop numerous bundles of actin filaments which are arranged parallel to the long axis of the cell, thus

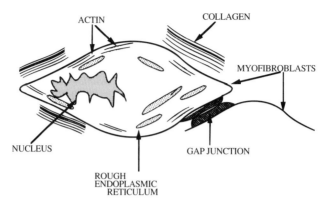

ACTIN

COLLAGEN

MYOFIBROBLASTS

NUCLEUS

GAP JUNCTION

ROUGH
ENDOPLASMIC
RETICULUM

Fig. 5.6   A myofibroblast (after Montandon).

resembling the structure of muscle cells (Fig. 5.6). The nucleus also develops multiple indentations, and intercellular connections are established between neighbouring myofibroblasts, referred to as gap junctions. In addition there is often a surface covering of material similar to basal lamina and where this occurs the resulting structure resembles hemi-desmosomes which attach cells to underlying basement membranes (Montandon et al 1977). The myofibroblast therefore possesses a contractile, motile property while still retaining the ability to synthesise and secrete necessary molecules. The ability of myofibroblasts to move over each other and contract is regarded as the major contributory factor in wound contraction (Gabbiani et al 1972).

Myofibroblasts deposit a wide variety of extracellular material, including a loose gel-like matrix largely composed of fibronectin (Popisilova et al 1986). Table 5.4 indicates the main components of the extracellular matrix.

Fibronectin is important in enhancing myofibroblast activity and, structurally, is crucial in assisting and directing the movement of fibroblasts into the area, since it provides a matrix on to which cells can rapidly adhere and detach, and thus move (Hsieh & Chen 1983). Thrombin and EGF are known to regulate production of fibronectin in the fibroblasts (Mosher & Vaheri 1978) and also during fibroplasia. In addition, fibronectin acts as a template for early collagen deposition (McDonald et al 1987).

A polysaccharide called hyaluronic acid (HA) is also part of the secreted ground substance. This is a linear polymer of repeating non-sulphated disaccharides grouped into a class known as the glycosaminoglycans (GAG). It can be observed relatively early in the healing process (4–5 days) and is later replaced by sulphated GAGs. HA has a role in fibroblast movement and proliferation (Clark 1988), facilitating the adhesion and detachment of cells and, as it is easily hydrated, HA can cause tissue swelling thus allowing cells to move into intercellular spaces (Toole 1981). As granulation tissue develops, HA is degraded by an enzyme, hyaluronidase,

Table 5.4   Components of the extracellular matrix (after Clark 1988)

Fibrous components	Structure and characteristics	
Collagens (70%)	Type I – adult dermis (80%) and bone	Triple helix, fibres 2–15 μm
	Type II – adult cartilage	
	Type III – embryonic connective tissue, aorta, dermis (15%)	Inelastic and inextensible
	Type IV – basement membrane	Loose network
	Type V – basement membrane	
Elastin (2%)		Extensible, wavy fibres, 1–3 μm
Reticulin		Very thin fibres, 0.2–1 μm, supports organs
Fibronectin and fibrin	Present in early healing, replaced by other fibrous components later	

Ground substance	Structure and characteristics	
Glycoproteins	e.g. Glycosaminoglycans chondroitin-4-sulphate, dermatan sulphate	Replace HA
Mucopolysaccharides		
Hyaluronic acid (HA)		Highest in early wounds

which cleaves glycosidic bonds (Bertolami & Donoff 1982). It is replaced by two other sulphated GAGs, chondroitin-4-sulphate and dermatan sulphate, after approximately 6–7 days (Hascall & Hascall 1981).

These substances belong to a family called proteoglycans which contain a protein core to which varying GAG chains are attached. Proteoglycans provide increased tissue resilience and hinder cell movement and proliferation. They are also concerned with regulation of collagen fibrillogenesis (McPherson et al 1988), and acceleration of polymerization of collagen monomers. Chondroitin-4-sulphate is involved with collagen deposition during the matrix remodelling stage of healing, whereas another proteoglycan, heparan sulphate, controls cell proliferation and division, as well as inhibiting smooth muscle cell growth (Kraemer & Tobey 1972, Castellot et al 1981).

Collagen is the next component of the ground substance to be synthesised by the myofibroblasts, at about the fifth day after initial myofibroblast migration. This provides the healing tissue with increased tensile strength and resilience. Collagen is a general term for a family of extracellular glycoproteins of five types, I to V. Types I and III are involved in wound healing: type III is synthesised to begin with and is gradually replaced by type I, as shown experimentally by Kurkinen et al in 1980. Collagen synthesis and degradation are important in matrix remodelling, so will be discussed further in another section.

The myofibroblast therefore initially secretes a matrix which encourages cell proliferation and is composed of fibronectin and hyaluronic acid, and follows with a matrix of proteoglycans that incite collagen deposition to increase tissue tensile strength.

Angiogenesis

The formation of new blood vessels in the healing tissue is vital in order to maintain a supply of oxygen and nutrients for regenerating tissue to attract cells such as macrophages and fibroblasts. The proposed stimuli for neovascularisation include various chemotactic and growth factors, in particular fibroblast growth factor, lactic acid (Imre 1964), biogenic amines (Zauberman et al 1969) and low oxygen tension (Remensnyder & Majno 1968). It has been proposed that endothelial cell migration is more important than proliferation in angiogenesis, so that chemoattractants such as fibronectin (Bowersox & Sorgente 1982), heparin (Azizkhan et al 1980) and platelet-derived factors (Wall et al 1978) would play a major role in angiogenesis. Consequently, an appropriate matrix for migration is essential. At the time of revascularisation, fibronectin is the predominant component of the extracellular matrix and acts as a guidance system. Furthermore, endothelial cells have been shown to produce fibronectin themselves (Clark et al 1982b). The free edge effect or loss of nearest neighbour cells is effectual here as endothelial cells actively move into the area.

Capillary endothelial cells are phenotypically altered and release the enzyme collagenase which breaks down collagen in the basement membrane to allow cytoplasmic extensions through into perivascular spaces. This occurs as early as the second day after wounding. Cells near the tip proliferate in response to stimuli and eventually buds are formed which branch at their tips and join to form a capillary loop. New buds emanate from these loops and a capillary plexus is quickly re-established in this way to supply nutrients and oxygen. Lymphatics also reform in the granulation tissue and are essential for proper drainage of oedematous fluid. As already indicated, the physical appearance of the superficial blood vessels is the reason for the term granulation tissue.

Wound contraction

Contraction is defined as the centripetal movement of pre-existing tissue in reducing the size of a wound and not the formation of new tissue. While it has been recognised for some time that forces produced by granulation tissue were responsible for the process of contraction, it is only relatively recently that actin-rich myofibroblasts have been demonstrated to be the cause (Majno et al 1971, Clark 1988). The abundance of actin equips these cells with both extensibility and contractility. They are aligned along wound contraction lines and contract in a way similar to muscle cells. Chemical mediators including serotonin, prostaglandin F_1, angiotensin, vasopressin, bradykinin, adrenaline and noradrenaline are involved in regulation of these contractions (Kloth et al 1990). Intercellular connections between myofibroblasts as well as links between cells and the extracellular matrix are necessary for contraction. The term fibronexus has been given to such contractile units.

The extracellular matrix components of a fibronexus include fibronectin (Singer 1979), types I and III collagen (Furcht et al 1980), while cytoplasmic actin (Singer 1979) and vinculin (Singer & Paradiso 1981) are recognised as intracellular factors. The rate of contraction is proportional to cell number (Bell et al 1979) and inversely related to collagen concentration. During contraction it has been noticed that healthy tissue surrounding the wound often increases its surface area, a process known as *intussusceptive growth* (Montandon et al 1977).

The end result of normal contraction is an area of scar tissue with little vascularisation since the newly formed capillaries retract during the contraction process. There are of course many extrinsic factors which may influence re-epithelialisation and contraction, including surgical techniques, infection, drugs, ulcers and various diseases (Kloth et al 1990); consequently agents for promoting re-epithelialisation and contraction are often useful.

MATRIX REMODELLING

Remodelling is the next overlapping stage of repair, beginning almost simultaneously with epithelialisation. It involves establishment of an equilibrium between collagen formation and lysis, which brings about the constant reshaping of the scar over the next few months.

As fibronectin is replaced by type III and eventually type I collagen fibrils, the scar gains increasing tensile strength. The strength of scar tissue will grow from only 5% of the original strength of the uninjured tissue to approximately 40% in about 1 month. However, even after a year and from then on, the wound tissue will never reach more than 80% of its original strength (Kanzler et al 1986). The gel-like matrix is replaced by more stable type I collagen fibrils which crosslink to provide additional strength. Other components, for example proteoglycans, are also constantly remodelled.

Collagen formation occurs in myofibroblasts, as well as in normal cellular fibroblast throughout life. Collagen comprises about 70% of the dry weight of the skin, so is manufactured in vast quantities. There are five major types of collagen: type I is located in dermal regions and bone; type II is found in cartilage; type III is found in wounds, the aorta and embryonic connective tissue; and types IV and V are in the basement membrane. These various types differ only in amino acid composition (Stryer 1988, Kloth et al 1990). The fibrils in type I have diameters of between 100 nm and 500 nm, whereas type III fibres are much smaller, only 40–60 nm in diameter (Fleischmajer 1986). The majority of dermal collagen is type I (80%) and the rest type III (Kloth et al 1990).

Collagen biosynthesis within the fibroblast leads to the formation of procollagen molecules (Fig. 5.7). These are modified extracellularly by peptidases to form tropocollagen. These tropocollagen molecules align in a staggered formation and are linked initially by hydrogen bonds. Subsequently, these relatively unstable bonds are replaced by stable covalent crosslinks and fibrils are created. Fibrils unite to form collagen fibres which are inherently inelastic and inextensible, and align along stress lines, allowing skin to stretch (Kloth et al 1990). Initially in the wound, fibrils are laid down in irregular bundles. Part of the remodelling process involves orientation and alignment of the collagen which increases mechanical strength and allows scars to stretch. The resorption of collagen takes place at various stages, is tissue-specific and is rigidly controlled by collagenases. During inflammation, macrophages engulf collagen and degrade it, releasing useful amino acids and other components for recycling. Tissue collagenase is synthesised mainly in mesenchymal, epithelial and inflammatory cells (Kanzler et al 1986).

Another component of the connective tissue reformed after wounding is elastin. It is, as the name suggests, extremely elastic and aids in providing extensibility of the newly formed tissue. It comprises a very small portion of dermal constituents, only approximately 2% (Braverman & Fonferko 1982).

Normal connective tissue formation is dependent on a number of factors including a good supply of vitamins (in particular vitamin C), minerals and amino acids which are essential for biosynthesis of collagen. Infection, drugs and disease may also impede normal processes.

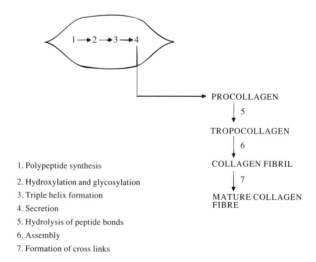

Fig. 5.7   Collagen formation within the fibroblast (after Stryer 1985).

Keloids and hypertrophic scars

Imbalances in the collagen formation/lysis equilibrium sometimes occur. Obviously synthesis is at a higher rate immediately following wounding, but it normally settles down after a few weeks and the reverse situation arises, with degradation exceeding formation. There are two types of imbalance which manifest as what are called keloids and hypertrophic scars. Keloids result from overdeposition of collagen in both injured and normal peripheral wound tissue. Hypertrophic scars are also a consequence of overproduction of collagen but only involve injured tissue. Histological examination of keloids reveals acellular, thick bundles of collagen, whereas whorled cellular structures are diagnostic of hypertrophic scars. The latter are thought to disappear in a short space of time, but without treatment keloids may persist for much longer.

One means of treatment for hypertrophic scars is the appliance of constant pressure, which is thought to realign the whorls into orderly parallel fibres. The theory behind this treatment relies on the fact that when stress is applied to collagen fibres they emit a small electrical voltage. This effect is termed *piezo-electric* and directly affects the production, alignment and lysis of collagen (Kloth et al 1990), leading to a normal, mature scar.

CELLULAR RESEARCH

Introduction

As already indicated in the introduction to this chapter, despite the popular use of low-intensity lasers for the treatment of open wounds, there remains a lack of basic information of the precise biological mechanisms by which lasers may stimulate the regenerative process. Although numerous studies have been conducted and several mechanisms of action have been proposed, the published information presents difficulties in its interpretation and integration owing to a wide diversity in experimental protocols. Such difficulties in comparison of the various studies make it difficult to identify reasons for success or failure and serve to reinforce the scepticism that has surrounded this area. However, research is necessary if we are to uncover the mysteries underlying the observed efficacy of low-intensity laser therapy for the treatment of open wounds.

Research findings to date based upon animal, human and most notably cellular studies have enhanced the establishment of LILT as an effective means of biostimulation for the wound healing process. Indeed, the study of the effect of low-intensity laser irradiation upon cell function is the most developed and systematic area of laser research (Basford 1989). When lasers were first introduced into medical practice, studies of the effect of laser on biological tissue were limited to in vitro experiments simply because, at that time, little was known about the possible side effects of such irradiation (Enwemeka 1988). Since then, numerous cellular studies have been carried out on a variety of cells related to the wound healing process including fibroblasts, lymphocytes and monocytes/ macrophages, as well as epithelial and endothelial cells.

Types of cell used in cellular research

Fibroblasts

As outlined previously, these cells are primarily responsible for wound healing, constituting a prominent part of reparative granulation tissue (Woolf 1977); thus photobiomodulation of wound healing by laser irradiation may be mediated through direct effects on fibroblasts (Wheeland & Walker 1986). In view of this, much of the in vitro experimental work to date in this area has focussed on fibroblasts (Abergel et al 1987, Bosatra et al 1984, Tocco et al 1985, Balboni et al 1986, Boulton & Marshall 1986, Glassberg et al 1988a, Colver et al 1989, Pourreau-Schneider et al 1990).

Lymphocytes

The immune system is an important and integral part of the healing process. It is particularly vulnerable to modulation by a variety of pharmacological and physical modalities (Anderson & Warner 1976, Ohta et al 1987). Lymphocytes in particular are responsible for the release of soluble mediators of immunity and of tissue repair. Consequently, by using human blood samples, lymphocytes have been separated out and investigated by several investigators to determine the effect of low-intensity lasers on the immune response (Mester et al 1978, Ohta et al 1987, Inoue et al 1989).

Monocytes/macrophages

Experimental evidence has shown that, when these cells are eliminated from a wound, healing is severely reduced and fibroplasia is greatly inhibited. They subserve multiple functions in the body such as killing of parasites, removal of unwanted debris and foreign material and regulation/ suppression of the immune response. Recently, a murine macrophage-like cell line and human peripheral blood mononuclear leukocytes have been used to investigate the mechanism underlying laser stimulated wound repair (Young et al 1989, Shields et al 1991).

Other cells

Monocytes and lymphocytes occur early in the healing process, while fibroblasts are particularly evident in the intermediate granulative stage. Other cells such as endothelial and epithelial cells are more prevalent in the later stages of repair and angiogenesis but have proved less popular in laser research studies (Glassberg et al 1988a, Colver et al 1989). Interestingly, Karu has successfully used a bacterial cell line (*Escherichia coli*) as a model for the investigation of the cellular effects of low-intensity laser, and her work on this cell line has made significant contributions to our understanding of the photobiomodulative effects of laser radiation (e.g. Karu 1985, 1988).

Research protocols

One would expect studies involving irradiation of cells in culture to share certain similarities with regard to materials and methods but, with the exception of the basic tissue culture techniques, this is unfortunately not the case.

Cell and tissue culture

In vitro experimental work is normally carried out under aseptic conditions within the confines of a laminar flow hood to minimise the risk of contamination. Cultured cells are maintained in a growth medium, supplemented with protein-rich serum and antibiotics. This medium nourishes the cells while an input of carbon dioxide and incubation at 37°C ensures an optimum growing environment. Cells are grown in a variety of sterile containers. In order to maintain a healthy population of cells, the cell samples are subcultured routinely depending on the doubling time of the cell line. Prior to irradiation, cell numbers are normally adjusted to particular concentrations using such techniques as centrifugation. Popular cell counting methods include the haemocytometer (Tocco et al 1985), Coulter counter (Hallman et al 1988, Colver et al 1989), radioisotope labelling (Ohta et al 1987, Inoue et al 1989), while electron microscopy has been used to examine ultrastructural changes in cells after laser irradiation (Bosatra et al 1984, Pourreau-Schneider et al 1990). In the literature reviewed above, these details have been well documented and are repeatable depending on the availability of materials and equipment.

Cell irradiation

While the cell and tissue culture protocols are usually well detailed in published papers, the same cannot, unfortunately, be said in respect of the specification of irradiation parameters used – e.g. type of laser used, dosage and irradiation time. Certainly the most popular laser in such studies to date has been the helium–neon (He–Ne) laser with a wavelength of 632.8 nm (Mester et al 1978, Abergel et al 1984b, 1987, Bosatra et al 1984, Lam et al 1984, 1986, Dyson & Young 1985, Tocco et al 1985, Balboni et al 1986, Boulton & Marshall 1986, Hallman et al 1988, Karu

1988, Quarto et al 1988, Colver et al 1989, Riceviuti et al 1989, Pourreau-Schneider et al 1990). The apparent effectiveness of the He–Ne laser as supported by earlier literature was instrumental in influencing Hallman's (1988) choice of laser and may perhaps have influenced others, although their reasons for selection of the He–Ne as the basis for their studies are not stated. In several studies the He–Ne has been used in conjunction with an infra-red laser, e.g. Space Mix 5, with the infra-red offering a range of pulsed frequencies (Dyson & Young 1985, Tocco et al 1985, Balboni et al 1986).

Semiconductor gallium aluminium arsenide (GaAlAs) lasers, which are more popular in clinical practice, have also been used, allowing the use of irradiation parameters which more closely reflect those used in clinical practice (Abergel et al 1987, Ohta et al 1987, Inoue et al 1989, Young et al 1989). Other less popular choices of laser have been the pulsed ruby laser (Hardy et al 1967) and the continuous-wave Nd:YAG (Castro et al 1983). In general, the selection criteria for the laser type in the studies carried out to date would seem to be a combination of ease of use, broader experimental background, low cost and availability (Basford 1989).

Laser output/waveforms

Waveforms can be either continuous or pulsed (see Ch. 2). He–Ne lasers typically offer continuous wave (CW) output, although in one study at least the investigators chose to pulse the output by 50% (Boulton & Marshall 1986). In contrast, the GaAlAs lasers used to date have typically been pulsed-output units. None of the authors venture to define the relative advantages of pulsed or continuous waveforms.

Laser dose/energy density

The greatest discrepancy among the existing literature lies in the wide variation of laser parameters employed, particularly dose and treatment time. The field of laser photobiomodulation is clouded by imprecise dosimetry (Meyers et al 1987). Furthermore, the inconsistency in terminology is confusing and somewhat laborious to the reader. Few authors describe accurately the laser parameters used in their respective studies. Where parameters are fully specified, this information gives the reader the opportunity to draw conclusions about the results, allows accurate repetition of the study and enables the clinician to apply the information to an in vivo situation. Unfortunately, however, most authors omit these vital details.

Although varying doses for different lasers have been effective, inducing changes within the cultured cells and consequently leading to an increased healing effect, the optimal dose for achieving this end has yet to be determined. According to Grosman (1976) 'the dominant factor for the effect of any sort of irradiation and thus also laser irradiation is the so called observed radiation dose'. If the power output of the laser, the area to be irradiated and the treatment time are known energy density or radiant exposure can be relatively easily calculated (see Ch. 4).

Treatment time and distance

In the literature published to date, treatment time and distance of sample from irradiation source are variable. Treatment times range from single 20 s exposures (Young et al 1989) to 15 min exposures over a 3-day period (Boulton & Marshall 1986). The distance the laser was placed from the cell samples ranges from 1 mm (Lam et al 1984) to 70 cm (Tocco et al 1985). The differences in treatment parameters as well as the lack of standardisation and basic information are evident throughout the published literature and serve to enhance the scepticism surrounding low-intensity laser therapy. Consequently repetition and comparison of previous studies is difficult and would be of only limited value.

Putative mechanisms of action

The published papers on cellular research present evidence for a variety of biological mechanisms by which low-intensity laser irradiation may stimulate the regenerative process. The most straightforward effect reported is proliferation of cells following irradiation, particularly where fibroblasts have been used (Hardy et al 1967, Abergel et al 1984a, Boulton & Marshall 1986). This would seem an acceptable mechanism of laser-stimulated healing in view of the role of these cells in the healing process. Using human embryonic foreskin fibroblasts and adult human skin fibroblasts, Boulton & Marshall (1986) reported an increase in cell proliferation following irradiation with a He–Ne laser. These authors admitted that their results were totally unexpected and statistically significant, but unfortunately did not attempt to explain their findings.

However, not all studies report an increase in fibroblast proliferation (Glassberg et al 1988a, Hallman et al 1988, Colver et al 1989). Using a 0.9 mW He–Ne source, Hallman et al (1988) found no alteration in proliferation of cultured human fibroblasts. Nevertheless, these authors do not overlook the fact that other studies did find a proliferative response, and suggest that if laser-stimulated proliferation does exist it may be that the specific laser irradiation parameters for successful treatment, e.g. wavelength, duration, power and intensity, need to be carefully established. If, however, proliferative effects do not arise from low-intensity laser stimulation, the acceleration reported in wound healing experiments must be attributed to other mechanisms.

Proliferation is not the only possible means by which low-intensity laser may accelerate wound healing, as other studies using fibroblasts have suggested alternative mechanisms of action. As already detailed above, fibroblasts are responsible for the production of collagen, which in turn is an important component of scar tissue formation. Using radioactive labelling as an index of collagen production, researchers at UCLA (Castro et al 1983, Abergel et al 1984b, Lam et al 1986, Lyons et al 1987) have found that laser irradiation (He–Ne and GaAlAs) stimulates the production of collagen by fibroblasts. While the mechanism by which these lasers may promote collagen production is not clear, the authors suggest that it may occur via collagen gene expression reflecting alterations in transcriptional or translational levels.

As outlined earlier in this chapter, myofibroblasts are modified fibroblasts that are directly involved in granulation tissue contraction. A study by Pourreau-Schneider et al (1990) found that He–Ne laser irradiation of fibroblasts transforms the cells into myofibroblasts, which the author suggests may set into motion the acceleration of the wound healing process which is typically observed in clinical practice after He–Ne laser treatment.

Other aspects of cell structure and metabolism have been investigated as to their possible role in laser-mediated acceleration of healing. Using electron microscopy, ultrastructural changes in irradiated human fibroblasts have been observed. Bosatra et al (1984) observed evident signs of protein synthesis leading to a more active synthesis of fibrillar material. Similarly, Tocco et al (1985), who found an increase in fibroblast proliferation using He–Ne and infra-red laser, also observed an increase in rough endoplasmic reticulum, suggesting stimulation of protein metabolism correlated with an increase in number and size of mitochondria in irradiated cells.

More recently, work in this area has been extended by the irradiation of isolated mitochondria (Karu 1988, Passarella 1988). Karu suggests that laser irradiation induces changes in cellular homoeostasis, which entails a whole cascade of reactions, and proposes that a number of the components of the respiratory chain (e.g. cytochromes, cytochrome oxidase and flavine dehydrogenases) are primary photoacceptors or chromophores and thus able to absorb laser light at appropriate wavelengths. This causes short-term activation of the respiratory chain leading to changes in redox status of both mitochondria and cytoplasm. The activation of the electron transport chain in this way in turn results in enhanced synthesis of ATP. Furthermore, laser irradiation also affects hydrogen ion levels in the cell. This coupled with an increase in ATP causes activation of other membrane ion carriers such as sodium and potassium and alters the flow of calcium between mitochondria and cytoplasm. The variation of such parameters is a necessary component in the control of proliferative activity of the cell.

However, the cascade does not end here. The changes in ion concentration further affect cell metabolism and developments by influencing cyclic nucleotide levels. These components are involved in events leading to initiation of DNA synthesis. Karu therefore believes that the action of visible light upon the cell might be mediated by regulation of cellular metabolism via this pathway. She concludes that more experimental data are needed to explain how light stimulus is converted into the type of chemical and electrical signals which may be understood by the cell, and how such signals can be detected and transmitted by subcellular components.

Thus it can be seen that much attention has been focussed on fibroblasts and to date the reported effects of laser irradiation on these cells has generally been favourable. In contrast, it would seem that laser irradiation of lymphocytes results in a decrease in proliferation of these cells (Mester et al 1978, Ohta et al 1987, Inoue et al 1989). Lymphocytes separated from human blood have been irradiated with a range of laser types, including diode lasers operating at 904 nm (Ohta et al 1987) and 780 nm (Inoue et al 1989); additionally Mester et al (1978) have used Argon and He–Ne gas lasers for the irradiation of lymphocytes. Cell proliferation for the purposes of these experiments was measured either by radioisotope incorporation or immunofluorescence.

Although these studies cannot be directly compared because of large variations in the laser parameters used and methods of irradiation employed, the results of each study indicate that the proliferation of human lymphocytes can be affected by low-intensity laser irradiation or, as Inoue et al (1989) suggest, low-intensity laser has the potential to interfere with the operation of the human immune system in vitro. In relation to wound healing, Mester et al (1978) suggest that laser might affect these immunocompetent cells by suppressing some undesirable immunoreaction and so contribute to the stimulation of wound healing. Both Mester et al (1978) and Inoue et al (1989) refer to the treatment of chronic wounds or inflammation by laser and the relative success of this treatment in clinical practice. They suggest that in these cases laser-mediated suppression and alteration of immune processes, which have a role in persistence of chronic wounds, may lead to an acceleration in healing.

Epithelial cells have been irradiated by Gross & Jelkmann (1990) in relation, not to wound healing, but to tumour growth. They found that certain energy densities decrease proliferation of cells in culture and suggest that laser irradiation could provide a useful tool for modulating cell cycle and subsequently cell proliferation. This group proposes the usefulness of investigating the effects of repeated and prolonged He–Ne irradiation on tumour growth in vivo. The bioinhibition of cell proliferation and hence healing observed in other studies (Castro et al 1983, Abergel et al 1984b, Dyson & Young 1985) using high energy levels is not considered a negative feature but rather is potentially of considerable therapeutic value. For example, in pathological situations where wound contracture would produce deformities as a result of excessive cell activity, laser therapy may yet have an important future role as a means of attenuating many distressing clinical conditions.

One of the most recently proposed mechanisms of laser photobiomodulation has been that laser radiation at appropriate wavelengths and energy densities stimulates the release of soluble factors from monocytes which induce cell proliferation. At Guy's Hospital in London, researchers have found that supernatant taken from an irradiated monocytic-like cell line can stimulate proliferation of fibroblasts in vitro.

These researchers propose that, following irradiation, the monocytic-like cell line releases a soluble factor which induces proliferation of the fibroblast cell line (Young et al 1989). Monocytes and macrophages have a central role in mediating the body's immune and inflammatory responses, largely through the release of a variety of substances. These substances include polypeptide growth factors and cytokines. When trauma occurs the haemostatic pathways and the immune response are activated, leading to the release of growth factors and cytokines respectively. These substances, many of which have already been identified, are implicated in immunity and tissue repair.

A recent study has provided more evidence that polypeptide growth factors are involved in laser-mediated wound repair. It has been shown that irradiated human mononuclear leukocytes release a factor which causes proliferation of a growth-factor-dependent cell line (Shields et al 1991). Further studies are ongoing to determine the nature of this factor.

Although many positive effects have been demonstrated in cellular experiments, a number of unresolved issues remain. In particular the putative relevance of such laser parameters as dose and treatment time present the greatest problems. Until these issues have been overcome the use of lasers for the treatment of wounds remains controversial. This controversy may be best resolved at a cellular level and the studies completed to date at least provide some scientific basis for the clinical use of such devices to promote wound healing; certainly if laser irradiation does accelerate wound healing then it must do so by affecting changes at the cellular level.

Applicability of cellular research to the clinical situation

How can research conducted at a cellular level be applied to conditions occurring in vivo? Certainly no laboratory study can accurately replicate the complex influences and interaction of wound healing; the living skin equivalent has its drawbacks and does not include a wound equivalent (Colver et al 1989). However, owing to the problems posed by in vivo experimental work such as standardisation, lack of controls and ethical considerations, cellular research offers a feasible alternative. This line of research allows adequately controlled, well standardised procedures to be carried out any number of times. How then can results and conclusions revealed by these studies be applied to the wound in vivo? A population of cells in suspension or in a monolayer present a different medium to the laser than the traumatised wound. When cells are irradiated the obvious barriers of skin, muscle, bone and vascular systems are absent. As a result, laser dosages used in the laboratory are considerably less than would be required for the same effect in vivo; therefore doses and times found to be effective in vitro need to be extrapolated for in vivo treatments.

Unfortunately, few authors are willing to define the clinical applications and implications of their respective studies. Inoue et al (1989), who found that laser irradiation decreased lymphocyte proliferation, speculate that clinical improvement of patients with rheumatoid arthritis could be obtained partially through an altered immune response using appropriate dosages of laser irradiation. Similarly, Ohta et al (1987) suggest that modulation (of immune response) could *potentially* occur in human subjects exposed to laser irradiation. Young et al (1989) conclude their published study by giving an overall picture of the benefit of using appropriate irradiation parameters to *optimise* the rate of repair, given the cost of treating injuries in terms of hospitalisation, as well the pain and incapacity suffered by the individual affected. Certainly, well designed cellular research provides an achievable means of realising this goal. However another possibility is research on animals and although not ideal, the problems of extrapolation encountered with cellular studies are considerably lessened.

STUDIES ON WOUND HEALING IN ANIMALS

Introduction

The animal studies completed to date on laser photobiomodulation of wound healing are largely anecdotal, diverse and singular with not all laser parameters clearly defined. The salient published papers are summarised in Table 5.5. There are also conflicting views as to low-intensity laser's efficacy in accelerating the wound healing process in animals and the suitability of animal research for extrapolation to human practice.

Small, loose-skinned rodents such as mice, rats or guinea pigs have been the animals most often used in such studies on wound healing (Table 5.5). This has been attributed to their relative ease of handling and examination, availability in large numbers, and low death risk upon anaesthesia. As previously described, wound healing is a complex process which occurs in many stages and involves a plethora of cellular and chemical mediators. There are therefore many variables which can be measured and are considered indicative of the rate and stage of the repair process. Herein lies one of the main problems associated with assimilation and comparison of results of animal trials: the use of diverse variables measured by disparate and often badly described methods.

Another dilemma is that, although rodent skins are suitable to a

Table 5.5 Examples of in vivo animal experiments

Author	Animal	Wound	Compared	Laser parameters		Effect
Mester (1971)	Mouse	Burn	Diameter	Ruby;	Power density (PD) not given 0.5, 1, 4, 5, 10 J/cm² twice weekly	1 J/cm² increased healing
Mester (1973)	Rat	Open skin	Complete wound and collagen synthesis	Ruby;	PD not given 1. 1 J/cm² on day 5 2. 4 J/cm² postoperatively and at 48 hours 3. 6 J/cm² postoperatively	4 J/cm² increased healing and collagen synthesis
Mester (1975)	Rat	Muscle injury	Regeneration of muscle	Ruby;	PD not given 1 J/cm² every 3rd day × 4	Immediate: irradiation increased regeneration but adverse effect with repeated irradiation
Haina (1981)	Rat	Open skin	Granulation tissue formation	HeNe;	PD = 50 mW/cm² 0.5, 1.5, 4, 10, 20 J/cm² once daily	Increase up to 4 J/cm² then decrease
Kana (1981)	Rat	Open skin	Rate of wound closure and collagen synthesis	HeNe;	PD = 45 mW/cm² 4, 10, 20 J/cm² once daily	None, but 4 J/cm² increased from 3–12 days
Surinchak (1983)	Rabbits	Open skin	Wound area, effect of eschar removal, tensile strength	HeNe;	PD variable 1. 1.1 J/cm² every 3rd day 2. 2.2 J/cm² twice daily 3. 4.5 J/cm² twice daily	None
Jongsma (1983)	Rats	Open skin	Wound area	Argon;	1. PD = 50 mW/cm², 1 J/cm² after 4 days then twice weekly 2. PD = 200 mW/cm², 4 J/cm² after 4 days then twice weekly	None
Mashiko (1983)	Guinea pig	Open skin	Wound area	830 nm;	PD = 17 mW/cm², 2 J/cm² every 2 days	Increased rate of healing

Table 5.5 (cont'd)

Author	Animal	Wound	Compared	Laser parameters	Effect
Hunter (1984)	Pig	Open skin	Wound area	He–Ne; PD = 64 mW/cm^2, 0.96 J/cm^2	None
McCaughan (1985)	Guinea pig	Open skin	Wound area	Argon; PD = 20 mW/cm^2, 2 J/cm^2 every 2–3 days	None
Mester (1985) (review)	Mice	Open skin	Wound area, cellular content of granulation tissue	Ruby; PD not given 1.1 J/cm^2 twice weekly	Increased rate of closure
Kokino (1985)	Rats	Tendons	Granulation tissue	Infra-red/ 800 Hz He–Ne	Increased rate of healing
Dyson (1985, 1986)	Mice	Open skin	Wound area, cellular content of granulation tissue	Infra-red/ 700 Hz and 1200 Hz He–Ne	Increased contraction with 700Hz
Lievens (1985)	Mice	Open skin, blood vessels, lymph vessel	Adhesion of eschar, oedema formation, regeneration of vein and lymph vessel	Infra-red/ 700 Hz He–Ne	Adhesion decreased, less oedema, faster regeneration
Abergel (1987)	Mice	Open skin	Wound area, collagen content, tensile strength	He–Ne; PD = 4.05 mW/cm^2, 1.22J/cm^2 every other day	Increased collagen and tensile strength
Abergel (1987)	Pig	Open skin	Procollagen levels	HeNe; PD = 1.56 mW/cm^2, 0.6 J/cm^2 three times a week	Increased levels
Lyons (1987)	Mice	Open skin	Wound area, tensile strength, collagen content	HeNe; PD = 4.05 mW/cm^2, 1.22J/cm^2 every other day	Increased collagen and tensile strength
Rochkind (1989)	Rats	Open skin, burns, peripheral and CNS	Wound area, action potential, neuron degeneration	HeNe; PD not given 1. 7.6 J/cm^2 daily for 21 days 2. 10 J/cm^2 daily for 21 days 3. 10 J/cm^2 daily for 20 days	Increased rate of healing, action potential increased and degeneration reduced

Table 5.5 (cont'd)

Author	Animal	Wound	Compared	Laser parameters	Effect
Braverman (1989)	Rabbits	Open skin	Wound area, tensile strength, epidermal thickness, collagen area	HeNe and infra-red 1. 1.65 J/cm² HeNe 2. 8.25 J/cm² IR	None, except increased tensile strength
Enwemeka (1990)	Rabbits	Tendons	Size, tensile strength, energy absorption, strain	HeNe;	1, 2, 3, 4, 5 m J/cm² daily	Size decreased, no other difference, but fibroblasts and collagen aligned
Zarkovic (1991)	Mice	Open skin	Wound area, serum lipoprotein content	GaAs; 50 W pulse power 210 s daily for 7 days	Increased rate of healing, decrease in LDLs
Urciuoli (1991)	Rat	Brain	Superoxide dismutase (SOD)	HeNe; PD = 5 mW, 1.08 J/cm²	Increased SOD

certain extent as models of wound healing, wound contraction plays a large part in the tissue repair of these animals. With human tegument, epithelialisation plays a much more significant role in healing. Consequently, it is often argued that pig skin represents a more suitable model for extrapolation to humans, since it is more similar in character to human skin (Hunter et al 1984, Basford 1986). There are some limitations in using pig skin however, in that it is often much thicker than its human equivalent, so that laser light penetration may be hindered and consequently light may not reach tissue other than that at the superficial wound site.

Animal models of wound healing

A wide variety of animal models of wound healing have been employed to assess the putative biostimulatory effects of low-intensity laser irradiation (Table 5.5). Professor Endre Mester began wound healing experiments using rats and mice during the 1960s and 1970s (Mester & Jaszsagi-Nagy 1973). These initial studies involved injecting rats with various radioisotopes which would be incorporated into healing tissue. Irradiation was with a pulsed ruby laser at radiant exposures of up to 4 J/cm^2 and applied at varying times after wound infliction. The animals were subsequently sacrificed and tissue was examined for uptake of radiolabelled amino acids.

These early studies thus attempted to link the biostimulatory effects of lasers to the biochemical events occurring during the repair process. The irradiation parameters used in these early experiments were not clearly defined and are often difficult to decipher, particularly as the majority are published in Hungarian. Further experimentation was conducted by Mester's group on the ability of laser irradiation to regenerate adductor muscles of rats (Mester et al 1975), again using a ruby laser.

Interestingly, tendon regeneration has also been studied in two groups of animals, rats (Kokino et al 1985) and rabbits (Enwemeka et al 1990). The earlier group incised and sutured the Achilles tendon in rats, and irradiated daily with a He–Ne laser, the parameters of which are not specified in their published report. After a period of time the rats were sacrificed and the tendons were removed, stained and examined histologically for cellular changes. By contrast, the second more recent investigation attempted to elucidate the ultrastructural and biomechanical changes induced by laser irradiation of rabbit tendons.

Rabbits have also been used in studies based upon skin wounds. Braverman and colleagues used infra-red and He–Ne laser irradiation individually and in combination to compare the relative effects of these two sources upon open skin wounds using well defined parameters (Braverman et al 1989). Photographic assessment of wound size, which is a popular method of measurement in animal studies on open wounds, was used for wound size comparisons at periodic intervals. Additionally the tensile strength of the healing areas was assessed posthumously using an automated gauge or tensiometer, while epidermal thickness and collagen content were measured in histological sections. This group also attempted to determine if there were any temperature changes in the skin both at the wound site and at a distant site; however this was discontinued as the needle thermistors used were found to be disruptive to the healing process.

Surinchak et al (1983) inflicted full skin thickness circular wounds on rabbits and irradiated with a somewhat complicated scanning He–Ne laser system which 'swept' over the area rather than irradiating a single point. A circular wound like this might be expected to close by means of contractual forces exerted by myofibroblasts and assisted by collagen synthesis. A straight line incision was made in rats to compare the effect of low level laser on such a wound, which may benefit more from collagen synthesis than contraction. Averbakh et al (1976) and Fangde et al (1980) used similar models but with relatively lower energy densities to irradiate full thickness defects in rabbits.

Undoubtedly the rate of closure of open skin wounds is one of the best studied aspects of animal healing in investigations of low-intensity laser photobiomodulation, possibly because it relates to a visible, easily measured process. The area of wound has been measured using various techniques ranging from tracing the wound on to paper for planimeter measurements to photography, and even computer-assisted image analysis. Kana et al (1981) subjected rats to irradiation with He–Ne (633 nm) and argon (514 nm) lasers and also monochromatic red and green light sources. The series of experiments were well planned and all the irradiation variables were identified so that wavelength specificity of any effect could be measured. The group also measured collagen hydroxyproline content periodically as a reflection of collagen synthesis.

Guinea pigs were used by McCaughan et al (1985) to determine the effect of Argon irradiation on the rate of wound closure. These animals had open circular wounds inflicted on their dorsal surfaces. These were traced on to glass microslides and the number of days required for 50% and 75% healing was determined. This study also assessed the effect of washing the wound with saline and peroxide every 2–3 days in parallel with irradiation. Mashiko et al (1983) also used guinea pigs to assess the effect of 830 nm irradiation applied at a radiant exposure of 2 J/cm^2 on alternate days upon the healing of complete thickness wounds.

Mice and rats appear to be the most frequently used animals in experimental studies of laser photobiomodulation of wound healing. Mester in particular carried out numerous wound healing trials on these small rodents. Apart from the previously reported radioisotope studies, which do not seem to have been replicated in any other of the published works, the cellular content of granulation tissue was assessed in further trials based upon ruby laser irradiation of total skin defects in mice.

Dyson & Young (1985) have carried out various well documented studies on wound contraction. Initially the effect of combined infra-red and He–Ne lasers on wound contraction and wound bed cellularity was investigated. Pre- and post-treatment wound tracings facilitated the computation of wound contraction rate. Furthermore, while Mester simply used microscopic examination and counted all dividing cells at the wound edge without indicating the type of cells observed, Dyson's group performed total and differential cell counts on areas of 8640 mm² centred on the middle of the wound bed using stained sections.

The following year the same group produced a further study on the effect of laser irradiation on wound contraction and cellularity in mice (Dyson & Young 1986). In this, they compared two pulse repetition rates: 700 Hz and 1200 Hz. This latter paper contained more experimental details than previously published work, and provided photographic evidence of cellular content of the tissue from the three groups used in their study (700 Hz, 1200 Hz and control). However, they admitted that this was a preliminary study, and that the frequencies studied (700 Hz and 1200 Hz) were chosen simply as they represented the available extremes on the infra-red laser unit used as the basis for their study.

Lyons et al (1987) appear to understand the need for complete specification of irradiation parameters and in their follow up study to the collagen content experiments already outlined above, such details are well set out. Using a rat model, this group investigated the effects of He–Ne laser irradiation upon tensile strength (measured by a tensiometer) and collagen deposition as reflected by hydroxyproline concentration.

Rochkind et al (1989) conducted one of the largest series of controlled animal trials on laser photobiomodulation. They investigated the effects of laser irradiation on the healing of cutaneous wounds and burns, as well as laser's effects upon normal and injured (crushed) peripheral and central nerves. Burn injuries were inflicted for the purposes of this study by applying water at 98°C to the hind legs of two of the experimental groups of animals. The energy densities applied to the animals in this series of trials were some of the highest in all such reports: up to 7.6–10 J/cm² daily for up to 20 days. Assessment of the effect of irradiation upon wound healing was by clinical/subjective observation and photography at periodic intervals to determine changes in rates of wound contraction.

In an effort to assess the neurophysiological effects of low-intensity laser irradiation on a daily basis using the parameters already outlined above, electrophysiological measurements were completed upon normal and injured (crushed) sciatic nerves on one group of rats. However, it was estimated by these researchers that the amount of radiation reaching the sciatic nerve was only 2–10% of the irradiance delivered to the skin. Recording of compound action potentials was performed on all rats for up to 360 days postoperatively and compared to initial pre-crush records.

The spinal cord is known to respond to injuries like nerve crushing, which trigger morphological and biochemical changes, by neuronal degeneration in the corresponding segment. Additionally, 14 days after the crush injury, a number of the rats were sacrificed and histological tissue sections were prepared to examine the effects of laser upon the spinal cord.

Animal research on laser photobiomodulation of wound healing has frequently focused on areas other than simple wound contraction per se and thus some other variable has often been examined in conjunction with measurements of 'healing rate'. For example, Lievens (1985) decided to investigate the influence of laser on the motricity of the lymph system, in parallel with healing of an abdominal incision in mice. The main artery, vein and lymph vessel were cut and examined for up to 6 months after surgery. An invasive technique involving transillumination microscopy was used to study the microcirculation along with photography and videotape recording. This study also looked at the effect of irradiation upon adhesion of the scar to the underlying tissue and local oedema, as well as regeneration of the vein and lymph vessel. In the control group, which did not receive any irradiation, evolution of scar tissue was observed and recorded. For the purposes of this study, the experimental group received daily irradiation from a mixed infra-red/He–Ne laser source with output pulsed at 700 Hz. Parameters such as distance from wound and treatment area were not specified in this report.

One of the most recent studies involving assessment of factors other than simple wound healing rates was carried out by a Yugoslavian team (Zarkovic et al 1991) who investigated the combined effect of GaAs laser irradiation and partial (30%) hepatectomy on murine open skin wound healing and lipoprotein composition. It is known that changes in plasma lipoprotein composition occur under various pathological conditions which cause tissue destruction (Cabana et al 1989), so the effects of laser on lipoprotein concentration were analysed in normal mice, those with either liver damage or skin wounds and those with both. Tracings were used to record changes in wounds during the 7-day period after surgery; plasma was also extracted after sacrifice and analysed for lipoprotein with a conventional system. Once again in this study, exact irradiation parameters were not specified, leaving reproducibility unattainable.

Skin flap survival rates after low-intensity laser irradiation have been extensively investigated and documented by Japanese scientists led by Professor Toshio Ohshiro. These studies are well described by Ohshiro & Calderhead (1990) along with other aspects of in vivo research. Skin flaps were raised on the backs of mice with treatment groups receiving laser either before or after flap elevation and suturing, or none in the case of controls.

It has already been indicated earlier that the healing process in pig skin is very similar to that in humans, as are dermal structure and turnover times. Unfortunately, relatively few studies have been carried out using swine models of wound healing and even with these there is wide variation in the reporting of experimental details and irradiation parameters. Hunter et al (1984) created open partial-thickness wounds on the dorsal surfaces of pigs and irradiated daily using a He–Ne laser at energy densities advocated by Mester for use in small rodents ($\leqslant 4\,J/cm^2$). In this study, the percentage of wound area that had healed over a fixed period of time was assessed. Basford et al (1986) monitored the effects of laser by determining the time to wound closure, wound strength and bacterial colonisation. Finally, two groups, Abergel et al (1987) and Glassberg et al (1988b) studied the effects of laser on procollagen levels in wounds; however the latter group did not indicate dosages thus preventing direct comparisons.

Overview of research findings

The results of all the studies outlined above reveal the problems inherent in in vivo trials using LILT: details of experimental and irradiation procedures are so numerous and variable that reproducibility and inter-trial comparisons are generally not practical. This is exacerbated by the variation in evaluation of efficacy and treatment in such studies, which has resulted in many (apparently) conflicting reports.

In general, research groups have either reported an acceleration or no effect on the healing process. Dyson & Young (1986) found that there was an increase in contraction and cellularity, the level of improvement being dependant on the pulsing frequency, with 700 Hz showing a greater improvement than 1200 Hz. However, there is some confusion as to whether this was a genuine pulse repetition rate (PRR) specific effect as irradiance varied with PRR on the laser employed in this trial. Haina (1982) noticed a laser-mediated stimulatory effect on the granulation tissue content of irradiated rats, with a steady dose-response relationship up to $4\,J/cm^2$. This energy density has been found to be effective by some others, most notably Mester & Jaszsagi-Nagy (1973) who concluded that it had the greatest effect on collagen production.

As has already been indicated, collagen content and tensile strength are two frequently used criteria of wound healing. Kana et al (1981) found that He–Ne laser irradiation had a statistically significant stimulatory effect on collagen synthesis in the wound, again with a maximum effect at $4\,J/cm^2$, which also increased the rate of wound closure. Interestingly, while argon laser irradiation also produced a significant increase in collagen content, wound healing rate was not accelerated by such treatment.

Lyons et al (1987) found a considerable improvement in tensile strength of irradiated wounds at 1 and 2 weeks postirradiation, with collagen content significantly increased after 2 weeks. Abergel et al (1987) also found improvement in tensile strength due to enhanced collagen accumulation in mice, and further showed that procollagen levels in irradiated pigskin were elevated.

Braverman et al (1989) reported a significant difference in tensile strength in all laser treated groups (i.e. both infra-red and He–Ne) in irradiated and, interestingly, non-irradiated contralateral wounds. On the basis of this, they concluded that laser irradiation may cause the release of tissue factors into the systemic circulation which increased tensile strength of non-irradiated wounds. However, in this study no differences in rate of wound healing or of collagen area were noticed.

Investigations into tendon regeneration stimulated by LILT (Kokino et al 1985, Enwemeka 1990) produced similar results, that laser was found to increase the rate of healing. The latter group found that although ultimate tensile strength, energy absorption and strain did not differ between treated and control tendons, laser-treated tendons were consistently smaller than controls. Muscle fibre regeneration was also found to be accelerated by laser (Mester et al 1975); it was further reported by this group that laser irradiation also produced a qualitative improvement in regeneration.

Investigations by Rochkind's group on the effects of laser on the peripheral and central nervous system, cutaneous wounds and burns, found highly beneficial effects as a result of LILT (Rochkind et al 1989). Wound healing rates in both irradiated and contralateral (non-irradiated) wounds were accelerated, as they were in cases of bilateral burns. The amplitude of action potentials in crushed sciatic nerve were raised substantially in irradiated groups, as well as in the opposite non-irradiated control legs of such animals. Finally, the systemic effect in corresponding spinal cord segments was noted. Laser treatment greatly reduced the degeneration of the motor neurons compared to control groups.

The parallel influences of laser irradiation upon the lymphatic system and wound healing as investigated by Lievens (1985) showed that adhesion to underlying tissue almost never occurred after laser treatment, whereas 100% adhesion appeared in control groups. In addition oedema disappeared more quickly as a result of laser treatment, while regeneration of vein and lymph vessels took place much sooner where LILT had been applied.

Zarkovic et al (1991) found that there was a significant increase in the speed of wound closure of irradiated mice, with or without hepatectomy. Furthermore lipoprotein composition was decreased in irradiated, operated mice, although in non-operated mice no such differences were found. They suggested that the biological effects of laser might involve non-specific changes in metabolism, of which lipoprotein composition could be of major importance. Hickman & Dyson (1988) also described an increase in angiogenesis following irradiation of wounds, which may also reflect a systemic effect.

However, not all results are so unequivocal; indeed there are a number of reports from such animal research which did not find any significant effect. For example, Surinchak et al (1983) found no significant difference between irradiated and control animals in the time required for

80% wound healing. McCaughan et al (1985) also reported no effect on wound closure as a result of argon irradiation. Jongsma et al (1983) indicated that there was no difference in the healing area between irradiated and control groups. Most interestingly of all, given the similarities with human wound healing processes, studies investigating laser photobiostimulation of wound healing in pigs have almost exclusively found no significant effects as a result of laser irradiation (e.g. Hunter et al 1984, Basford 1986).

Summary

Perhaps the main lesson to be gained from the in vivo animal trials on laser photobiostimulation conducted to date is that proper reporting of treatment parameters is important for continuance of this type of study, and essential if results from such research are to be extrapolated for application in human research trials or clinical practice. Furthermore, it becomes difficult to ethically justify any research, especially where experimental lesions are inflicted upon laboratory animals, if the methodology is so poor or the published report so scant that the results cannot be relied upon.

STUDIES ON WOUND HEALING IN HUMANS

This chapter has already outlined the research that has been and is currently being completed in a number of laboratories into the effects of laser upon wound healing, both at the cellular and whole animal level. These laboratory studies are gradually developing a physiological basis for the actions and continued clinical application of low-intensity laser therapy for wound repair. However the literature reviewed indicates that much work needs to be done to substantiate the claimed physiological effects of low-intensity lasers and to find the optimal conditions under which they may occur. Alongside the type of laboratory work on cell lines and animals outlined above, research on human subjects is necessary; not least because clinical trials are essential in order to discover the extent to which it is possible to reproduce the generally positive effects seen in the laboratory. In extending such work to the clinical setting, the results obtained in well controlled laboratory studies can play an essential part in formulating the necessary hypotheses for clinical trials (Kitchen & Partridge 1991).

   That the laser is a popular modality for the treatment of wounds in the clinical situation has been well shown by Baxter et al (1991). In a questionnaire survey of physiotherapy departments in Northern Ireland, analysis of responses revealed therapeutic laser to be the most popular modality for the treatment of wounds; indeed 62.1% of respondents indicated wounds of various aetiologies as conditions which 'responded well' to LILT. Thus photostimulation of wound healing remains the cardinal indication for therapeutic laser in physiotherapy. In this, laser therapy has come to be recognised by many therapists as superior to a range of other alternative electrotherapeutic modalities such as ultrasound, interferential and shortwave. For this reason laser therapy is often the physiotherapeutic modality of choice in a variety of conditions including trophic, diabetic and decubitus ulcers, particularly where these have become chronic and/or unresponsive to other treatment approaches. In addition cases of necrosis, burns and postoperative wounds would also seem to respond favourably to low-intensity laser treatment. The use of laser has also extended to areas such as plastic surgery and gynaecology with some promising results.

Such popularity of therapeutic laser in the clinical field reinforces the importance of well controlled clinical research on human subjects. Unfortunately, relatively little well controlled and reported research has been completed to date in this area. However, the published studies that are available demonstrate the clinical potential of this modality in the treatment of various wounds.

As far back as the 1960s Professor Endre Mester was treating open wounds with laser. These wounds were mainly chronic ulcers which had proved unresponsive to other treatment regimes. Mester's work, spanning 25 years and including over 1000 patients, has demonstrated considerable success, with 50–100% healing rates achieved depending on the type of lesion. Although Mester's literature lacks some detail of procedure and dosage, as is perhaps understandable in the circumstances, all patients were reported as receiving an energy density of 4 J/cm^2 (Mester & Mester 1989).

Ulcers of various aetiologies have been used by other investigators to study the effect of laser therapy in the clinical situation. Ulcers are a predictable lesion in particular client groups, e.g. elderly and diabetic patients, which makes them relatively common and thus available for research. Ulcers are normally treated with compression bandaging, local dressings, bed rest and limb elevation. This conventional regime has changed little in 20 years and ulcers remain a significant cause of patient morbidity and financial strain on the health services (Sugrue et al 1990).

To assess the potential role of laser therapy in the management of such conditions, Sugrue and colleagues (1990) chose 12 patients suffering from chronic protracted venous ulcers; using two laser systems for treatment: an Endolaser (GaAlAs, 780 nm, continuous wave, 0–2 mW) and a Space Mid Laser IR (GaAs, 904 nm, pulsed 4000 Hz, 3 mW). In this trial, patients had a maximum treatment of 20 minutes duration, three times per week for 12 weeks. Objective measures included wound size assessed using photographic measurements, percentage granulation floor area, depth of wound, PaO$_2$ and tissue biopsy. Patients' pain intensity was also assessed subjectively using a Visual Analogue Scale.

The results of this group demonstrated a significant decrease in ulcer size, increased granulation tissue and epidermal growth, an increase in PaO_2 in one patient, increased capillary density and a significant decrease in pain. On the basis of these results Sugrue et al (1990) suggest that there may be a role for low-intensity laser therapy in the management of venous ulcers, particularly where these are painful and unresponsive to other treatments.

A number of groups, including Vertyanov et al 1982, Fenyo 1984, Santioanni et al 1984, Karu 1985 and Robinson & Walters 1991, also looked at the effect of laser on a variety of ulcerated lesions. A range of laser devices and models were used in these studies including Evolite (Fenyo 1984), Biotherapy 3ML (Robinson & Walters 1991) and an He–Ne (Santioanni et al 1984, Karu 1985). The diversity continues with regard to treatment parameters and as with the cellular and animal studies outlined earlier, there is a lack of detail in these reports which frustratingly does not allow the studies to be easily compared and/or replicated. While exact laser irradiation parameters such as power, wavelength, area irradiated and energy density are generally well described, other important aspects of the treatment regime such as length of treatment times and duration of the course of treatment are poorly documented. One study describes a one-treatment-per-day regime (Fenyo 1984) while another describes a regime of 56 sessions with no indication of the time involved or the duration of treatment until healing was completed (Karu 1985).

It appears that the most straightforward, and therefore popular, way to assess healing is to measure differences in wound size over time (Fenyo 1984, Santioanni et al 1984, Robinson & Walters 1991). Other objective measurements of treatment outcome include assessment of epithelialisation and granulation, amount of secretions and the haemodynamic state of the wound (Fenyo 1984). However, pain and psychological state of the patient represent other justifiable and measurable outcomes of treatment and have been assessed in a number of studies (Fenyo 1984, Wilder-Smith 1988, Sugrue et al 1990).

The overall results from the reviewed literature in general show a favourable response of ulcers to laser therapy. Fenyo (1984) cites the case of one subject with a 15-year problem with ulcers in whom, after 2 months of laser therapy, the ulcers had healed. Robinson & Walters (1991) saw a dramatic increase in healing with laser and consequently this resulted in a decreased workload for the physiotherapy department concerned, allowing more time to be spent on individual patients. On the other hand, Santioanni et al (1984) found no difference between laser-treated groups and control groups – therefore laser had no advantage over standard local treatments. However they are prudent enough to suggest that this may be connected with the schedules and protocols employed in their study. An interesting study by Karu (1985) found that phototherapy was 85% effective in healing gastric and duodenal ulcers. However there was no difference found in results obtained with coherent light (laser) and those obtained with incoherent monochromatic light sources. Karu also observed that higher doses were required to produce such in vivo clinical effects than those commonly used for in vitro research. This serves to emphasise the point that extrapolating too rapidly from cellular and animal studies to human clinical practice is unwise.

In gynaecology, Kovacs (1981) investigated the effect of He–Ne laser (5 mW, 632.8 nm, 124 cm distance from treatment site, 1 cm^2 irradiated area) on cervical erosion and ectopium. He reports a 90% increase in epidermal growth within a short time and an increase in connective tissue metabolism. The advantages of this treatment in gynaecology are numerous and Kovacs maintains that this method is promising in the outpatient treatment of ectopium.

Other wounds which have been treated with laser include skin grafts, burns, amputation injuries, infected wounds and trapping injuries (Cabrero et al 1985). After laser therapy, Cabrero et al (1985) found increased rates and quality of healing in all such cases. Interestingly, they also found that young patients healed better than old patients and thus pose the question of whether there is a better biological response in the young individual than in the old. From a single case study involving skin grafts Cabrero found an increase in healing in both donor and grafted area even though only the donor area was irradiated. Interestingly, another study by this same group revealed that laser decreased activity of bacterial culture in parallel with a laser-mediated increase in rates of healing, suggesting a potential and selective bioinhibitory effect of laser upon wound infections.

Using a Nd:YAG laser, Abergel et al (1984a) tested the efficacy of laser as a non-destructive treatment for keloids (see p. 109). The treatment resulted in a flattening and softening of the lesions, supporting the possibility that laser might prove an effective modality for treatment and prevention of keloids. While its mode of action in such cases may be unclear, it might reasonably be suggested that these could involve selective bioinhibition of the fibroblast functions within the tissue.

How useful then is this literature to the physiotherapist or practitioner in the clinical field? Although it is difficult to identify consistent use of particular irradiation parameters or regimes in the studies completed to date, these are certainly useful as a starting point. For example, Mester quotes 4 J/cm^2 as the optimal radiant exposure for treatment of wounds; thus this figure represents a useful baseline dosage for the treatment of open wounds. If unsuccessful, the clinician can feel confident that this dose can safely be increased.

In general, energy densities used to treat open wounds will vary from those used to treat closed wounds. The very fact that they are open removes the barriers of skin layers and so the energy density can be reduced. However, open wounds tend to be treated with a non-contact method to avoid cross-infection and patient discomfort. In such cases, the distance between light source and treatment area will increase the area being irradiated and thus decrease the energy density on the target tissue. This should be taken into account when planning and recording treatment (see p. 189). Other factors such as ischaemia and swelling can also affect the dose applied to an open wound. Blood proteins absorb light within the therapeutic wavelengths (Ohshiro & Calderhead 1990; see p. 70) and thus the state of the blood supply to the treatment area needs careful consideration in the planning of laser treatments. Finally, the state of the skin is important in that swollen, shiny areas will reflect light and therefore the energy density used in such cases should be increased.

The overall picture of the importance of laser for the treatment of open wounds in the clinical field is one of promise and, with further research in this environment to optimise and standardise the protocols of treatment, this new and exciting modality can be used with confidence and success.

SUMMARY OF KEY POINTS

1. Wound healing is a complicated series of processes which consist of three overlapping processes:
   a. inflammation
   b. re-epithelialisation and contraction
   c. matrix remodelling.
2. The initial inflammatory phase of wound healing is characterised by an immediate vascular response (vasodilation) and oedema formation.
3. During the inflammatory phase of wound healing, a variety of cells arrive at the wound site. These include:
   a. neutrophils
   b. macrophages
   c. lymphocytes, eosinophils and basophils
   d. platelets.
4. A host of biochemical mediators are important during the early phase of wound repair including:
   a. cytokines
   b. histamine
   c. bradykinin
   d. serotonin
   e. prostaglandins
   f. complement components.
5. Re-epithelialisation and contraction is the proliferative stage of wound repair, also comprising fibroplasia and angiogenesis. The most important cells during the phase are fibroblasts, myofibroblasts and macrophages.

6. Matrix remodelling is the establishment of an equilibrium between collagen formation and lysis, resulting in the constant reshaping of the scar over several months.

7. In assessing the potential modulative effects of low-intensity laser irradiation upon the wound healing process, research to date has been completed at three levels:
   a. at the cellular level
   b. using animal models of wound healing
   c. clinical trials on humans.

8. In all three areas, comparison of research findings is frustrated by the variety of irradiation parameters and measurement techniques employed, as well as the scant reporting of research protocols.

9. Cellular research has typically been completed on macrophage- and fibroblast-like cells and cell lines and has generally demonstrated a positive effect as a result of laser irradiation. Based upon such research, a number of putative mechanisms of action of laser-mediated photobiomodulation have been postulated. These include cellular proliferation, enhanced collagen synthesis and conversion of fibroblasts into myofibroblasts as well as direct stimulation of the respiratory/electron transport chain leading to enhanced ATP synthesis.

10. Animal studies have been diverse in terms of wound healing models used and research findings. These have typically been conducted on rats and mice, in which positive findings are generally reported. In contrast, studies on wound healing in pigs, whose skin has more in common with that of humans, have typically yielded negative results.

11. Given the problems in extrapolating irradiation parameters and findings from cellular and animal research to human practice, trials in humans are essential. To date, a number of such trials have been completed, primarily on the laser photobiostimulation of ulcers. While findings to date have been encouraging and typically positive, further research is required to effectively determine optimal treatment parameters/regimes.

REFERENCES

Abergel R P, Dwyer R M, Meeker C A et al 1984a Laser treatment of keloids: a clinical trial and an in vitro fibroblast study with Nd-YAG laser. American Society for Lasers in Medicine and Surgery, Abstracts, 329

Abergel R P, Meeker C, Lam T et al 1984b Control of connective tissue metabolism by laser. Recent developments and future prospects. Dermatologic Surgery 11: 1142–1150

Abergel R P, Lyons R F, Castel J C 1987 Biostimulation of wound healing by lasers:

experimental approaches in animal models and fibroblast cultures. Journal Dermatological Surgery Oncology 13: 127–133

Anderson R E, Warner N L 1976 Ionizing radiation and the immune response. Advanced Immunology 24: 215–335

Averbakh M M, Sorkin M Z et al 1976 The effect of helium neon laser on the healing of aseptic experimental wounds. Eksperimentalna Khirurgiia Anesteziologiia 3: 56

Azizkhan R G, Azizkhan J C, Zetter B R 1980 Mast cell heparin stimulates migration of capillary endothelial cells in vitro. Journal of Experimental Medicine 152: 931–944

Balboni G G, Zonefrati R, Brandi M L et al 1986 Effects of He–Ne/IR laser irradiation on two lines of normal human fibroblasts in vitro. Archivio Italiano Anatoma Embriologia 91(3): 179–188

Banda M H, Hunt T K, Silver I A 1985 Fibrosis. Clinical Symposia 37: 12

Basford J R 1986 Low-energy laser treatment of pain and wounds: hype, hope or hokum? Mayo Clinic Proceedings 61: 671–675

Basford J R 1989 Low-energy laser therapy: Controversies and new research findings. Lasers Surgery Medicine 9: 1–5

Bassett E G, Baker J R, DeSowza P 1977 A light microscopical study of incised dermal wounds in rats. With special reference to eosinophil leucocytes and to the collagenous fibres of the periwound areas. British Journal Experimental Pathology 58: 581

Baxter G D, Bell A J, Allen J M et al 1991 Low level laser therapy. Current clinical practice in Northern Ireland. Physiotherapy 77: 171–178

Bell E, Ivarsson B, Merrill C 1979 Production of a tissue-like structure by contraction of collagen lattices by human fibroblasts of different proliferative potential in vitro. Proceedings of the National Academy of Sciences USA 76: 1274–1278

Bertolami C N, Donoff R B 1982 Identification characterisation and partial purification of mammalian skin wound hyaluronidase. Journal of Investigative Dermatology 79: 417–421

Bosatra M, Jucci A, Olliano P et al 1984 In vitro fibroblast and dermis fibroblast activation by laser irradiation at low energy. Dermatologica 168: 157–162

Boulton M, Marshall J 1986 He–Ne laser stimulation of human fibroblast proliferation and attachment in vitro. Lasers in Life Sciences 1: 125–134

Bowersox J C, Sorgente N 1982 Chemotaxis of aortic endothelial cells in response to fibronectin. Cancer Research 42: 2547–2551

Braverman I M, Fonferko E 1982 Studies in cutaneous ageing: 1. The elastic fiber network. Journal Investigative Dermatology 78: 434–443

Braverman B, McCarthy R J, Ivankovich A D et al 1989 Effect of helium neon and infra-red laser irradiation on wound healing in rabbits. Lasers Surgery Medicine 9: 50–58

Brown G L, Curtsingel L, Brightwell J R et al 1986 Enhancement of epidermal regeneration by biosynthetic epidermal growth factor. Journal Experimental Medicine 163 (5): 1319–1324

Bullough W S, Lawrence C B 1961 The study of mammalian epidermal mitosis in vitro. A critical analysis of technique. Experimental Cell Research 24: 287–297

Cabana V G, Siegel J N, Sabesin S M 1989 Effects of the acute phase response on the concentration and density distribution of plasma lipids and apolipoproteins. Journal of Lipid Research 30: 39–49

Cabrero M V, Failde J M G, Mayordomo O M 1985 Laser therapy as a regenerator for healing wound tissues. International Congress on Laser in Medicine and Surgery, June 26–28, 187–192

Castellot J J, Addonizio M L, Rosenberg R et al 1981 Vascular endothelial cells produce a heparin-like inhibitor of smooth muscle growth. Journal of Cell Biology 90: 372–379

Castro D J, Abergel P, Meeker C et al 1983 Effects of Nd-Yag laser on DNA synthesis and collagen production in human skin fibroblast cultures. Annals of Plastic Surgery 11(3): 214–222

Clark R A F 1985 Cutaneous tissue repair: basic biologic considerations. Journal of the American Academy of Dermatology 13: 701–725

Clark R A F 1988 Overview and general considerations of wound repair. In: Clark R A F, Henson P M (eds) 1988 The molecular and cellular biology of wound repair. Plenum Press, New York, p 3–33

Clark R A F, Lanigan J M, Dellapelle P et al 1982a Fibronectin and fibrin provide a provisional matrix for epidermal cell migration during wound reepithelialization. Journal of Investigative Dermatology 70: 264–269

Clark R A F, Quinn J H, Winn H J et al 1982b Fibronectin is produced by blood vessels in response to injury. Journal of Experimental Medicine 156: 646–651

Cohen S 1965 The stimulation of epidermal proliferation by a specific protein (EGF). Developmental Biology 12: 394–407

Collins P D, Jose P J, Williams T J 1991 The sequential generation of neutrophil chemoattractant proteins in acute inflammation in the rabbit in vivo. Relationship between C5a and proteins with the characteristics of IL-8/ neutrophil-activating protein 1. Journal of Immunology 146(2): 677–684

Colver G B, Priestly G C 1989 Failure of He–Ne to affect components of wound healing in vitro. British Journal of Dermatology 121: 179–186

Deuel T F, Senior R F, Sanhuang J et al 1982 Chemotaxis of monocytes and neutrophils to platelet-derived growth factor. Journal of Clinical Investigation 69: 1046

Dyson M, Young S 1985 The effect of laser therapy on wound contraction. International Congress Laser Medicine Surgery 215–219

Dyson M, Young S 1986 The effect of laser therapy on wound contraction and cellularity in mice. Lasers in Medical Science 1: 125–130

Enwemeka C S 1988 Laser biostimulation of healing wounds: Specific effects and mechanisms of action. Journal of Orthopedic and Sports Physical Therapy 9(10): 333–338

Enwemeka C S, Rodriquez O, Gall N G et al 1990 Correlative ultrastructural and biomechanical changes induced in regenerating tendons exposed to laser photostimulation. Lasers in Surgery and Medicine (Suppl 2): 12

Fangde H, Pingan O, Haiyun K 1980 Irradiation effect of low power laser on the healing of experimental animal wounds. Laser Journal 7: 53

Fenyo M 1984 Theoretical and experimental basis of biostimulation by laser irradiation. Optics and Laser Technology, August: 209–215

Fernandez H N, Henson P M, Otani A et al 1978 Chemotactic response to human C3a and C5a anaphylatoxins. I: Evaluation of C3a and C5a leukotaxis in vitro and under simulated in vivo conditions. Journal of Immunology 120: 109–115

Fleischmajer R 1986 Collagen fibrillogenesis: a mechanism of structural biology. Journal of Investigative Dermatology 5: 553–554

Furcht L T, Wendelschafer-Crabb G, Mosher D F et al 1980 An axial periodic fibrillar arrangement of antigenic determinants for fibronectin and procollagen and ascorbate treated human fibroblasts. Journal of Supramolecular Structure 13: 15–33

Gabbiani G, Hirschel B J, Ryan G B et al 1972 Granulation tissue as a contractile organ. A study of the structure and function. Journal of Experimental Medicine 135: 719–734

Gabbiani G, Chapponnier C, Huttner I 1978 Cytoplasmic filaments and gap junctions in epithelial cells and myofibroblasts during wound healing. Journal of Cell Biology 76: 561–568

Gipson I K, Grill S M, Spurr S J et al 1983 Hemidesmosome formation in vitro. Journal of Cell Biology 97: 849–857

Glassberg E, Lask G P, Tan E M L et al 1988a Cellular effects of the pulsed tunable dye laser at 577 nanometres on human endothelial cells, fibroblasts and erythrocytes. Lasers in Surgery and Medicine 8: 567–572

Glassberg E, Lask G P, Uitto J 1988b Biological effects of low-energy laser irradiation. Lasers in Surgery and Medicine 8: 126

Grosman Z 1976 Effect of laser irradiation on different cell structures. S B Omik Vedeckych Praci Lekarske 19: 3–4

Gross A J, Jelkmann W 1990 Helium-Neon laser irradiation inhibits the growth of kidney epithelial cells in culture. Lasers in Surgery and Medicine 10: 40–44

Grotendorst G R, Seppä H E, Kleinman H K et al 1981 Attachment of smooth muscle cells to collagen and their migration toward platelet-derived growth factor. Proceedings of the National Academy of Sciences of the USA 78: 3669

Haina D, Brunner R, Landthaler M et al 1982 Animal experiments in light induced wound healing. Laser in Basic Biomedical Research 22: 1

Hallman H O, Basford J R, O'Brien J F et al 1988 Does low energy He–Ne laser irradiation alter in vitro replication of human fibroblasts? Lasers in Surgery and Medicine 8: 125-129

Hardy L B, Hardy F S, Fine S et al 1967 Effect of ruby laser radiation on mouse fibroblast culture. Federal Proceedings 26: 668

Hascall V C, Hascall G K 1981 Proteoglycans. In: Hay E B (ed) Cell biology of extracellular matrix. Plenum Press, New York

Hickman R A, Dyson M 1988 The effect of laser therapy on angiogenesis during dermal repair. Lasers in Surgery and Medicine 8: 186

Hoffbrand A V, Pettit J E 1984 Essential haematology, 2nd edn. Blackwell Scientific, London

Hsieh P, Chan L B 1983 Behavior of cells seeded on isolated fibronectin matrices. Journal of Cell Biology 96: 1208–1217

Hugli T E, Muller-Eberhard H J 1978 Anaphylatoxins, C3a and C5a. Advances in Immunology 26: 1–53

Humes J L, Bonney R J, Pelus L et al 1977 Macrophages synthesize and release prostaglandins in response to inflammatory stimuli. Nature 269: 149–151

Hunter J G, Leonard L G, Snider G R et al 1984 Effects of low-energy laser on wound healing in a porcine model. Lasers in Surgery and Medicine 3: 328

Imre G 1964 Role of lactic acid. British Journal of Ophthalmology 48: 75–82

Inoue K, Nishioka J, Hukuda S 1989 Altered lymphocyte proliferation by low dosage laser irradiation. Clinical and Experimental Rheumatology 7: 521–523

Jongsma F M H, van de Bogaard A E J M, van Gemert M J C et al 1983 Is closure of open skin wounds in rats accelerated by argon laser exposure? Lasers in Surgery and Medicine 3: 75–80

Kana J S, Hutschenreiter G, Haina D et al 1981 Effect of low power density laser radiation on healing of open skin wounds in rats. Archives of Surgery 116: 293–296

Kanzler M H, Gorsulowsky D C, Swanson N A 1986 Basic mechanisms in the healing cutaneous wound. Journal of Dermatologic Surgery and Oncology 12: 1156–1164

Karu T I 1985 Biological action of low-intensity visible monochromatic light and some of its medical applications. International Congress on Lasers in Medicine and Surgery, June 26-28, p 25–29

Karu T I 1988 Molecular mechanism of the therapeutic effect of low intensity laser irradiation. Lasers in the Life Sciences 2: 53–74

King P R 1989 Low level laser therapy: a review. Lasers in Medical Science 4: 141–150

Kitchen S S, Partridge C J 1991 A review of low level laser therapy. Physiotherapy 77: 161–168

Kloth L C, McCulloch J M, Feedar J A 1990 Wound healing, alternatives in management. F A Davis, Philadelphia

Knighton D R, Silver I A, Hunt T K 1981 Regulation of wound healing angiogenesis – effect on oxygen gradients and inspired oxygen concentration. Surgery 90: 262

Knighton D R, Hunt T K, Thakral K K et al 1982 Role of platelets and fibrin in the healing sequence. Annals of Surgery 196: 379

Kokino M, Tozun R, Alatli M et al 1985 Effect of laser irradiation on tendon healing. International Congress Laser Medicine Surgery 405–411

Kovacs L 1981 The stimulatory effect of laser on the physiological healing process of portio surface. Lasers in Surgery and Medicine 1: 241–252

Kraemer P M, Tobey R A 1972 Cell-cycle dependent desquamation of heparin sulfate from the cell surface. Journal of Cell Biology 55: 713–717

Kurkinen M, Vaheri A, Roberts P J et al 1980 Sequential appearance of fibronectin and collagen in experimental granulation tissue. Laboratory Investigations 43: 47–51

Lam T, Abergel P, Meeker C et al 1984 Low-energy lasers selectively enhance collagen synthesis. Lasers in Surgery and Medicine 3: 328

Lam T, Abergel P, Meeker C et al 1986 Low-energy lasers selectively enhance collagen synthesis. Lasers in the Life Sciences 1: 61–77

Laub R, Huybrechts–Godin G, Peeters–Joris C et al 1982 Degradation of collagen and proteoglycan by macrophages and fibroblasts. Biochimica Biophysica Acta 721: 425

Liebovich S J, Ross R 1975 The role of macrophages in wound repair. A study with hydrocortisone and antimacrophage serum. American Journal of Pathology 78: 71

Lievens P 1985 The influence of laser irradiation on the motricity of lymphatical system and on the wound healing process. Proceedings International Congress Laser Medicine Surgery 171–174

Lyons R F, Abergel R P, White R A et al 1987 Biostimulation of wound healing in vivo by a helium neon laser. Annals of Plastic Surgery 18: 47–50

McCaughan J S, Bethel B H, Johnston T et al 1985 Effect of low-dose argon irradiation on rate of wound closure. Lasers in Surgery and Medicine 5: 607–614

McDonald J A, Quade B J, Broekelmann T J et al 1987 Fibronectin's cell-adhesive domain and an amino-terminal matrix assembly domain participate in its assembly into fibroblast pericellular matrix. Journal of Biological Chemistry 262: 2957–2967

McPherson J M, Sawamura S, Condell R A et al 1988 The effects of heparin on the physicochemical properties of reconstituted collagen. Collagen Related Research 8(1): 65–82

Majno G 1979 The story of the myofibroblasts. American Surgery and Pathology 3: 535–542

Majno G, Gabbiani G, Hirschel B J et al 1971 Contraction of granulation tissue in vitro: Similarity to smooth muscle. Science 173: 548–550

Martin W J, Gadek J E, Hunninghake G W et al 1981 Oxidant injury of lung parenchymal cells. Journal of Clinical Investigation 68: 1277–1288

Mashiko S, Shimamoto M, Inaba H et al 1983 Effect of near infra-red light irradiation on wound healing using high power light emitting diodes. Journal of the Japanese Society of Laser Medicine 4: 187–192

Mester A F, Mester A 1989 Wound healing. Laser Therapy 1: 7–15

Mester E, Jaszsagi-Nagy E 1973 The effect of laser radiation on wound healing and collagen synthesis. Studia Biophysica 35: 227–230

Mester E, Korenyi-Both A, Spiry T et al 1975 The effect of laser irradiation on the regeneration of muscle fibers. Zeitschrift für Experimentelle Chirurgie 8: 258–262

Mester E, Mester A F, Mester A 1985 The biomedical effects of laser application. Lasers in Surgery and Medicine 5: 31–39

Mester E, Nagylucskay S, Tisza S et al 1978 Stimulation of wound healing by means of laser rays. Acta Chirurgica Academiae Scientiarum Hungaricae Tomus 19: 163–170

Meyers A, Joyce J, Cohen J 1987 Effects of low watt He–Ne laser radiation on human lymphocyte cultures. Lasers in Surgery and Medicine 6: 540–542

Michaeli D, Hunt T K, Knighton R D 1984 The role of platelets in wound healing: demonstration of angiogenic activity. In: Hunt T K et al (ed) Soft and hard tissue repair. Biological and clinical aspects. Praeger, New York, p 392

Montandon D, d'Andiran G, Gabbiani G 1977 The mechanism of wound contraction and epithelialization. Clinics in Plastic Surgery 4: 325–346

Mosher D F, Vaheri A 1978 Thrombin stimulates the production and release of a major surface associated glycoprotein (fibronectin) in cultures of human fibroblasts. Experimental Cell Research 112: 323–334

Nourshargh S, Williams T J 1990 Evidence that a receptor-operated event on the neutrophil mediates neutrophil accumulation in vivo. Journal of Immunology 145: 2633–2638

Ohshiro T, Calderhead R G 1990 Low level laser therapy: a practical introduction. Wiley, Chichester

Ohta A, Abergel R P, Vitto J et al 1987 Laser modulation of human immune system: Inhibition of lymphocyte proliferation by Gallium-Arsenide laser at low energy. Lasers in Surgery and Medicine 7: 199–201

Olsen C E 1984 Macrophage factors affecting wound healing. In: Hunt T K et al (ed) Soft and hard tissue repair. Biological and clinical aspects. Praeger, New York, p 343

Passarella S 1988 Recent discoveries on mitochondria bioenergetic mechanisms after low power laser irradiation. Abstract: Omega Laser Conference, London

Peacock E E 1984 Wound repair, 3rd edn. W B Saunders, Philadelphia

Polverini P J, Cotran P S, Gimbrone M A J et al 1977 Activated macrophages induce vascular proliferation. Nature 269(5631): 804–806

Popisilova J, Riebelova V 1986 Fibronectin – its significance in wound epithelialization. Acta Chirurgica Plastica 28: 96–102

Postlethwaite A E, Kang A H 1976 Collagen and collagen peptide-induced chemotaxis of human blood monocytes. Journal of Experimental Medicine 143: 1299–1307

Postlethwaite A E, Snyderman R, Kang A H 1976 Chemotactic attraction of human fibroblasts to a lymphocyte-derived factor. Journal of Experimental Medicine 144: 1188–1203

Postlethwaite A E, Keski-Oja J, Moses H L et al 1987 Stimulation of the chemotactic migration of human fibroblasts by transforming growth factor b. Journal of Experimental Medicine 165: 251–256

Pourreau-Schneider N, Ahmed A, Soudry M et al 1990 He–Ne laser treatment transforms fibroblasts into myofibroblasts. American Journal of Pathology 137: 171–178

Quarto E, Martino G, Michelini G 1988 Succinic oxidase activity in He–Ne laser irradiated mitochondria. Bollettino Societa Italiana Biologia Sperimentale 129–133

Remensnyder J P, Majno G 1968 Oxygen gradients in healing wounds. American Journal of Pathology 52: 301–319

Riceviuti G, Mazzone A, Monaia C et al 1989 In vivi and in vitro He–Ne laser effects on phagocyte function. Inflammation 1395: 507–527

Robinson B, Walters J 1991 The use of low level laser therapy in diabetic and other ulcerations. Journal of British Podiatric Medicine 46: 10

Rochkind S, Rousso M, Nissan M et al 1989 Systemic effects of low power laser irradiation on the peripheral and central nervous system, cutaneous wounds and burns. Lasers in Surgery and Medicine 9: 174–182

Roitt I, Brostoff J, Male D 1985 Immunology. Churchill Livingstone, Edinburgh

Rouzer C A 1988 Secretion of leukotriene C and other arachidonic acid metabolites by mouse pulmonary macrophages. Journal of Experimental Medicine 155: 720–733

Santioanni P, Monfrecola G, Martellotta D et al 1984 Inadequate effect of Helium-Neon laser on venous leg ulcers. Photodermatology 1: 245–249

Seppa H E J, Grotendorst G R, Seppa S I et al 1982 Platelet-derived growth factor is chemotactic for fibroblasts. Journal of Cell Biology 92: 584–588

Shields T D, O'Kane S, Leckey D et al 1991 The effect of laser irradiation upon human mononuclear leukocytes in vitro (article in preparation)

Shimokado K, Raines E W, Madtes D K et al 1985 A significant part of macrophage-derived growth factor consists of two forms of PDGF. Cell 43: 277–286

Silver I A 1984 Oxygen and tissue repair. In: Ryan T J (ed) An environment for healing: the role of occlusion. Royal Society of Medicine International Congress and Symposium Series No. 88: 18

Simon R H, Scoggin C H, Patterson D 1981 Hydrogen peroxide causes fatal injury to human fibroblasts exposed to oxygen radicals. Journal of Biological Chemistry 256: 7181–7186

Simpson D M, Ross R 1972 The neutrophilic leucocyte in wound repair. A study with antineutrophilic serum. Journal of Clinical Investigation 51: 2009

Singer I I 1979 The fibronexus: a transmembrane association of fibronectin-containing fibers and bundles of 5 nm filaments in hamster and human fibroblasts. Cell 16: 675–685

Singer I I, Paradiso P R 1981 A transmembrane relationship between fibronectin and vinculin (130kd protein): Serum modulation in normal and transformed hamster fibroblasts. Cell 24: 481–492

Sporn M B, Roberts A B 1986 Peptide growth factors and inflammation, tissue repair, and cancer. Journal of Clinical Investigation 78: 329–332

Sporn M B, Roberts A B, Wakefield L M et al 1986 Transforming growth factor β. Biological function and chemical structure. Science 233: 532–534

Stimler N P, Bach M K, Bloor C M et al 1981 Release of leukotrienes from guinea pig lung stimulated by C5a des arg anaphylatoxin. Journal of Immunology 128: 2247–2257

Stryer L 1988 Biochemistry, 3rd edn. W H Freeman, New York

Sugrue M E, Carolan J, Leen E J et al 1990 The use of infra-red laser therapy in the treatment of venous ulcerations. Annals of Vascular Surgery 4: 179–181

Surinchak J S, Alago M L, Bellamy R F et al 1983 Effects of low-level energy lasers on the healing of full-thickness skin defects. Lasers in Surgery and Medicine 2: 267–274

Tocco G, Le Borgne De Kaouel C, Aubert C 1985 He–Ne and I.R. mid-laser influences in skin cells in vitro-preliminary results. Proceedings International Congress Lasers Medicine Surgery, p 175–182

Toole B P 1981 Glycosaminoglycans in morphogenesis. In: Hay E B (ed) Cell biology of extracellular matrix. Plenum Press, New York

Tsukamoto Y, Hesel W E, Wahl S M 1981 Macrophage production of fibronectin, a chemoattractant for fibroblasts. Journal of Immunology 127: 637

Turk J L, Heather C J, Diengdoh J V 1976 A histochemical analysis of mononuclear cell infiltrates of the skin with particular reference to delayed hypersensitivity in the guinea pig. International Archives of Allergy and Applied Imunology 29: 278–289

Vertianov V, Khanian A G et al 1982 Treatment of trophic ulcers with lasers. Khirurgiia 8: 19–22

Wahl L M, Wahl S M, Mergenhagen S E et al 1974 Collagenase production by endotoxin-activated macrophages. Proceedings of the National Academy of Sciences of the USA 71: 3598

Wall R T, Harker L A, Striker G E 1978 Human endothelial cell migration. Stimulated by a released platelet factor. Laboratory Investigations 39: 523–529

Wheeland R, Walker N P J 1986 Lasers – 25 years later. International Journal of Dermatology 25: 209–215

Wilder-Smith P 1988 The soft laser: therapeutic tool or popular placebo. Oral Surgery Oral Medicine Oral Pathology 66: 654–658

Wilkerson G B 1985 Inflammation in connective tissue: etiology and management. Athletic Training Winter: 298

Winter G D 1972 Epidermal regeneration studied in the domestic pig. In: Maibach H I, Rovee D T (ed) Epidermal wound healing. Year Book Medical Publishers, Chicago

Woolf N 1977 Cell tissue and disease. The basis of pathology. Baillière Tindall, London

Young S, Bolton P, Dyson M et al 1989 Macrophage responsiveness to light therapy. Lasers in Surgery and Medicine 9: 497–505

Zarkovic N, Saltzer B, Hrzenjak M et al 1991 The effect of gallium arsenide laser irradiation and partial hepatectomy on murine skin wound healing and lipoprotein composition. Period Biology 93: 359–361

Zauberman H, Michaelson I C, Bergman F et al 1969 Stimulation of neovascularization of the cornea by biogenic amines. Experimental Eye Research 8: 77–83

Zetter B R, Chen L B, Buchanan J 1976 Effects of protease treatment on growth, morphology, adhesion, and cell surface proteins of secondary chick embryo fibroblasts. Cell 7: 407–441

6. Low-intensity laser therapy for pain relief

INTRODUCTION

The manufacturers of therapeutic lasers have used the analgesic potential of such devices as a major selling point for their wares. However, the extravagance of some claims has, perhaps understandably, led to a certain amount of scepticism within the medical community regarding the analgesic potential of LILT, especially as the possible mechanism of any such effect remains unclear (Siebert et al 1987, Basford 1989, Hansen & Thoroe 1990, Devor 1990). Despite this scepticism, such use has been recommended by a number of authors (Seitz & Kleinkort 1986, Ohshiro 1988, Walker 1988, Woolley-Hart, 1988, Zhou Yo Cheng 1988, Kert & Rose 1989).

The analgesic efficacy of therapeutic laser would also seem to be supported by the experience of clinicians as summarised by the results of a recent survey, the most salient findings in this respect being:

1. LILT achieved the premier overall ranking for relief of pain compared with the other listed electromodalities
2. Painful conditions figured prominently as 'indications for laser treatment' and as conditions identified as 'responding particularly well' to such treatment
3. While rated overall as only giving 'variable results' in the treatment of low back pain, laser therapy was rated overall as 'effective' for myofascial and post-operative pain (Baxter et al 1991).

The relief of pain would therefore appear to be an important treatment objective in physiotherapists' use of low-power lasers. This positive experience on the part of clinicians canvassed in the survey is underpinned by a range of published reports and abstracts, examples of which are summarised in Table 6.1. However, although apparently extensive, two points need to be made with respect to these publications. In the first instance, findings are not exclusively positive: a number of groups have failed to demonstrate any analgesic or antinociceptive effect with such devices (e.g. Haker and Lundeberg 1990) Secondly, the deficiencies and criticisms identified in previous chapters apply equally to the

Table 6.1 Laser-mediated analgesia: overview of clinical findings. This table is not intended to be exhaustive, merely to provide an indication of the scope of the papers published in this area.

Reference	Laser	Treatment	Diagnosis	n	D	P	Eff	Measure	Comments
Atsumi et al (1987)	830	60 mW, CW & pulse	RA pain	163	Y	Y	82%*	report	[Ab] *40% placebo
Basford et al (1987)	632.8	0.9 mW, 90 s, CW × 3 pw, 3/52, T	OA thumb pain	81	Y	Y	ns	numeric*	* + ROM, strength etc.
Bieglio & Bisschop (1987)	632.8	N + IR	Radicular pain	?	?	?	+ve*	report	*inflamm phase; ?neural/vasc mechanisms
Bliddal et al (1987)	632.8	10 mW, 5 min, × 3 pw, 3/52, T	RA pain	17	Y	Y	ns	VAS*	* + EMG etc; ?systemic effects
Burgudzhieva et al (1985)	632.8	T	Postop pain (gynae)	179	–	Y	+ve	report	[FLA]
Choi et al (1986)	904	<1 mW, 60 s, × 2 pw, Acu	Painful elbow	1	N	N	67%	report*	* + glucocorticoid excretion
Dubenko et al (1976)	?	?	Tri neuralgia	106	–	–	+ve	report	[FLA]
Emmanouilidis & Diamantopoulos (1986)	820	15 mW, 90 s, CW × 5 pw, 2/52, T	Sports injuries	62	Y	Y	90%*	Scot/VAS**	Cumulative effect *25%; placebo, ** + thermography
England et al (1989)	904	3 mW, 5 min, 4000 Hz, T, × 3 pw, 2/52	Tendinitis	30	Y	Y	+ve*	VAS**	*p < 0.001; ** + goniometry
Galperti et al (1987)	632.8	<60s, <7.2 J/cm²	PA pain	60	–	–	+ve	quest	
Gartner et al (1987)	IR	10–20 min, × 5 pw, 4/52, T	AS, PA, LBP, etc	546	–	–	87%	report*	* + functional; cumulative effect
Glykofridis & Diamantopoulos (1987)	632.8; 660–950	<25 mW, var time, CW, × 5 pw, T	Locomotor pain	200	N	N*	+ve	numeric	* Comparative study; ? analysis
Gussetti et al (1986)	904/632.8	5–20 min, × 5 pw, T	PA shoulder	30	–	–	80%	report*	* + X-ray invest

Table 6.1 *cont'd*

Reference	Laser	Treatment	Diagnosis	n	D	P	Eff	Measure	Comments
Jensen et al (1987)	904	0.3 mW, 30 min, 250Hz, ×5 pw, T	PA knee	29	Y	Y	nil	report*	cross over study; * + drug intake
Kamikawa & Kyoto (1986)	IR	×14 Rx, T	Various	60	–	Y	79%*	numeric	*46% 'effective'/34% fair
Kats et al (1985)	632.8	?	Oral pain*	88	?	?	+ve	report	[FLA], *sialidenitis
Kreczi & Klinger (1986)	632.8	2 mW, 30 s, 100 Hz, 1 Rx, Acu	Radicular pain	21	N	Y	+ve*	Adapt VAS	*$p < 0.001$, max post 1 h; effects <9.6 h
Lonauer (1986)	632.8/IR*	10 min, 15/365, T	OA pain hand	40	N	Y	+ve**	?	*combination preferable; ** + grip strength etc
Lukashevich (1985)	632.8	T	PHN	150	–	–	+ve*	report	[FLA] * versus alternatives
Martino et al (1987)	CO_2	5 mW, CW?, <20 min, ×5 pw, 3/52, N+T	Mastalgia	50	–	–	32%	Keele/Lasa/Map	[Ab]
Mayordomo et al (1986)	CO_2	<25 W, scan, 5–10 min, ×3 pw	Locomotor pain	82	?	N	<80%	numeric*	* + thermography
Mester & Mester (1987)	Clust	50 mW	Wound pain	?	?	?	+ve		[Ab]
Morselli et al (1985a)	CO_2	<25 W, scan, CW, 5–10 min, ×3 pw	OA Pain	200	N	N	>70%*	?	[Ab], *62% acute effect; effects extend >1 h
Morselli et al (1985b)	CO_2	<25 W, scan, CW?; 10–15 min, ×2 pday	Sports injuries	>100	–	–	+ve	report	[Ab]
Roumelidis et al (1985)	820	15 mW, CW, <25 min, ×5pw, 2/52, T	Sports injuries	31	N	Y	+ve	VAS*	[Ab] * + thermography
Shiroto et al (1986)	830	<30 s/pt, <7 min, TP+Acu	Various pain	1600	N	N	85%	report	[Ab]

Table 6.1 cont'd

Reference	Laser	Treatment	Diagnosis	n	D	P	Eff	Measure	Comments
Siebert et al (1987)	632.8; 904	<30 mW, 1200 Hz, 15 min, 10/365, T	Tendinopathies	64	Y	Y	ns	numeric*	* + thermography; ?placebo ?10 cm distance
Simunovic (1987)	632.8	?	Oral pain	?	–	–	+ve	report*	[Ab]
Ternovoy (1984)	632.8	T + TP	Locomotor pain	400	–	–	+ve	report*	[FLA] * + thermography
Vidovitch et al (1987)	CO_2	1 mW	RA pain	272	–	–	75%	VAS*	[Ab] * + drug intake etc
Walker (1983)	632.8	1 mW, <30 s, 20 Hz, ×3 pw, 10/52, N + T	Chronic pains	36	Y	Y	73%	VAS*	Chronic effect,* + 5-HIAA
Walker et al (1986)	632.8	1 mW, ×3 pw, 10/52	RA pain	64	S	Y	+ve*	VAS**	*$p < 0.001$ ** + drug intake
Willner et al (1985)	904	60 s, 1000 Hz, ×3pw, 3/52, TP	OA pain hands	67	?	Y	62%	MPQ*	[Ab], + drug intake
Zhou Yo Cheng (1987)	CO_2	30 mW, Acu	Minor surgery	40	–	–	95%	report*	[Ab], * + drug intake

Abbreviations: D = double-blind; P = placebo-controlled; Eff = efficacy; Measure = pain measurement method used; RA = rheumatoid arthritis; [Ab] = abstract; pw = per week; 3/52 = 3 weeks; T = topically applied/to lesion; ns = non-significant findings; ROM = range of movement; N = applied to nerves/nerve roots; VAS = visual analogue scale; EMG = electromyography; [FLA] = foreign language abstract; Acu = applied to acupuncture points; Tri = trigeminal; PA = periarthritic pain; AS = ankylosing spondylitis; LBP = low back pain; Rx = treatment; OA = osteoarthritis; PHN = postherpetic neuralgia; scan = laser used in conjunction with scanning device; 10/365 = 10 days; 5-HIAA = 5-hydroxyindoleacetic acid; MPQ = McGill Pain Questionnaire published reports within this field (Basford 1986, 1989, Siebert et al 1987, Devor 1990, Kitchen & Partridge 1991).

For example, few of the completed studies would conform to the rigorous standards outlined by Walker (1988) or more recently by Max et al (1991), especially with regard to algesimetry. Algesimetry is a particularly important consideration in such studies as pain is by definition a psychological event (Merskey 1979), and thus can only be measured directly by psychometric means (Chapman & Loeser 1989). Algesimetric methods commonly employed in human studies include simple visual analogue scales (VAS; Huskisson 1983) upon which subjects or patients may rate pain intensity, or more complex pain questionnaires comprising various scales, the best known of which is the McGill Pain Questionnaire (MPQ; Melzack 1975).

Given the controversy surrounding such use, the current chapter will concentrate on the analgesic effects of low-intensity laser therapy. The chapter begins with an extensive review of the clinical research completed to date in this area, followed by an overview of laboratory findings using experimental pain. To conclude the chapter, the evidence for neurophysiological and neuropharmacological substrates of the clinically observed effects of laser are outlined.

CLINICAL STUDIES ON LASER-MEDIATED ANALGESIA

Overview of literature

The majority of publications in this area are available only either as conference abstracts, or alternatively are English abstracts accompanying foreign language papers (e.g. Ternovoy 1984a, b, Lukashevich 1985). Consequently, these only provide scant details of the protocols and methodology used. This serves to reduce the detail and extent of the published database on LILT-mediated analgesia, at least for Anglophone researchers and clinicians. The picture is also confused by the wide range of conditions treated and the diversity of treatment parameters employed (see Table 6.1), making it difficult for the clinician or researcher to generalise findings from these reports.

The preferred method of assessment of the clinical potential and efficacy of any treatment modality or drug is the clinical trial, the so-called stage III trial being the most rigorous test (Friedman et al 1983, Pocock 1987). However, the vast majority of the publications on laser-mediated analgesia are either empirical or anecdotal reports based upon the authors' clinical experiences with a particular machine or treatment (e.g. Ternovoy 1984a, Morselli et al 1985b, Shiroto et al 1986, Wilder-Smith 1988), or are reports of the results of small-scale investigations (Kreczi & Klinger 1986, Bliddal et al 1987), a sizable proportion of which are badly designed or controlled. A number of comparative clinical studies have also been completed on laser therapy for pain relief: comparing various wavelengths (e.g. Lonauer 1986), laser acupuncture and conventional treatments including physiotherapy (Choi et al 1986, Glykofridis & Diamantopoulos 1987) and comparing laser versus traditional acupuncture (Lundeberg et al 1987b, Haker & Lundeberg 1990).

The bulk of the remaining relevant publications do not document analgesic trials of laser, but rather report studies in which pain relief represents but one of a number of indices upon which the efficacy of LILT is judged for a particular condition. Relatively few are based upon trials in which LILT has been assessed specifically as an antinociceptive or analgesic modality (Walker 1983). This distinction is important, especially as the latter type of study is usually more carefully controlled and reported in respect of algesimetry. The paucity of published clinical trials of laser-mediated analgesia is therefore a serious deficiency in the literature and represents one important area for future research efforts.

However, while some of the criticisms levelled at the published clinical reports may be justifiable, two points can be made. Firstly, laser therapy is still a relatively new modality (at least in the West), so that a certain number of anecdotal reports are to be expected as for any new application. Secondly, laser research has to be seen in context: large stage III, multicentre trials are expensive to implement and conduct. The funding for such research usually comes from the pharmaceutical companies who develop and consequently profit from the products. With a few notable exceptions, research funding from laser manufacturers has been non-existent.

Conditions treated

Therapy using various types of laser system has been used to treat a range of conditions in which pain plays a significant part in the clinical presentation.

Rheumatoid arthritis

In the Northern Ireland survey, LILT was rated by respondents as 'effective' for the treatment of rheumatoid arthritis. This rating is corroborated by a range of reports from the Soviet Union and eastern Europe, which testify to the apparent efficacy and popularity of He–Ne lasers for the treatment of rheumatic pain in these countries (e.g. Bulakh et al 1983, Yakovenko & Simoonova 1985, Soroka 1989). A number of clinical trials, both controlled and uncontrolled, of laser therapy for rheumatoid arthritis have been completed in the West and Japan, the majority of which have shown positive effects on a number of indices, including pain.

In an early American study using a low-output Nd:YAG laser, Goldman and colleagues found that laser irradiation of painful rheumatic joints in the hand resulted in significant abatement of reported pain and inflammation (Goldman et al 1980). Similarly positive results with this type of laser system have subsequently been reported by Vidovich & Olson (1987) in a treatment group ($n = 272$) which included a majority of rheumatoid arthritis patients. These investigators found that 80% of the rheumatoid patients treated with an Nd:YAG laser operating in the milliwatt range showed 'good' pain relief, assessed by means of VAS and reduced oral analgesic intake. These positive effects upon pain were paralleled by similar improvements in functional status (Vidovich & Olson 1987).

Equally encouraging results have been demonstrated with other laser systems, operating at wavelengths more commonly found in routine physiotherapeutic practice. Walker's group in California have reported a highly significant difference ($p < 0.001$) in levels of reported pain and analgesic drug intake between treatment and control groups after a 10-week course of treatment with a 1 mW He–Ne unit (Walker et al 1986, 1987a). More recently, Palmgren and colleagues at the University of Copenhagen have demonstrated a significant effect on reported pain in a placebo-controlled, double-blind study ($n = 35$) using an 820 nm continuous wave diode (3.58 J/cm^2) to treat the small joints of the hand (Palmgren et al 1989). The other indices used in this trial (grip strength, swelling, range of movement and early morning stiffness) showed concomitant improvements with laser treatment.

In a larger, uncontrolled trial on 170 patients using an 830 nm, 60 mW, continuous wave infra-red laser diode, Asada and colleagues at Osaka City University found that 90% of all patients so treated reported some degree of pain relief on a three-point scale ranging from 'excellent' through 'good' to 'unchanged'. Almost 60% of these patients reported 'excellent' pain relief following such laser treatment (Asada et al 1989). Interestingly, reductions in VAS scores following irradiation with a 30 mW, 830 nm laser system in 19 rheumatic patients were found to correlate with thermograph changes by Obata and colleagues (1990). Thermography has been used by a number of groups as an objective measure to substantiate subjective patient pain reports with similar results (see below). The putative alteration in autonomic nervous system function suggested by such findings may represent one possible mechanism of laser-mediated pain relief, at least in cases of rheumatic pain.

The characteristic pattern of exacerbation and remission found in rheumatoid arthritis can make it difficult to assess the efficacy of any drug or modality tested as a potential treatment for the condition. Under these circumstances, it could be argued that the improvements reported in the above studies represent no more than expected remission observed as part of the pathological process, especially as a number of the studies are open or uncontrolled. However the fact that control groups, whose members did not show similar improvements to those in the laser treated groups, were employed in some of these studies would tend to preclude spontaneous remission as a major factor in the reported positive results.

Despite these generally positive results, Bliddal and colleagues (1987) found only a slight decrease in VAS pain ratings, using a 10 mW He–Ne laser for a total treatment time of 5 minutes. Furthermore, neither early morning stiffness nor joint function were found to be significantly improved by treatment. This rather disappointing finding may be in part explained by the research protocol employed in that study. Treating the small joints of the hand of 17 patients, this group irradiated one hand and used the other as control. In these circumstances, any generalised, systemic effects of laser (so called 'secondary effects'; Ohshiro & Calderhead 1988) will influence the control limb as well as the irradiated limb. Furthermore, the use of such a protocol disregards the possibility of contralateral analgesic effects. Acupuncturists routinely utilise such contralateral effects and may needle one limb to induce analgesia in the contralateral limb (Chaitow 1983). If such mechanisms are responsible for the results found by Bliddal et al, there are important implications for both clinical practice and research.

Osteoarthritis

In assessing the efficacy of LILT for osteoarthritis, a number of clinical studies have indicated a positive effect on pain relief. Morselli et al (1985b), using a relatively high-power (< 25 W) continuous wave (CW) CO_2 laser in open trial, in conjunction with a scanning device, found that 70% of patients so treated experienced good pain relief, which lasted over 1 month. Other investigators have used systems more commonly found in clinical practice (Willner et al 1985, Lonauer 1986, Trelles et al 1990). Willner et al (1985), in a placebo-controlled trial completed on 67 subjects suffering from osteoarthritic hand pain, found that 60 seconds' irradiation of the affected joints with a 904 nm diode, three times per week, resulted in significant decreases in MPQ scores and analgesic drug use. Trelles et al (1990) report that, in an open trial of laser treatment (830 nm, 60 mW, CW) of osteoarthritic knees, patients' pain was markedly reduced after a 4-week course of therapy, and that such reductions in pain were found to be accompanied by increases in ROM and other indices of treatment efficacy. Unfortunately, this particular report lacks detail, notably the numbers involved in the trial and any indication of the extent of success with treatment: it is hard therefore to come to any opinion as to the significance of their reported findings.

Similarly positive results were found by Lonauer (1986) in a placebo controlled trial, using He–Ne and infra-red diode lasers individually and in combination to irradiate affected joints. Interestingly, Lonauer notes that the best treatment effects were obtained where the two different lasers were used in combination. While this observation would tend to provide support for the use of multi-wavelength, multi-diode arrays, the use of relatively low numbers in such a comparative trial ($n = 40$) and insufficient detail in the published abstract do not allow any categorical conclusions on such devices to be drawn.

Whereas the abstracts reviewed above would suggest that laser therapy has a part to play in the management of osteoarthritic pain, the non-significant findings of Basford and colleagues (1987) indicate that the evidence is far from unequivocal. Basford's group confined its study to irradiation of osteoarthritic thumbs. Their study can be criticised because of the power and energy levels used (0.9 mW and 0.081 J respectively), which are well below those recommended for clinical applications (see Ch. 7). Furthermore, the He–Ne laser used in this trial possesses the least penetration of those laser systems routinely used in LILT. This lack of penetration, coupled with the relatively small dosage levels used, may explain the non-significant effect reported in this case.

Periarthritis and other arthritic conditions

Periarthritis and other arthritic conditions in various presentations have proved to be popular conditions with investigators. As with rheumatoid and osteoarthritis, the majority have found beneficial effects on pain with laser therapy. Gussetti et al (1986) found in 30 cases of periarthritis of the shoulder that therapy lasting between 5 and 20 minutes using a He–Ne laser together with a 904 nm infra-red source led to a reduction in pain report in 80% of the patients so treated. The English abstract accompanying this foreign language paper is unfortunately not sufficiently detailed to allow comment upon the dosages nor the research design employed in this trial. Despite this, it is interesting to note another instance of positive results using a combination of visible and infra-red laser radiation for treatment (see also Lonauer 1986).

Similarly positive results in the reduction of periarthritic pain have been reported using He–Ne and infra-red diode lasers in isolation (Galperti et al 1987, Gartner et al 1987). Galperti et al (1987) used an He–Ne source to irradiate the affected joints of 60 female patients suffering from shoulder periarthritis as a complication of breast surgery for cancer. Using an algesimetric questionnaire to assess the efficacy of such laser therapy, they reported a significant reduction in pain as a result of treatment with dosages of up to 7.2 J/cm². In common with the Gussetti study above, the lack of detail in this group's abstract precludes further comment upon the research design employed in this study. In an apparently open trial on 546 patients suffering from pain due to a variety of conditions including ankylosing spondylitis and low back pain as well as periarthritis, Gartner et al (1987) found that 87% of patients reported significant pain reduction with infra-red laser therapy. While the comments regarding detail made on the above papers apply equally here, it is interesting to note from this abstract that, in common with the study by Gussetti et al (1986), rather long treatments (i.e. 10–20 min) given five times per week would seem to give positive results, apparently without the danger of overtreatment cited by some authors (Kitchen & Partridge 1991).

However, in contrast to the above, the solitary double-blind, crossover study on periarthritic pain that has been completed to date (Jensen et al 1987) failed to show any significant differences in pain report or analgesic drug intake between laser treated patients (904 nm) and controls. As with the investigation by Bliddal and colleagues discussed above, this study would seem to be flawed by the relatively low power levels used (0.3 mW), and possibly because of the employment of a crossover design. Such designs are popular in clinical trials as they provide a practical means of matching treatment and control groups, particularly in trials based upon smaller sample sizes. However, in using this design, investigators make a number of assumptions: most importantly that the effect of the drug or modality used in the treatment condition can be 'washed out' during the crossover period (Friedman et al 1983, Pocock 1987). The results of Walker (1983), Gartner et al (1987) and Shiroto's group (1989) would indicate that the analgesic effects of laser are, at least in some circumstances, both cumulative and long-lasting, so that no such assumption is warranted. The implication of this is that crossover designs may not be the most appropriate research design in analgesic trials of LILT.

Musculoskeletal pain and sports injuries

A number of Russian and eastern European language papers have reported the apparent efficacy of laser therapy (usually with He–Ne systems) in the relief of a range of painful musculoskeletal syndromes (e.g. Ternovoy 1984, b). This is supported by the report of at least one Chinese group, in which up to 82% of patients treated with laser therapy (He–Ne/CO_2) in open trial demonstrated 'very good' results (Li 1990). Several trials have been completed in Western Europe which would tend to bear out the positive results reported in these Chinese and Russian papers (Mayordomo et al 1986, Glykofridis & Diamantopoulos 1987). In an open trial with a 25 W, CW CO_2 source equipped with a scanner, Mayordomo et al (1986) found that just under 80% of treated patients reported good pain relief measured by a numeric rating scale and corroborated with thermograph findings. Glykofridis & Diamantopoulos, in one of the very few trials completed with such devices, compared laser irradiation with a CW multiwavelength multidiode array with a prescribed, standardised 'physiotherapy' regime, which did not include LILT, in 200 patients suffering from various musculoskeletal syndromes in open trial, and found that LILT compared favourably with the standardised physiotherapy regime in terms of pain relief.

In comparing laser therapy with such a standardised regime of physio-therapy (which excluded LILT), this trial is not unique. Kumar and colleagues (1988) reported interim findings from an ongoing comparative study that LILT was apparently superior to *their* 'physiotherapy' regime in the management of inversion injuries of the ankle, based upon a number of indices including pain relief (Kumar et al 1988). It must be stréssed, however, that the validity of such comparative studies can be questioned on the grounds that in practice physiotherapy is not applied in a standard-ised, prescribed regime to all patients presenting with a given condition or range of conditions.

A number of reports document the apparent efficacy of LILT in the reduction of pain associated with sports injuries (Morselli et al 1985a, Emmanoulidis & Diamantopoulos 1986, Roumeliotis et al 1987, see also Ohshiro 1988). Morselli et al (1985a), as in the other study by this group on osteoarthritis reported above, used a relatively high-power (25 W) CO_2 CW laser with scanner for a 10–15 min treatment given twice daily. In this (apparently) open trial, good pain relief was reported in over 100 patients so treated (Morselli et al 1985a). In a placebo-controlled, double-blind trial, Emmanoulidis & Diamantopoulos (1986) found decreases in measured pain in 90% of the athletes treated with an 820 nm CW diode (15 mW) for 90 s each working day for 2 weeks. The single-blind study of sports injuries by Roumeliotis et al (1987) used the same delivery system for a much longer treatment time (< 25 min), with an identical pattern of treatment (five times per week for 2 weeks) and found good analgesic effects in the 31 athletes so treated. Interestingly, in common with the study of Obata et al (1990) already considered above, pain reduction was found in both these studies to be accompanied by de-creases in thermograph readings (Emmanoulidis & Diamantopoulos 1986, Roumeliotis et al 1987).

In laser treatment of the pain associated with tendonopathies, England and colleagues (England et al 1989) found significant pain reduction with the use of an 904 nm infra-red source (0.9 J/point, ~7.2 J/cm²) on the points of maximum tenderness in a group of 30 patients suffering from either bicipital or supraspinatus tendonitis. In contrast, another study by Siebert et al (1987) with a larger group ($n = 64$) found no significant difference in reported levels of tendon pain between laser-treated patients and controls. Despite being highly critical of the standard of previous laser research, these investigators employed a non-contact technique in their trial, irradiating patients' skin from a distance of 10 cm. Given the beam divergence of clinical LILT apparatus, the use of such a distance would appear to be inappropriate, producing minimal power and energy den-sities on the irradiated tissue. This, coupled with apparent inaccuracies in calculation of dosage (by a factor of 10), casts serious doubts upon the reliability and validity of the reported findings. In the final analysis the study is flawed by the use of almost negligible energy densities.

The efficacy of laser therapy in the treatment of lateral humeral epicondylitis/epicondylalgia (tennis elbow) has been investigated by several groups with conflicting findings: some reporting positive effects (Choi et al 1986, Li 1990, Terashima et al 1990), while others have failed to show any benefit with laser therapy (Lundeberg et al 1987a, Haker & Lundeberg 1990). Using a single subject design, Choi et al (1986) compared laser therapy, TENS and acupuncture in the treatment of the condition. While this group reported finding comparable levels of analgesia with the three modalities tested, their study can be criticised for the lack of wash-out allowed between conditions. Despite this, the study did find that all three modalities produced increased levels of glucocorticoids. This finding is interesting as it implicates serotonin metabolism as one possible mechanism of laser-mediated analgesia, and that this mechanism might be common to the three modalities tested. As one potential mechanism of laser-mediated analgesia, serotonin metabolism is considered further below. However it is useful to note here that single-subject designs have traditionally been frowned upon by the medical community, the clinical trial being considered the most appropriate test of the efficacy of a particular treatment (see above). From this perspective, the study by Choi et al can at best be considered a pilot and needs to be replicated with a larger sample.

Terashima et al (1990) found, in an open trial on 23 patients suffering from tennis elbow and 40 patients suffering from de Quervain's disease, that 50% of all patients treated with a GaAlAs diode for 10–20 s per tender point, three to four times per week experienced lasting pain relief. Results from digital plethysmography and thermography investigations completed on some of the patients in this study indicated an increase in local blood flow as a result of laser irradiation (Terashima et al 1990). Similarly, Li (1990) reports 'very good' results in 84% of tennis elbow patients ($n = 25$) treated with a combination CO_2/He–Ne unit in the Xia-Guan Laser Hospital in Nanjing City, China.

In contrast, Eva Haker's group at the Karolinska Institute in Sweden have published results from two double-blind, placebo-controlled studies in which they failed to show any effect with laser acupuncture treatment of tennis elbow (Lundeberg et al 1987a, Haker & Lundeberg 1990). Given the positive results of Choi et al (1986), Li (1990) and Terashima et al (1990), it is important to consider the possible reasons for the non-significant effects reported by this group in more rigorous double-blind, controlled trials.

In the first instance acupuncture points were used as the site of irradiation by Lundeberg et al, which may or may not be appropriate in this condition. Indeed, this group's most recent findings on tennis elbow show highly significant ($p < 0.01$) improvements in a number of objective indices including vigorometer and strength tests after a course of ten laser treatments (904 nm, 0.36 J/point) applied *directly* to six points over the painful site (Haker 1991). Furthermore, the dosages used in their earlier acupuncture study were very low: 0.004 (904 nm) and 0.093 (632.8 nm) J/point (Lundeberg et al 1987a). Having admitted that these were rather low, the group's later acupuncture publication was still based upon a laser acupuncture treatment of 0.36 J/point (Haker & Lundeberg 1990). Despite being fourfold greater than the higher dose used in the previous study, this can still be regarded as much lower than is commonly used in clinical practice, at least in the UK.

This criticism can also be levelled at the study by Waylonis and colleagues, which found non-significant results in the He–Ne laser acupuncture treatment of 62 cases of chronic myofascial pain (Waylonis et al 1988). While details of the irradiation parameters are not fully specified by these authors, the maximal energy used apparently did not exceed 0.012 J per acupuncture point (Waylonis et al 1988). Under these circumstances the integral non-laser 'point finder' photodiode could well have been supplying similar levels of irradiation to the placebo treated controls in this placebo-controlled double-blind trial. The possible relevance of energy densities in analgesic laser therapy is considered further below.

Neuropathic/neurogenic pain

In the previously cited survey (Baxter et al 1991), respondents rated laser overall as 'effective' for the treatment of post-herpetic neuralgia (PHN), an application which is supported by a number of anecdotal reports from eastern Europe (e.g. Lukashevich 1985) and the West (Corti et al 1988). Moore et al (1988a) have investigated the efficacy of laser in the treatment of this condition in a double-blind, crossover trial on 20 patients with apparently significant reductions in pain after laser treatment. The laser used in this study was a 60 mW CW GaAlAs system operating at 830 nm (Moore et al 1988a), which has also been successfully employed in open trial by Hong and colleagues (1990). Of 20 patients treated for between 5 min and 10 min with this unit, 60% achieved either 'excellent' or 'good' results (Hong et al 1990).

Similarly positive results have also been reported by McKibben & Downie in Canada, who found significant ($p < 0.05$) and lasting (> 1 year) pain relief in an open trial on 39 patients (McKibben & Downie 1990). The system used in this study was a single wavelength (904 nm) multidiode array, delivering 7 J per treatment, which the authors found represented a practical method of treating the extensive areas usually affected in the condition (McKibben 1991). Nanjin et al (1990) investigated the incidence of PHN after laser treatment of herpes zoster in 101 patients. In this single-blind comparative study, He–Ne laser treatment of the affected nerve roots was found to significantly lower the incidence of PHN compared to existing (pharmacological) treatments (Nanjin et al 1990). Laser treatment was also observed to have significantly shortened the pathogenesis of the herpes zoster in this study.

Trigeminal neuralgia has also apparently been successfully treated by

He–Ne laser by at least one centre in eastern Europe (Dubenko et al 1976). Several research reports on the laser treatment of this painful condition have been published by Walker's group (Walker et al 1987b, Walker 1988). Using a relatively low-power 1 mW He–Ne system to deliver 20 s treatments to each nerve, and treatments of between 30 s and 90 s to the painful areas on the face, this group applied treatments three times per week for a total of 10 weeks. In the 35 patients studied in this double blind placebo-controlled trial, Walker's group found a significant difference in VAS ratings between active and placebo treated patients.

Several groups have investigated the efficacy of laser therapy in the treatment of radicular and pseudoradicular pain syndromes (Bieglio & Bisschop 1986, Kreczi & Klinger 1986, Mizokami et al 1990). All reported positive effects on pain. Kreczi & Klinger (1986) found a highly significant ($p < 0.001$) difference between VAS scores for laser treated patients and controls ($n = 21$) in the treatment of radicular pain syndromes, after a single treatment of the appropriate acupuncture point with a 2 mW He–Ne unit for 30 s. The report by Bieglio & Bisschop (1986) lacks detail, other than that these investigators apparently obtained a good result using a combination of He–Ne and infra-red diode systems in the treatment of radicular pain, which was most pronounced in the early 'inflammatory' phase. The group ($n = 206$) studied in the open trial reported by Mizokami et al (1990) included not only patients suffering from occipital neuralgia, but also cases of neurogenic neck, shoulder and back pain. The laser used was a CW GaAlAs diode system operating at 60 mW. While the poorest results were obtained for the back pain subgroup, over 80% of patients with occipital neuralgia reported 'excellent' or 'good' pain relief (Mizokami et al 1990).

Operative and postoperative pain

Given the nature of the early work of Endre Mester and his colleagues, it is perhaps not surprising that low-power laser has been used in the treatment of various types of surgical wound. In addition to promoting wound healing, laser seems also to produce an analgesic effect in such patients (Mester & Mester 1987, Simunovic 1987, Abe 1990). The published accounts of this application of LILT are almost exclusively in abstract form. A number of reports from Burgudjieva's group in Hungary document the use of He–Ne units for photobiostimulation of postoperative wounds in obstetrics and gynaecological practice. These reports have included reference to the pain relief experienced by laser-treated patients (Burgudjieva et al 1985).

Several trials have been completed in this area with encouraging results (Martino et al 1987, Moore et al 1988b, 1990). Martino et al (1987) found in an open trial on 50 patients that irradiation of (postmastectomy) mastalgia with a CW CO_2 unit operating at 5 mW at unspecified intervals over a 3-week period led to significant pain reduction in one third of cases. In double-blind trials on postoperative pain following herniorrhaphy and cholecystectomy procedures, Moore and colleagues in Oldham found that 6–8 min irradiation of the operative wound with a 60 mW, 830 nm, CW diode resulted in significant reductions in pain. Pain was assessed for the purposes of these studies by numerical rating scales and decreased oral analgesic request (Moore et al 1988b, 1990).

Low-power laser has also apparently been successfully used as a means of inducing preoperative anaesthesia, both in veterinary practice and in humans, in whom success rates of 95% have been reported using various devices ranging from a 2 mW He–Ne laser system to more powerful CO_2 systems (Zhou Yo Cheng 1988). Some of the most interesting reports of this application describe the apparent anaesthetic efficacy of laser acupuncture for minor oromaxilofacial operations in dental practice (Zhou Yo Cheng 1984, 1987). Dental surgery is one of the most popular areas for low-power laser application (Christensen 1989, Hansen & Thoroe 1990), with pain relief frequently being cited as one of the benefits of such therapy (Kovacs 1987, Simunovic 1987). Kats and colleagues also report positive results in cases of sialoadenitis (inflammation of the salivary glands), with decreased levels of pain being reported by patients irradiated with He–Ne laser (Kats et al 1985).

However the use of lasers in dentistry is still subject to intense debate. Despite the positive experiences of clinicians, usually reported in the Russian and eastern European literature, recent controlled studies in the West and Japan have yielded contradictory results (e.g. Hansen & Thoroe 1990, Harazaki et al 1990). Harazaki et al (1990) found a significant analgesic effect on post-dental-surgery pain in 81 patients recruited for their single-blind, placebo-controlled trial. In contrast, a double-blind, placebo-controlled, crossover study on 40 patients with chronic orofacial pain by Hansen & Thoroe (1990) failed to find any significant difference in reported pain between laser-treated patients and controls. Using a 904 nm diode, these investigators used a dosage of between 2.35 J/cm^2 and 4.7 J/cm^2 on the affected sites, which would appear to be well within the range routinely used by physiotherapists for laser treatments. While further consideration of the application of low-power lasers in dentistry is beyond the scope of the current text, it would appear that the conflict between clinical experience and the findings from the relatively few trials completed to date in this area would indicate further investigation as being necessary before any definitive statement can be made on the role of LILT in the management of pain in dentistry.

Studies with non-homogeneous populations

A number of studies have been more generalised and have assessed the effectiveness of LILT for pain relief in patients suffering from a range of painful conditions (e.g. Kamikawa & Kyoto 1985). Several of these have defined inclusion criteria on the basis of chronicity (Walker 1983, Atsumi et al 1987). Others represent reports of retrospective studies of efficacy (e.g. Shiroto et al 1986). The study by Kamikawa & Kyoto (1986) investigated the efficacy of laser therapy for pain relief, using a numeric algesimetric rating scale. The percentage experiencing pain relief was similar to that found by Walker (1983) at 80%. However, of this figure 34% reported only 'fair' (versus 'effective') pain relief. Consequently, the statistical significance of these results is unclear. Indeed, no evidence of the use of any statistical test of significance is presented by these researchers. This criticism is, unfortunately, not unique to this study.

Walker's often cited early study (Walker 1983) used 36 patients suffering an assortment of chronic pain syndromes apparently unresponsive to other therapy. Based upon patients' estimates of pain, Walker found that 73% of the treatment group reported decreases in estimated pain. Walker's study is interesting for two very different reasons. Firstly, Walker noted an increase in urinary 5-hydroxyindoleacetic acid (5-HIAA) in those patients experiencing analgesia. This increase was not found in placebo-treated subjects. This would seem, as in the study by Choi et al discussed above, to implicate an alteration in serotonin metabolism as one mechanism of LILT-mediated analgesia. Also interesting was the lack of any placebo effect among placebo-treated controls, especially in the light of the placebo potential of lasers. This finding is almost, if not entirely, unique: the extent of placebo-induced analgesia is usually estimated as being approximately 50% of that expected from the active treatment (Evans 1974).

Similarly positive findings have been reported by Atsumi and colleagues in a double blind, placebo-controlled trial on chronic pain: the percentage of patients reporting pain relief (82%) after laser treatment with an 830 nm CW/pulsed diode system operating at 60 mW was found to be just over twice that among placebo-treated subjects (40%) (Atsumi et al 1987). Included in the treatment group of this study were patients suffering chronic lumbago, arthritic and neurogenic pain.

Shiroto and colleagues in their various publications (e.g. Shiroto et al 1986, 1989, Shiroto & Sato 1990a, b) report ongoing successes with infra-red laser acupuncture treatment in several thousand patients suffering from various pain syndromes. The authors cite positive results in between 76% and 83.3% of the patients so treated. While essentially uncontrolled and retrospective in nature, the large numbers involved in these studies represent an important body of anecdotal evidence of laser's potential as an analgesic modality. Perhaps the most interesting finding in these reports is the duration of laser-mediated analgesia indicated by the results of the questionnaire studies (Shiroto et al 1989, Shiroto & Sato 1990b). This, rather than the subjective impressions of improvement described by patients (Shiroto & Sato 1990b) would tend to discount placebo reactions as a basis for the observed analgesic effect of laser therapy.

Treatment parameters

It would seem that there has been a certain amount of confusion, and possibly even ignorance, regarding the importance of the treatment parameters used in laser therapy, both in routine clinical practice and in the studies reviewed above. In fact some authors do not even specify in their abstracts the wavelength of the laser used (Dubenko et al 1976), while others merely describe the source as 'infra-red' (e.g. Kamikawa & Kyoto 1986, Bieglio & Bisschop 1986, Gartner et al 1987). More frequently, details given are insufficient to calculate energy dosages (e.g. Kats et al 1985) and consequently it is impossible to replicate the work either clinically or experimentally.

This lack of detail in reporting can be attributed to three factors. In the first instance, the clinical significance of factors such as wavelength, pulsing frequency etc. is still largely unknown. Indeed the importance of specifying treatment parameters such as energy dosage has only recently been realised and stressed by clinical investigators (Calderhead 1990). This is to be expected to a certain extent, since LILT is a relatively new treatment modality whose mechanisms of action are still poorly understood. Secondly, the investigators involved in laser research have apparently not always been sufficiently knowledgable nor experienced regarding the basic physical principles of laser. Inappropriate treatment techniques and inaccuracies in calculations of energy dosage (e.g. Siebert et al 1987) are an example of this. Finally, in historical or anecdotal reports based upon relatively large numbers of patients it is frequently not practical to specify the precise parameters used, unless a rather artificial treatment 'prescription' has been employed in all cases. This is particularly so where such reports are in abstract form. However, the specification of the rationale behind selection of treatment parameters in such reports is to be expected and would be useful, not least for clinicians.

Wavelength

He–Ne lasers (632.8 nm) have been the single most popular laser source with investigators, with almost half of all published studies reporting use of these devices. The reason for this is twofold: firstly He–Ne lasers were the first devices to be available for therapeutic clinical use. It was only with later developments in semiconductor diode opto-technology that infra-red sources became commercially available. Additionally, there has been some delay in the granting of licences for the use of diode units in the USA because of stringent Food and Drug Administration rules (Ohshiro 1990).

Interestingly, of the studies reviewed above which found non-significant results with laser therapy, the majority used He–Ne sources (either in isolation or in combination with infra-red) (Basford et al 1987, Bliddal et al 1987, Lundeberg et al 1987a, b, Siebert et al 1987, Waylonis et al 1988). The relative lack of penetration with such sources may have played a part in the apparent failure of laser therapy to produce analgesia in these cases. However, the situation is not straightforward, as other studies using He–Ne sources have produced positive findings (e.g. Bieglio & Bisschop 1986, Kreczi & Klinger 1986, Galperti et al 1987). The inference is that other treatment parameters may play an important role in the efficacy of clinical laser treatment.

Carbon dioxide laser sources have also been popular with investigators (Martino et al 1987, Vidovich & Olson 1987); although these are rarely used in routine clinical practice, at least in the UK. These sources have found medical applications in such areas as surgery and photodynamic therapy for a number of years. Producing infra-red radiation at 10 600 nm, such devices produce photothermal effects on irradiated tissues, even when delivered in relatively low dosages (Carruth & McKenzie 1986). Consequently they have tended to be used with a scanning device to keep power densities low (Morselli et al 1985a, b, Mayordomo et al 1986). Alternatively, optical power outputs have been kept low (Vidovich & Olson 1987), or the sources have been used on acupuncture points with extremely short irradiation times (Zhou Yo Cheng 1987). Based upon the publications reviewed here, CO_2 lasers appear to be an effective modality for pain relief. Despite this, such lasers do not represent a practical option as a laser source for physiotherapeutic applications of LILT.

The other wavelengths used are to be found in the 820–950 nm part of the spectrum, and are thus classed as near infra-red. These wavelengths are invariably produced by diode lasers, and their use in clinical research reflects a shift in practice from more traditional laser technology using largely gaseous media (He–Ne, CO_2). Negative results were found with these lasers by Jensen et al (1987) and Siebert et al (1987), each using 904 nm wavelength sources (the latter study in conjunction with a He–Ne unit). However, as already indicated above, these studies appear to be inappropriately designed, so that the negative results may have little or nothing to do with the choice of wavelength per se.

Only one study (Mester & Mester 1987) reports use of a multiwavelength, multidiode 'cluster' array for pain relief. Such units are offered by a number of manufacturers (see Appendix I), and have proved popular among clinical practitioners. While Mester & Mester (1987) report positive effects on wound pain, further work is necessary to establish the advantages (if any) that such units offer over standard treatment diodes.

Power output and energy densities

From Table 6.1 it is apparent that a wide range of power and energy settings have been used in the studies completed to date. Once again, a number of reports provide only scant details of the dosages used (Kamikawa & Kyoto 1985, Simunovic 1987, Vidovich & Olson 1987). In those publications where relevant details are provided, power outputs ranged from 0.3 mW (Jensen et al 1987) to 25 W (Morselli et al 1985), with the majority being in the 1–30 mW range, which largely reflects current clinical practice. Lower-power sources have tended to be used, although not exclusively, for laser acupuncture treatments (e.g. Kreczi & Klinger 1986), while the high-power CO_2 units have been used with a scanning device to spread the incident power over a greater area, and thus keep energy densities low (Morselli et al 1985a, b). Interestingly, scrutiny of the treatment regimes used in the various trials reviewed here would suggest that low power densities (and consequently energy densities) may represent one contributory factor in the non-significant findings reported by some groups (Basford et al 1987, Jensen et al 1987, Siebert et al 1987, Waylonis et al 1988). If this is the case, there are important implications for clinical practice and research. These are considered below.

As already indicated in Chapter 4, energy density is an important consideration in laser therapy, the calculation of which requires specification of the size of irradiated (treatment) area, power output and time of irradiation. Unfortunately, few of the studies cited specify all of the details necessary (e.g. Galperti et al 1987), so that energy densities can, at best, only be estimated. As with power outputs, low energy densities associated with relatively short treatment times (< 1 min) and low-power outputs would seem to have been employed successfully in laser acupuncture therapy (Choi et al 1986, Shiroto et al 1986). However, relatively low energy densities have also produced positive results when used directly on the painful site (Vidovich & Olson 1987), or in conjunction with irradiation of the associated nerve (Walker 1983). It is, unfortunately, impossible to infer more than this, due to the lack of details presented in the publications reviewed.

The same lack of information also precludes much assessment of the possible clinical significance of pulse repetition rate. In the papers reviewed, a range of pulsing frequencies were employed, ranging from continuous wave (e.g. Emmanoulidis & Diamantopoulos 1986, Basford 1987) to over 1000 Hz (e.g. Willner et al 1985, Siebert et al 1987).

Frequency of treatment and length of treatment course

Treatment regimes vary considerably, from a single laser acupuncture treatment lasting 30 s (Kreczi & Klinger 1986) to thrice weekly treatments for 10 weeks (Walker 1983), with no obvious differences in efficacy between regimes regardless of regularity of treatment or length of treatment course. In the studies where these are specified, the most popular regimes tend to incorporate treatment regimes of up to five times per week (e.g.

Gartner et al 1987, Martino et al 1987) for periods of 2–4 weeks (Willner et al 1985, Roumeliotis et al 1987).

LABORATORY STUDIES OF LASER MEDIATED ANALGESIA

Based upon the review presented in the preceding section, it is apparent that, while numerous anecdotal accounts and reports of open trials would support the clinical application and efficacy of LILT as an analgesic modality, more carefully controlled and reported studies have yielded equivocal findings. Apart from the lack of an obvious underlying mechanism of action, research on laser-mediated analgesia is confounded by uncertainty surrounding the possible relevance of treatment/irradiation parameters, which may or may not be a contributory factor in some of the negative findings reported. While the ideal method of establishing such relevance would be via a series of clinical trials in which a particular treatment parameter was systematically manipulated while others were fixed (Kitchen & Partridge 1991), economic, practical and ethical constraints render this approach unfeasible.

Alternatively, the identification and development of a suitable experimental model of pain in humans would allow the systematic investigation of laser treatment parameters in a controlled environment without recourse to clinical subjects, and the inherent variability found in any clinical population. Additionally, laboratory investigations of pain have a number of other advantages over clinical studies, not least of which is the ability to investigate effects at minimal and maximal pain intensities within the same experimental session (Wolff 1983). Laboratory-based studies on humans have already been successfully used in the assessment of the relevance of stimulation frequencies in electro-mediated analgesia (Ashton et al 1984, Johnston et al 1989). The application of such an approach within the LILT field could potentially yield useful information for clinical practice, and upon which to design better future clinical trials. The aim of this section of the current chapter is therefore to review the literature on laboratory investigations of laser-mediated analgesia.

Investigations of laser-mediated analgesia in animals

In contrast to the numerous clinical studies of laser-mediated analgesia reviewed in the preceding chapter, relatively few laboratory studies of laser-mediated analgesia have been completed. With few exceptions (see below), animal models of pain have been used in these investigations. Of these, a sizable proportion have been completed in China using a variety of experimental animals including rabbits, rats, sheep, goats and horses. Zhou Yo Cheng (1988) provides an overview of the findings of these Chinese studies, which include significant increases in pain thresholds and tolerances after relatively short periods of laser acupuncture using He–Ne laser systems. Unfortunately as no English abstracts nor translations of this work are available, it is impossible to comment further upon these apparently positive findings.

The studies published in English have reported more variable findings. Wu (1983) used a He–Ne system to deliver 0.216 J/cm^2 to the tails of experimental rats, which were then assessed against controls using a tail flick methodology (D'Armour & Smith 1941). In such investigations, noxious thermal stimulation is applied to the tails of experimental animals and any observed increases in latency to tail flick (i.e. withdrawal) is taken as indicative of raised pain threshold, and thus of the analgesic efficacy of the drug or procedure under study. In the Wu study, two levels of noxious stimulation, described merely as 'high' and 'low', were investigated. Laser irradiation was found to significantly increase the latency to tail flick at the lower level of noxious thermal stimulation. However, at the higher level of stimulation, laser irradiation was only effective when delivered at a 'higher' pulse repetition rate. While this report provides evidence of a laser-mediated hypoalgesic effect, the magnitude of which is apparently frequency-dependent, the actual pulse repetition rates were unfortunately not specified.

Ponnudurai and colleagues have provided further evidence of frequency-dependent hypoalgesia in rats, again using the tail flick methodology (Ponnudurai et al 1987). These investigators found that a low pulsing frequency (4 Hz) produced an immediate hypoalgesic effect of short duration, 60 Hz a delayed but longer-lasting effect and that 200 Hz was apparently ineffective. This finding may explain the insignificant results in a similar study on rats reported by Lundeberg's group in Sweden (Lundeberg et al 1987b). Using relatively long irradiation times of up to 30 min and a source pulsed at 73 Hz, Lundeberg et al failed to find any hypoalgesic effect, apparently *immediately* after laser irradiation.

Ponnudurai's group has subsequently investigated the mechanism of the hypoalgesic effect which they had found at 4 Hz (Ponnudurai et al 1988). In this later study, hotplate tests (Woofle & McDonald 1944) were used to supplement the tail flick methods they had previously used. While hotplate tests, like tail flick methods, rely upon latency to an observed behaviour as an estimate of induced analgesia, in this technique the behaviours used as the end points are usually foot licking or limb withdrawal (Bonnett & Peterson 1975). In both the experimental models used in this study, latencies were found to increase significantly after laser treatment; this effect lasting for up to 24 h after irradiation (Ponnudurai et al 1988). Moreover, it was further found that naloxone, a potent opiate antagonist (Jacob & Ramabadran 1978) had no effect upon this laser mediated hypoalgesia, either in terms of magnitude or duration. This would suggest that the analgesic effect observed at 4 Hz was not mediated by endogenous opiates (see below) and that some other neurophysiological or neurochemical substrate was responsible for the observed hypoalgesia.

A more recent study by Zhu and colleagues has assessed the efficacy of He–Ne laser acupuncture in the treatment of experimental arthritis in rats, using a number of indices including pain threshold assessments and an unspecified pain scale (Zhu et al 1990). In this study, vocalisation and limb withdrawal were used to assess the hypoalgesic effects of such laser acupuncture treatment. Vocalisation in response to noxious stimulation is a commonly used laboratory technique which is considered by some authors to be a good measure of the affective components of pain in experimental rodents (Chapman et al 1985). In the study by Zhu et al, no significant differences were found between controls and irradiated rats in terms of either measure of pain threshold, whereas significant improvements were noted in joint swelling and 'pain scale' readings as a result of laser acupuncture treatment.

Unfortunately, the lack of detail provided in this abstract on the pain scale used precludes further comment on this aspect of the reported results. However, and more interestingly, while *routine* testing of pain thresholds as described (i.e. limb withdrawal and vocalisation) showed no significant differences between the experimental groups used in this study, pain thresholds estimated by latency to vocalisation assessed *immediately after laser* in irradiated rats were found to be significantly raised. These results would suggest that while laser irradiation may be effective in reducing the signs and symptoms of experimental arthritis in rodents in the short term, it apparently does not have *lasting* effects on pain threshold. However, while the immediate laser-mediated hypoalgesia detected by the vocalisation technique in this study is apparently in keeping with the broad findings of Wu (1983) and Ponnudurai et al (1987, 1988), it is unclear as to why the limb withdrawal reflex also used in this study failed to show any alteration in threshold. As already stated, vocalisation techniques are thought to better reflect the affective components of an animal's pain. In these circumstances, and given that no placebo/sham irradiated group was used in this study, it could be argued that the observed differences in latency to vocalisation resulted from placebo-like effects in the irradiated animals, similar to those described by McKibben (1988).

In contrast to the generally positive findings outlined above, one group has reported an apparent laser-mediated *hyper*algesia in experimental mice using a hotplate technique (Zarkovic et al 1989). While this finding apparently contradicts those of the studies already reviewed above, and indeed the authors' own experiences in human patients, it may in part be explained by the experimental paradigm, and particularly the irradiation parameters employed by this group. It is useful to note for instance that Zarkovic and colleagues used a 904 nm infra-red system to deliver an energy density of 0.00041 J/cm^2 to the feet of experimental mice used in the study. Given the use of such an exceptionally low dosage in this investigation, the relevance of these results to clinical practice

are unclear. The decreased latency to jumping demonstrated by irradiated animals represents an enhanced nociception at the energy density
used, which may (or may not) be reversed at higher power and energy
densities.

Laboratory studies of laser-mediated analgesia in humans

Despite the generally encouraging findings in animals, the difficulties and
problems of extrapolating the findings of such work to humans remain.
In addition to problems such as species differences, there are a number
of limitations to the use of laboratory studies on animals for the assessment of analgesic effects in humans. The most obvious of these is that
human pain is a multidimensional, subjective *psychological* event (Merskey
1979); consequently the use of animal behaviours such as withdrawal
can represent only a poor model of the human pain experience. This is
particularly so of the reflex-type behaviours (such as tail flick) which rely
upon neural function at spinal/segmental level with minimal (if indeed
any) influence from more rostral centres in the neuraxis. Furthermore,
and in spite of their wide use, a recent evaluation of such methods suggests that they are relatively insensitive even to systemic administration
of morphine (Vierck et al 1982).

These limitations notwithstanding, few published papers to date have
reported investigations of the analgesic effects of laser in humans using
laboratory techniques (Seibert & Gould 1984, Brockhaus & Elger 1990,
King et al 1990). Using a pulsed He–Ne laser with a maximum power
output of 10 mW, Brockhaus & Elger irradiated the *hegu* (dorsum of
hand) and *jianqian* (clavicle) acupuncture points bilaterally for a total
of 1 min per point and compared the effects of this laser acupuncture
with traditional (needle) acupuncture upon thermal pain threshold. While
laser acupuncture was found to have an insignificant effect upon thermal
pain threshold in the 39 subjects studied by Brockhaus & Elger, their
study can be criticised on a number of points, not least of which is
the use of relatively low levels of incident energy on the irradiated acupuncture points (< 0.6 J/point). Additionally, these investigators used a
psychophysical approach by employing the estimation of thermal pain
threshold, but ignored other easily quantifiable variables which are usually measured in such studies (e.g. pain tolerance, pain sensitivity range
etc.; Chapman et al 1985, see below). This, taken in conjunction with
the relatively low energy levels employed, casts doubts over the validity
of the findings in this study.

In contrast, thermal pain threshold was found to be significantly increased after only 35 s of 1 mW laser irradiation by Seibert & Gould
(1984). Hypoalgesic effects have also been reported by King and colleagues at the University of Alabama in a single-blind, placebo-controlled
study using laser acupuncture treatment of auricular acupuncture points.

After treating four points in the ipsilateral ear for 30 s per point (0.03 J/point, ~0.3 J/cm²), increases in electrical pain thresholds measured at the wrist were found in irradiated subjects. These increases in irradiated subjects ($n = 41$) were significantly greater than those in unirradiated controls (King et al 1990). While providing further evidence of the analgesic potential of laser, the relevance of these results to clinical practice is somewhat limited, as laser irradiation of auricular acupuncture points is not a part of routine clinical practice, at least in the British Isles. These results would, however, indicate that the use of such treatment techniques may represent a useful therapeutic technique for the relief of pain. This notwithstanding, the several studies completed to date (Seibert & Gould 1984, Brockhaus & Elger 1990, King et al 1990), would all appear to be flawed by the sole use of pain threshold as a means of quantifying analgesic effect; this would tend to limit the applicability and relevance of these studies to clinical practice.

THE NEUROLOGICAL EFFECTS OF LILT: CURRENT FINDINGS

Introduction

The findings from the clinical and laboratory studies as outlined above provide evidence of the analgesic potential of low-power laser; these are therefore in broad agreement with the experiences of clinical practitioners. However the mechanism(s) of action underlying such analgesic effects remain unclear, despite extensive conjecture in the literature, often apparently based upon scant evidence (Milani & Roccia 1982, Choi et al 1986, Kemmotsu et al 1990). The identification of underlying mechanisms of action therefore represents an important field for investigation, especially in light of the scepticism surrounding this area (Devor 1990), and the obvious placebo potential of laser. While the identification of potential mechanism(s) of action is not essential to the establishment of clinical efficacy, the lack of such knowledge renders the evaluation of apparently conflicting results difficult, if not impossible (Basford 1986). The remainder of this chapter therefore reviews the work currently completed to date in this area.

Background: an overview of the neuropharmacology and neurophysiology of pain

The neurophysiological and neuropharmacological substrates of pain have been extensively reviewed elsewhere (e.g. Bowsher 1988, Baldry 1989, Melzack & Wall 1989). Walsh (1991) has recently provided a succinct review of the neurophysiological substrates and the relevance of these to physiotherapeutic practice. These are briefly overviewed here as background to the reviews presented below.

The small diameter fibres of the peripheral nervous system (Aδ and C fibres; Williams et al 1989) carry nociceptive information from the site of peripheral injury to the dorsal spinal cord, from where two distinct but complementary systems conduct the information to the most rostral levels of the nervous system (Bond 1984; Fig. 6.1). The first of these, travelling via the lateral spinothalamic tract, is principally a fast-conducting system concerned with sensory-discriminative aspects of the pain experience. In contrast, the second system, known as the multisynaptic ascending system, is more diffuse, with numerous collaterals. The latter is thought to be more important in mediating the motivational-affective components of pain through brain centres such as the brain stem and limbic system.

While this may appear to be a straightforward system in which tissue injury invariably leads to the perception of injury and pain, the lack of a simple relationship between the extent of injury and the degree of pain experienced is well recognised (Merskey 1979) and is usually explained, in theoretical terms at least, by the so-called gate control theory of

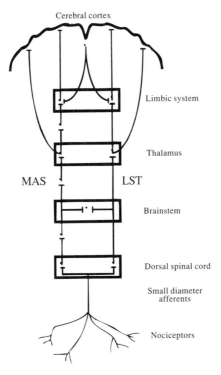

NB: MAS=Multisynaptic ascending system
LST =Lateral spinothalamic tract

Fig. 6.1 Nociceptive pathways (after Walsh 1991).

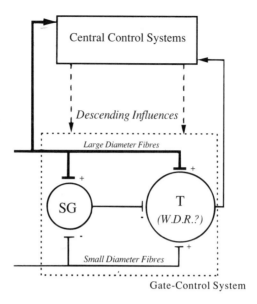

Fig. 6.2 Gate-control theory (Melzack & Wall 1989). SG = Substantia gelatinosa; T = 'T' cell; thought to be wide dynamic range (WDR) cell.

Melzack & Wall (Fig. 6.2). This proposes the existence of a neural circuit, in the substantia gelatinosa of the dorsal spinal cord, which allows modulation of afferent (incoming) activity at spinal level and before onward transmission to more rostral levels of the neuraxis. At segmental level, such modulation depends upon the total level of afferent activity (i.e. spatial and temporal summation effects), as well as the *relative* activity in large and small diameter afferents, with a net balance in favour of small diameter fibres 'opening the gate' for onward pain transmission and vice versa for large diameter afferents (Melzack & Wall 1989). Furthermore, descending influences from higher centres are proposed as being able to significantly modulate the operation of the gate and thus block (or enhance) nociceptive transmission at the level of the primary synapse.

While the theory has not been without its critics, its contribution to pain research and clinical practice has been inestimable, not least because of the incorporation of physiological and affective processes within the same theoretical framework.

In terms of pharmacology, while substance P has been recognised as an important nociceptive neurotransmitter since the 1930s, the isolation of a morphine-like peptide from pig brains by Hughes & Kosterlitz in 1975 provided the first neuropharmacological evidence of an endogenous pain *control* system (Bond 1984). Subsequent research has identified a range of such endogenous opiates, including β-endorphin and dynorphin, which are implicated in the modulation of pain at both spinal and more

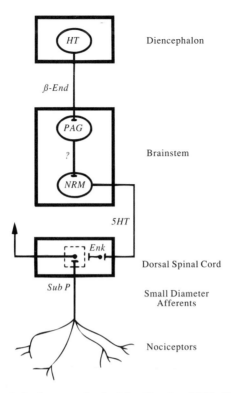

Fig. 6.3 Neurochemical substrates of pain (after Bowsher 1988). HT = Hypothalamus; PAG = Periaqueductal grey; NRM = Nucleus raphe magnus; β-End = β-endorphin; ? = Substance unknown; 5-HT = Serotonin; Enk = Enkephalin; Sub P = Substance P.

rostral centres (Baxter 1988, Bowsher 1988). Another substance which has become closely associated with pain modulation is serotonin (5-hydroxytryptamine; 5-HT) an endogenous amino acid which has also been implicated in the regulation of temperature, mood and particularly depression; increases in levels of 5-HT in the brain have been correlated with pain relief (Mannheimer & Lampe 1984). The source and site of action of these various neurochemicals are summarised in Figure 6.3.

Given their apparent importance in the perception and modulation of the pain experience, a range of clinical and laboratory studies of pain and analgesia have attempted to use some correlate of the activity, or levels, of neurochemicals such as substance P, 5-HT and the endogenous opiates to corroborate subjective or observed behavioural responses. In particular, a number of studies have examined the neuropharmacological effects of laser irradiation. These are reviewed below.

Neurological effects of laser irradiation: historical perspective

Studies of the effects of lasers upon the central nervous system began in the mid 1960s in the USA, using relatively high energy fluences ranging from 50–200 J on experimental animals (Earle et al 1965, Liss & Roppel 1966, Fox et al 1967, Hayes et al 1967). These studies superbly demonstrated the ability of high power laser to lesion selected areas of brain to such an extent that the animals used in these experiments invariably perished. The fact that military personnel were involved in a large proportion of the studies, some of which were apparently performed in defence research establishments, would suggest that military applications were the primary interest of at least some of these early investigators. Later studies, although using lower so-called 'non-lethal' power and energy levels (< 7 J), still tended to concentrate on the potentially destructive effects of laser irradiation on the nervous system (Yew & Chan 1977).

With the development of LILT applications came a renewed interest in laser–tissue interaction, including the effects of low-power (athermic) laser upon nervous tissue. In contrast to those already identified, the focus of more recent studies has generally been upon the photobiomodulatory effects of laser upon neural function, particularly in relation to laser's putative analgesic action. These studies can usefully be considered under two headings, those investigating the neuropharmacological effects of laser and those investigating the neurophysiological effects of laser.

Neuropharmacological effects of laser

There is evidence to suggest that LILT may have significant effects on the synthesis, release and metabolism of a range of neurochemicals, including serotonin and acetylcholine.

Serotonin

Walker, in her previously reported study on chronic pain patients, found an increase in urinary excretion of 5-hydroxyindoleacetic acid (5-HIAA), a metabolite of 5-HT, in those patients experiencing pain relief as a result of laser treatment (Walker 1983). Given these findings, altered serotonin metabolism would apparently represent one potential neuropharmacological substrate of laser-mediated analgesia. Despite this, while the increases in urinary 5-HIAA reported by Walker would suggest increased turnover of 5-HT, this cannot be taken as demonstrative of increased 5-HT activity in the brain: urine levels of 5-HIAA also reflect the rate of 5-HT metabolism at other sites throughout the body. However, given the corroborative findings in animals (Zarkovic et al 1989, Lombard et al 1990), the possibility that brain-specific 5-HT activity may be affected by laser irradiation cannot be ignored. Zarkovic et al (1989) reported a hyperalgesic effect accompanied by decreased potency of intraperitoneal morphine in mice as a result of laser irradiation, which would indicate a *decrease* in serotonin neurotransmission. More recently,

Professor Lombard's group in Torino has demonstrated a range of central neuropharmacological effects in albino rats as a consequence of low-energy (1.08 J per animal) He–Ne laser irradiation of the sinciput (Lombard et al 1990). These effects included significant increases in the levels of 5-HT in the striatum and hippocampus of irradiated rats, some evidence of increase in gamma-aminobutyric acid (GABA) levels, as well as parallel decreases in glutamic acid (an immediate precursor for GABA). Taken together, these studies would indicate the potential of laser to produce significant alterations in 5-HT synthesis and metabolism. However, the results of Zarkovic et al (1989) would further suggest that at specific parameters, laser irradiation may also produce significant decreases in serotonin metabolism.

The results are not exclusively positive, as several investigators have failed to find evidence of any significant laser-mediated effect upon the serotoninergic system. Hansen & Thoroe (1990), in their study on orofacial pain, failed to find any significant increase in urinary 5-HIAA in patients treated with laser. However, it should be stressed that these investigators also failed to find a significant analgesic effect, which may be the primary reason for this apparently conflicting result. Similar non-significant findings on serotoninergic metabolism have also been reported in experimental rats (Amemiya et al 1990). In this study, laser irradiation at unspecified parameters, while significantly increasing the latency to threshold in tail flick tests, failed to produce any significant effects upon levels of 5-HT or 5-HIAA in the hypothalamus, midbrain or medulla of irradiated animals (Amemiya et al 1990). Unfortunately, the lack of detail in this abstract, particularly concerning irradiation parameters, does not permit conjecture as to the possible reasons for this apparently non-significant finding.

Despite these negative reports, the findings of Walker (1983), Zarkovic et al (1989) and Lombard's group (1990) would suggest that laser has the potential, at least under some circumstances, to significantly alter serotonin metabolism.

Acetylcholine

Acetylcholine (ACh) is widely distributed throughout the central and particularly the peripheral nervous system, notably at neuromuscular junctions and the terminals of the parasympathetic autonomic nervous system (Iversen & Iversen 1981). ACh has been recognised as a potent algesic agent in experimental studies since the late 1940s (Brown & Gray 1948, Keele & Armstrong, 1964); however its role in pathogenic pain is less clear. A number of animal studies have shown significant effects on the cholinergic system after low-power laser irradiation. In one of the earliest of these, Vizi and colleagues found that laser irradiation using a ruby source enhanced release of ACh in isolated Auerbach's plexus preparation (Vizi et al 1977). Even though a ruby laser was used in this study, the observed effect was not accompanied by any discernible increase in temperature, nor indeed can such an effect be mediated by temperature elevation.

Subsequent work has largely been completed using He–Ne systems. A sizable proportion of this has been published in eastern Europe, particularly the former USSR, with equally interesting results. In a study on rats using laser acupuncture, Lupyr & Sergienko (1986) found increased acetylcholinesterase activity in the spinal cord, duodenum and liver after irradiation with a He–Ne system. Interestingly, direct irradiation of the organs involved produced no such change in metabolism, neither were these seen in blood erythrocytes during the laser acupuncture treatments. This provides evidence of the capacity of laser acupuncture to produce significant neurochemical effects at sites distant to the point of irradiation. Zynanova and co-workers (1987) found similar increases in acetylcholinesterase activity after He–Ne laser irradiation of rat brain, and that such irradiation also altered the noradrenaline/adrenaline balance. However, in this case the observed neurochemical effects were as a result of the direct irradiation of brain tissue. This would suggest that under appropriate circumstances similar net results in the central nervous system, at least in terms of altered neurochemistry, may be achieved with quite disparate irradiation regimes. However, more studies would appear to be warranted to identify the precise effects of low-power laser irradiation on cholinergic systems and the relevance (if any) of these to laser-mediated analgesia.

Other neuropharmacological effects at central levels

Apart from the putative effects on the serotoninergic and cholinergic systems outlined above, several studies have investigated alternative neuropharmacological effects of laser in the central nervous system. In the previously reported study by Choi and colleagues (Choi et al 1986), laser acupuncture was seen to induce similar increases in urinary glucocorticoid levels to that produced by transcutaneous electrical nerve stimulation and electroacupuncture. Furthermore, the lower of the two laser pulsing frequencies used by this group (2 Hz) was found to produce higher levels of urinary glucocorticoids than the higher (64 Hz) frequency. Unfortunately the rather rudimentary algesimetric techniques used by this group did not allow the possible correlation between level of pain relief and glucocorticoid excretion to be assessed (Choi et al 1986). These authors suggested endogenous opiate release as a probable mechanism of laser-mediated analgesia, possibly as glucocorticoids can inhibit the synthesis of β-endorphin, one of the better characterised endogenous opiates (see Mannheimer & Lampe 1984). However, Ponnudurai's group found that the hypoalgesia produced by low-power laser irradiation of experimental rats was not naloxone reversible and therefore that such hypoalgesia was apparently not opiate-mediated (Ponnudurai et al 1988). The evidence for an endogenous opiate substrate of laser-mediated analgesia is therefore equivocal.

Several reports suggest a broad spectrum of central neuropharmacological effects of laser irradiation under certain circumstances. In addition to laser-mediated increases in 5-HT levels in irradiated rats, Lombard et al (1990) also found parallel increases in levels of the central inhibitory neurotransmitter gamma-aminobutyric acid (GABA) coupled with decreased levels of its immediate precursor glutamic acid, which is additionally recognised as an important excitatory neurotransmitter in its own right (Iversen & Iversen 1981). Interestingly, this group also noted a significant decrease in levels of glycine, which like GABA is an inhibitory central neurotransmitter, in parallel with the other reported neuropharmacological effects. In the study by Amemiya et al (1990) already outlined above, levels of the catecholamine neurotransmitter dopamine (DA) in the midbrain and medulla (but *not* the hypothalamus) were found to be significantly reduced by laser irradiation. The direct relevance of these findings to the putative analgesic effects of laser is unclear.

Taken together, these findings from human and animal studies provide evidence of the potential of low-power laser irradiation to produce significant alterations in CNS neurochemistry. This is an interesting consideration, as evidence suggests that alterations in the levels of CNS transmitters such as 5-HT may have profound behavioural effects.

Peripheral pharmacological effects and nociception

In addition to these findings, predominantly at central levels, several studies have investigated the effects of laser irradiation upon the pharmacology of nociceptive processes at the level of the primary receptor. Maeda & Ohshiro (1990) found in Wistar rats that laser irradiation using unspecified parameters produced significant reduction of mitochondrial density in axons of the trigeminal nerve injected with bradykinin, a potent algesic agent (Keele & Armstrong 1964). The density of mitochondria in the laser irradiated group was further found to be not significantly different from saline injected controls (Maeda & Ohshiro 1990). In these circumstances, any increase in mitochondrial density in injected nerves is thought to reflect the level of ectopic signals generated by the afferent; thus the authors proposed that their findings indicated another possible mechanism of LILT-mediated analgesia in vivo.

In investigations on mouse tongues, Trelles and colleagues found significant decreases in histamine levels and mast cell numbers after a course of irradiation (2.4 J/cm^2) with a He–Ne unit (Trelles et al 1989). As mast cells are rich in histamine, a well characterised, powerful inflammatory and algesic agent, their apparent destruction/degranulation as a result of laser irradiation in this study could also suggest a net hyperalgesic effect. In spite of these rather ambiguous findings, these investigators insist that such degranulation of mast cells as a result of laser irradiation represents a possible mechanism of laser-mediated pain relief. However, such a conclusion would apparently not be warranted on the basis of their results; rather, additional work would appear to be indicated to further investigate the effect of laser radiation upon histamine and (ideally) prostaglandin release.

Neurophysiological effects of laser

The use of neurophysiological recording techniques enables accurate measurements of amplitudes and conduction latencies to be made and thus can allow objective assessment of the neurophysiological effects of laser (Basford 1989). There are essentially two types of such study: those in which spontaneous electrical activity is monitored (e.g. electroencephalography), or studies in which electrical stimuli applied to a nerve are used to elicit a series of (synchronised) compound action potentials which are recorded at some other site in the neuraxis (e.g. nerve conduction studies). A range of electrophysiological studies have been completed to date in animals and humans to investigate the neurophysiological effects of laser, with some interesting if contradictory findings.

Animal investigations

A range of basic in vitro research has investigated the potential neurophysiological effects of low-intensity laser. In one of the earliest studies of its kind, irradiation with low-power argon laser was found to alter firing patterns in isolated abdominal ganglion cells from *Aplysia* in response to stimulation (Fork 1971). Interestingly, these alterations were found not to be due to a photothermal effect, as they occurred before any measurable temperature elevation was possible in the in vitro preparation. Furthermore, heating the preparation apparently failed to produce similar effects.

Olson and colleagues used cell monolayers derived from neonatal rat cerebella to investigate the effects of a tunable dye laser at a range of wavelengths (490–684 nm) and energy densities (0–100 J/m^2) upon excitability to extracellular electrical stimulation (Olson et al 1981). They found that all laser pulses, above a certain (wavelength specific) energy threshold, reduced the excitability of the nerve cells to electrical stimulation.

More recently, Mezawa and colleagues (1988) reported that in 11 nociceptors which they identified on the tongues of anaesthetised cats, 904 nm laser irradiation dramatically reduced the firing patterns in response to noxious thermal stimulation. This reduction in firing pattern was found to be dosage-dependant, with a plateau in effect after 10 min (equivalent to 0.73 J, 3040 Hz) of irradiation. At the lowest energy used by this group (0.073 J, 3040 Hz), only 60% of the nociceptors investigated displayed any such reduction in elicited activity (Mezawa et al 1988).

Despite the above, findings from several recent studies would suggest that the evidence is far from unequivocal (Lundeberg et al 1988, Lundeberg & Zhou 1988, Jarvis et al 1990). Using nociceptors isolated from the medical leech (*Hirudo medicinalis*) Lundeberg et al (1988) studied the neurophysiological effects of low-power He–Ne and GaAs (904 nm) lasers at incident energies ranging from 0.0042–0.936 J. With the irradiation parameters stated, these investigators failed to find any apparent changes upon a range of electrophysiological measures including resting membrane potential, mechanical stimulation threshold and evoked response.

One possible reason for the negative findings reported by Lundeberg et al might be the use of a 73 Hz pulsing frequency with the diode laser employed in this study. Lundeberg and colleagues completed neurophysiological testing 10 min immediately after laser irradiation which, from the results of the laboratory pain studies of Ponnudurai's group (Ponnudurai et al 1987, 1988), may be too early to assess the effects of laser radiation at this pulsing frequency. However, even if this were so, this could not explain the findings for the CW He–Ne system also used in this study. What is not entirely clear from the authors' rather ambiguous report is how they irradiated four nociceptors using six different irradiation regimes and what statistical tests (if any) they used to analyse their experimental data (Lundeberg et al 1988). The absence of such information casts some doubt over the significance and validity of the published findings.

Similar criticisms can be levelled at this group's complementary study on a single isolated stretch receptor and associated sensory neuron from *Astacus fluviatilis* (Lundeberg & Zhou 1988). In this study, the authors employed eight separate irradiation regimes using either He–Ne or GaAs laser and energy levels of up to 1.87 J. No detectable changes in the resting membrane potential of the sensory neuron, or in the receptor potential generated in response to stretch stimulation, were found as a result of laser irradiation.

In contrast to these studies in invertebrates, Jarvis and colleagues used samples from rabbit cornea to investigate the effects of He–Ne laser upon Aδ and C fibres in vitro (Jarvis et al 1990). In this study, prolonged electrophysiological recording (120 min) of Aδ and C fibre activity after irradiation (1 mW, 0.3 J) showed no significant differences between laser and control data for spike amplitude, discharge frequency, instantaneous discharge frequency or interspike intervals. In addition to these neurophysiological recordings, these investigators also used mathematical modelling to assess if low-power He–Ne laser irradiation (1 mW, 0.004 J) could stimulate human thermoreceptors in vivo (Jarvis et al 1990). Such stimulation (i.e. depolarisation) was found to be impossible at these irradiation parameters using their modelling technique, which is hardly surprising given that therapeutic laser is athermic by definition and, with very few exceptions, produces no subjective sensation on the part of patients even at dosages tens of thousands of times higher than the one used by these investigators.

At more central levels, the effect of laser irradiation upon electrically evoked potentials recorded from the dorsal spinal cord has been investigated in experimental cats by Rusakov (1987). Irradiation at unspecified parameters was found to maintain the amplitude of the repetitively evoked potential over time, leading the author to suggest that irradiation somehow stimulated the replenishment of neurotransmitter at synaptic level and thus mitigated the fatigue effects commonly observed in (non-irradiated) controls (Rusakov 1987). Further studies by Rusakov & Klering have apparently found structural alterations and enhanced subcellular function in spinal cord neurons irradiated with low intensity He–Ne laser (Rusakov & Klering 1986, Rusakov et al 1987).

More recent work by Wesselmann's group (1990) on cats and rats investigated the effect of Q-switched (pulsed) Nd:YAG laser (1064 nm, 10 Hz pulsing frequency) irradiation upon nerve conduction and evoked potentials recorded from the dorsal roots and dorsal spinal cord. In studying the effect of laser upon the electrically evoked potential recorded from the dorsal spinal cord of rats, Wesselmann et al applied laser for 5 min directly to the dorsal column white matter at progressively increasing power and energy levels, starting with 10 mJ pulses and increasing up to 100 mJ pulses within a 5 min period of irradiation (Wesselmann et al 1990). The average energies delivered during these experiments were therefore in the region of 30–300 J, which is somewhat higher than in the majority of other studies completed in this area.

Using this regimen, these investigators found that the negative components of the evoked potential (N_1 and N_2) were selectively reduced in amplitude by laser irradiation: the larger positive component of the potential (P_1) being unaffected. Furthermore, the reduction in amplitude observed in the negative components of the evoked potential was found to occur in a progressive but non-uniform fashion depending upon dose (Wesselmann et al 1990). This implicated selective blocking of small diameter fibres as the reason for the observed reductions in amplitude, which the authors subsequently investigated by means of evoked potential recordings at the dorsal root of cats and nerve conduction studies in the sciatic nerve of rats. The irradiation regimen used in these studies was identical to that used in the investigation on spinal cord evoked potentials. The results of these studies confirmed the hypothesis of selective blocking of small diameter fibre activity, with slower conducting fibres being found to be most affected by such laser irradiation. These investigators also found some evidence of laser-mediated inhibition of large diameter fibres coupled with increased conduction latencies, but only at the higher dosages used (~300 J; Wesselmann et al 1990).

While interesting, the direct relevance of these results to LILT applications is limited, as the possibility of a photothermal mechanism underlying the observed effect cannot be discounted. Indeed, the authors themselves consider this the most likely explanation for their findings, given the 'substantial' temperature increases which they measured during laser irradiation. Despite this, the fact that *increased* conduction latencies were found at higher energy densities would tend to discount photothermal effects as an underlying mechanism of action, as increased latencies are associated with *decreases* in temperature (Ma & Liveson 1983).

Nonetheless, this group has further examined the laser-mediated effects upon nerve conduction in the rat sciatic nerve by analysis of the distribution of nerve conduction velocities (Lin et al 1990). Once again, the pattern of selective laser-mediated effects upon the slower-conducting fibres at low energies was found, together with suppression of faster-conducting fibres at the highest energy densities. In this report, the authors specify the temperature elevation measured close to the site of irradiation as being between 5°C and 22°C, equivalent to temperatures of 41–56°C. This would certainly imply that the observed effects were photothermal in origin, especially as heat block in mammalian myelinated nerves has been reported at temperatures of between 41°C and 51°C (Klumpp & Zimmerman 1980); however the possibility that photochemical mechanisms also played a part in the observed effects cannot be discounted (Lin et al 1990).

In addition to these studies on various aspects of neural function, the potential of laser acupuncture to produce alterations in the electrocardiogram has also been investigated. Using the *neiguan* point in cats (situated on the volar surface of the forelimb), bilateral He–Ne laser acupuncture (3 mW, 2.7 J/point) was found to produce decreases in heart rate and in the shape of the recorded ECG. The reason for referring to this report here is that neural substrates were found to be implicated in the effects demonstrated in this study, which disappeared after bilateral transection of the animals' median nerves and resumed when the proximal end of the transected nerves was irradiated (Zhang et al 1986).

The work of Rochkind's group in Israel on laser-mediated stimulation of experimental nerve injury is referred to in Chapters 5 and 8. The results are also worthy of mention here because of the findings of increased amplitude of recorded compound action potential (CAP) in *non-injured* rat sciatic nerves after He–Ne laser irradiation delivered either transcutaneously (Rochkind et al 1987) or directly (Rochkind et al 1988) to the nerve. The laser used in the former study was a 16 mW CW unit, delivering an energy density of 10 J/cm² to the shaven skin of experimental rats. In the second study, the increase in CAP amplitude was seen as a result of direct irradiation with a 0.3 mW CW unit, delivering approximately 0.2 J/cm² of incident energy to the intact but dissected nerves (Rochkind et al 1988). While these power and energy densities are significantly different, these investigators consider that attenuation due to overlying tissues where transcutaneous irradiation is applied results in similar net energy densities being delivered to the nerve in each case (Rochkind et al 1988). While no data or results for latencies is presented by these investigators, the findings of increased CAP amplitude provides further evidence of the potential of low-power laser to significantly alter the neurophysiology of irradiated neural tissue.

Human studies

A number of human studies have been completed in this area, findings from which are contradictory and provide no clear, coherent picture of laser's putative neurophysiological effects in vivo.

Judith Walker in Los Angeles has reported the potential of He–Ne laser (1 mW, 20 Hz) to completely suppress ankle clonus in paraplegic patients after only 40 s bilateral irradiation of the radial, median and saphenous nerves (Walker 1985). No such suppression was observed in sham irradiated controls nor in controls who received irradiation at alternative (non-neural) sites. This effect was further found to be dose-dependent and, at 40 s of irradiation, equivalent to 1 h of electrical stimulation (Walker 1985, Walker & Katz 1979). Walker subsequently took out a US patent on the associated laser treatment (Walker 1987). The observed laser-mediated suppression was suggested by Walker to be due to some direct effect upon the irradiated nerves which she proposed were 'photosensitive' and thus capable of generating action potentials in response to laser irradiation at appropriate parameters (Walker 1985).

Walker's group subsequently assessed this hypothesis by means of evoked potential (EP) techniques (Walker & Akhanjee 1985). These studies showed a small but reproducible potential at Erb's point in response to short bursts of laser from a 1 mW He–Ne unit pulsed at 3.1 Hz, suggesting that irradiation at these parameters may have a *direct* stimulatory effect on peripheral nerves, as the latencies quoted by Walker & Akhanjee (mean 9.659 ms) effectively preclude anything other than a direct effect upon nerve endings or axons. These results further implicate large-diameter myelinated afferents as being photosensitive, as the conduction velocities quoted by Walker & Akhanjee (70–80/ms) are within the upper range of these fibres (Williams et al 1989).

This would suggest, in view of the types of cutaneous receptor subserved by such large-diameter afferents (i.e. mechanoreceptors), that laser irradiation should produce some discernible sensation on the part of the subject. Walker & Akhanjee reported that subjects in their investigation experienced no laser-mediated sensation(s). This is in common with the experiences of clinicians and of researchers and authors who do not report concomitant sensations in irradiated patients, notable exceptions being Woolley-Hart (1986) and Zarkovic et al (1989), and these (perhaps significantly) used infra-red units. This evoked potential in the absence of any associated sensation is a novel finding, especially as intraneural microstimulation of even single large-diameter afferents is sufficient to produce a distinct, specific sensation in subjects (Torebjork et al 1987).

In addition to this apparent photosensitivity of peripheral nerves, Walker & Akhanjee also noted a gradual decrease in the amplitude of the laser-evoked response over time, in contrast to electrically evoked potentials which were invariably stable (Walker 1988). This decrement would suggest that low-power laser also has the potential to produce fatigue or habituation effects even at relatively low dosage levels. While similar findings, both in terms of laser-evoked potentials and decrement in amplitude over time, have subsequently been reported after irradiation with a nitrogen laser operating at 337.1 nm, (Czopf et al 1987), the irradiation parameters used cannot exclude the possibility of photothermal effects giving rise to the EPs observed in this latter study.

Given the remarkable findings detailed above, the protocol used by Walker & Akhanjee was replicated by Wu and colleagues at three different centres in the USA. These investigators found no evidence of the photosensitivity described by Walker's group (Wu et al 1987). Interestingly, and in contrast to the earlier study, Wu et al specify that a range of laser pulse lengths were used (50–150 ms). This is certainly comparable with commercially available units but, as Walker & Akhanjee do not specify these parameters in their report, direct comparison is somewhat limited. With constant pulse repetition rates (3.1 Hz in this case) varying pulse width can produce wide variations in dosage. This may represent one possible explanation of the inability of Wu et al to replicate the earlier study, as it may be possible that the dosages used in the Walker & Akhanjee study were many times greater.

It is also possible that some form of electrical artifact was responsible for the findings reported by Walker & Akhanjee, due either to the signal used by Walker's group to trigger the recording apparatus, or perhaps the 'shutter' on the laser. It is worthy of note that Wu et al used a variety of different methods to trigger the recorder, and indeed to 'chop' the laser. It is conceivable that these variations in experimental procedure could have been responsible for the exclusions of artifact(s) which were unwittingly present in the Walker & Akhanjee study. However the elaborate measures taken by Walker & Akhanjee to exclude such artifacts would suggest another possible explanation for the discrepancy in findings: that the trigger and shutter artifacts in the later study served to drown the (small) laser-evoked potential with electrical noise. The importance and implications of a possible photosensitivity of peripheral nerves mean that further investigation of this phenomenon is warranted.

In contrast to these investigations of putative photosensitivity in peripheral nerves, Andreeva & Minenkova (1981) have reported the possibility of laser-mediated alterations in electroencephalograms recorded from patients treated with He–Ne laser. Paucity of detail in this abstract unfortunately precludes further comment or consideration of these apparently interesting findings.

Wu (1983) has subsequently used somatosensory evoked potential (SEP) techniques to investigate the potential neurophysiological effects of laser acupuncture in two separate experiments. For these, a He–Ne unit (0.7 mW, CW) was used to deliver 30 min of irradiation (i.e. 1.26 J) to the *ho-ku* and *neikwan* points unilaterally and median nerve stimulation to generate an SEP recorded from the scalp at four points (C_3, C_4, P_3 and P_4). In the first study ($n = 6$), 50% of the experimental subjects showed a decreased amplitude in the late positive components of recorded SEPs. This was found to be associated with a generalised change in the shape of the SEP. Furthermore, this effect was ipsilateral to the site of irradiation, and was found to fade after 60 min.

Because of the involvement of late components and the fact that only 50% demonstrated such (apparently) laser-mediated effects, Wu performed a second experiment based upon a 19-site recording technique and an enhanced blinding procedure (Wu 1983). Based upon the results of this second experiment, Wu claims (but does not adequately prove) that the changes observed in SEPs can be completely accounted for by psychological events such as anticipation and habituation. Despite the negative comments of Wu, the findings of this rather ambiguous report would suggest that additional studies are required before the possibility of laser-mediated effects at central levels can be discounted.

More peripherally, the neurophysiological effects of laser have been investigated using conduction studies with contradictory findings (Greathouse et al 1985, Bieglio & Bisschop 1988, Snyder-Mackler & Bork 1988, Basford et al 1990). Greathouse and colleagues completed their study on the radial nerve of 20 subjects and apparently failed to show any significant effect of GaAs (904 nm) irradiation at two different dosage levels: 20 s and 120 s to each of five centimetre squares marked over the course of the nerve. Unfortunately these authors do not specify the power output of the laser used, nor do they give any estimate of the energy delivered during their irradiation procedure. Interestingly, the results of this group showed a significant increase in latency of about 0.2 ms in the group receiving the higher level of irradiation (120 s). However, the authors argued that this was as a result of the significant temperature decrease also observed in this experimental group, rather than any possible neurophysiological effects of irradiation (Greathouse et al 1985). While this contention is certainly feasible, given the sensitivity of nerve conduction velocity to temperature change (Bolton et al 1981), the fact that no such temperature decrease was seen in the other two groups used in this study is puzzling.

In contrast, Snyder-Mackler & Bork (1988) found a significant increase in radial nerve conduction latency (mean = 0.37 ms) in 24 subjects irradiated for 20 s with a continuous wave 1 mW He–Ne laser at six points along the course of the nerve. No such increase was seen in sham irradiated controls ($n = 16$). The energy delivered at each point was 0.02 J which, assuming an irradiated area of 0.1 cm^2, would be equivalent to an energy density of approximately 0.2 J/cm^2 immediately under the treatment probe used in this study (Snyder-Mackler 1990). Given the importance of these findings, Basford et al (1990) have subsequently attempted to replicate this study and establish the duration of the observed latency shift. In contrast, this group found no significant increases in conduction latencies as a result of irradiation performed identically to that described for the Snyder-Mackler & Bork study. The evidence from conduction studies in the human radial nerve is thus contradictory and on balance would suggest that laser at the energy densities specified has no significant effect upon conduction latency.

This is in broad agreement with the findings of Bieglio & Bisschop (1988), who used H- and T-reflex studies in the posterior tibial nerve and soleus muscle to assess the neurophysiological effects of laser irradiation. These reflexes are so-called late responses, essentially due to segmental reflexes; the H-reflex in particular is thought, at least in diagnostic terms, to reflect the state of the S$_1$ nerve root (Ma & Liveson 1983). Using both He–Ne and infra-red units to deliver 10 min of irradiation at unspecified power and energy densities, Bieglio & Bisschop reported no significant alterations in nerve conduction velocity. In contrast, these investigators did find an increase in the amplitude of the so-called M response (resulting from the direct orthodromic stimulation of the motor nerve), coupled with significant *decreases* in the amplitude of both the H- and T- reflexes (Bieglio & Bisschop 1988). This is particularly interesting, as it would suggest that effects of low-power laser at spinal level may be very different to the direct effects of such irradiation.

In summary, it can be seen that findings of the neurophysiological studies completed to date in humans are contradictory. Thus, while a range of studies at both peripheral and central levels have been completed, further work is indicated to establish definitively the neurophysiological effects of low-level laser irradiation in vivo.

SUMMARY OF KEY POINTS

1. The use of lasers in clinical practice for the relief of pain of various aetiologies is based upon an extensive published database. However, in common with other areas of LILT application, the quality of these publications is highly variable, with few properly controlled clinical trials of laser being reported, leading to a certain amount of criticism from some quarters.

2. The efficacy of laser for the relief of pain has been investigated in a range of conditions, principally rheumatoid, osteo- and poly-

arthroses, musculoskeletal and sports injuries as well as a number of neurogenic/neuropathic pain syndromes including postherpetic neuralgia and radicular pain.

3. A bewildering range of permutations of wavelength, power and energy density, pulse repetition rate, frequency and duration of treatment have been employed in the trials reviewed. Without the benefit of results from a series of trials in which the treatment parameters employed are systematically varied and investigated, it is almost impossible to make any definitive statements regarding optimum parameters for treatment in a given condition.

4. A number of publications have reported non-significant findings with laser. Of these, the majority were completed using He-Ne sources, possessing the least penetration of any therapeutic laser source. Power outputs and energy dosage in these studies also tended to be low in comparison to the other studies reviewed. The implication is that, in some circumstances at least, a combination of shorter wavelengths and lower power (and energy) densities may compromise the analgesic potential of laser treatment. Furthermore, the appropriateness of research designs used in some of these studies is open to question.

5. The lack of an obvious modus operandi of laser-mediated analgesia is a contributory factor to the confusion over the relevance of irradiation parameters as well as the scepticism surrounding the area. Although such knowledge is not essential to the routine clinical use of analgesic laser in physiotherapy, it would help in the determination of optimal parameters and methods for analgesic laser treatment. Furthermore, an understanding of the mechanisms of action may indicate additional potential applications.

6. While the findings from those laboratory investigations of laser-mediated analgesia completed to date are contradictory, the positive results seen in such studies would suggest that, under certain circumstances, laser irradiation at appropriate energy densities and treatment parameters has the potential to significantly alter pain threshold. It would further appear from those animal studies completed to date that pulse repetition rate has a profound influence on the latency to onset of the observed hypoalgesic effects, with relatively low frequencies mediating an immediate but short-term analgesia. This finding in particular has potentially important implications for clinical practice.

7. Problems and limitations arise in attempting to extrapolate findings in animals directly to humans. However, the extension of laboratory-based work on laser-mediated analgesia to humans has to date only been attempted by a few groups, most using He–Ne systems at relatively low power and energy densities and with contradictory results.

8. A range of studies have indicated the apparent potential of low intensity laser radiation to significantly alter the neurochemistry of the central and peripheral nervous system, sometimes at centres quite remote from the site of irradiation. These findings further suggest the possibility of a neuropharmacological substrate of laser-mediated analgesia.

9. Neurophysiologically, while some studies have suggested that laser irradiation may alter endogenous electrophysiology, others have demonstrated the ability of such irradiation to significantly affect electrically evoked potentials, in terms of both latency (or velocity) and amplitude. However, these studies are conflicting and frequently contradictory in nature: in the superficial radial nerve, reports of laser-mediated latency shifts are counterbalanced by reports of non-significant findings using similar protocols.

REFERENCES

Abe T 1990 Orthopaedic surgical aspects of low reactive level laser therapy (LLLT). Laser Therapy 2: 15

Amemiya R, Hasegawa H, Takeda H et al 1990 Effects of low level laser irradiation on thermal nociception-induced amine dynamics changes in rat brain regions. Laser Therapy 2: 45

Andreeva V M, Minenkova A A 1981 Effect of low-intensity laser radiation on the functional state of the central nervous system and cerebral circulation in patients with hypertensive disease. Voprosy Kurortologii Fizioterapii Lechebnoi Fizioheskoi Kultury 6: 12–16

Asada K, Yutani Y, Shimazu A 1989 Diode laser therapy for rheumatoid arthritis: a clinical evaluation of 102 joints treated with low reactive laser therapy (LLLT). Laser Therapy 1: 147–151

Ashton H, Ebenezer I, Golding J F et al 1984 Effects of acupuncture and transcutaneous electrical nerve stimulation on cold induced pain in normal subjects. Journal of Psychosomatic Research 28: 301–308

Atsumi K, Fujimasa I, Abe Y et al 1987. Biostimulation effect of low-power energy of diode laser for pain relief. Lasers in Surgery and Medicine 7: 77

Baldry P E 1989 Acupuncture, trigger points and musculoskeletal pain. Churchill Livingstone, Edinburgh

Basford J R 1986 Low energy laser treatment of pain and wounds: hype, hope or hokum? Mayo Clinic Proceedings 61: 671–675

Basford J R 1989 Low energy laser therapy: controversies and new research findings. Lasers in Surgery and Medicine 9: 1–5

Basford J R, Sheffield C G, Mair S D et al 1987 Low energy helium–neon laser treatment of thumb osteoarthritis. Archives of Physical Medicine and Rehabilitation 68: 794–797

Basford J R, Daude J R, Hallman H O et al 1990 Does low-intensity Helium–Neon laser irradiation alter sensory nerve action potentials or distal latencies? Lasers in Surgery and Medicine 10: 35–39

Baxter G D, Bell A J, Allen J M et al 1991 Low level laser therapy. Current clinical practice in Northern Ireland. Physiotherapy 77: 171–178

Baxter R 1988 Neuropharmacology of the pain pathway. In: Wells P E, Frampton V, Bowsher D (ed) Pain: management and control in physiotherapy. Heinemann Physiotherapy, London

Bieglio C, Bisschop G de 1986 Physical treatment for radicular pain with low-power laser stimulation. Lasers in Surgery and Medicine 6: 173

Bieglio C, Bisschop G de 1988 Low-power laser action in humans on nerve fibres and monosynaptic reflex arc. Lasers in Medical Science, Abstracts Issue, July 1988: 283

Bliddal H, Hellesen C, Ditlevsen P et al 1987 Soft laser therapy of rheumatoid arthritis. Scandinavian Journal of Rheumatology 16: 225–228

Bolton C F, Sawa G M, Carter K 1981 The effects of temperature on human compound action potentials. Journal of Neurology Neurosurgery and Psychiatry 44: 407–412

Bond M R 1984 Pain: its nature, analysis and treatment. Churchill Livingstone, Edinburgh

Bonnett K A, Peterson K E 1975 A modification of the jump-flinch technique for measuring pain sensitivity in rats. Pharmacology Biochemistry and Behaviour 3: 1–47

Bowsher D 1988 Central pain mechanisms. In: Wells P E, Frampton V, Bowsher D (ed) Pain: management and control in physiotherapy. Heinemann Physiotherapy, London

Brockhaus A, Elger C E 1990 Hypoalgesic efficacy of acupuncture on experimental pain in man. Comparison of laser acupuncture and needle acupuncture. Pain 43: 181–186

Brown G L, Gray J A B 1948 Some effects of nicotine-like substances and their relation to sensory nerve endings. Journal of Physiology 107: 306–317

Bulakh A D, Derzhavin A E, Korolik I M et al 1983 Laser therapy of the lumbar pain syndrome in patients with rheumatoid arthritis. Abstracts, 10th European Congress of Rheumatology, Moscow 704: 211

Burgudjieva T, Katranushkova N, Blazeva P 1985 Laser therapy of complicated wounds after obstetric and gynaecologic operations. Akusherstvo I Ginekologiia 6: 60–69

Calderhead R G 1990 On the importance of the correct reporting of parameters and the adoption of a standard terminology in clinical papers on Low reactive Level Laser Therapy (LLLT). Abstracts, 'Laser 90' Manchester, UK

Carruth J A S, McKenzie A L 1986 Medical lasers: science and clinical practice. Adam Hilger, Bristol

Chaitow L 1983 The acupuncture treatment of pain: safe and effective methods for using acupuncture in pain relief, 2nd edn. Thorsons, Wellingborough

Chapman C R, Loeser J D 1989 Issues in pain measurement. Raven Press, New York

Chapman C R, Casey K L, Dubner R et al 1985 Pain measurement: an overview. Pain 22: 1–31

Choi J J, Srikantha K, Wu W-H 1986 A comparison of electroacupuncture, transcutaneous electrical nerve stimulation and laser photobiostimulation on pain relief and glucocorticoid excretion. International Journal of Acupuncture and Electrotherapeutics Research 11: 45–51

Christensen P 1989 Clinical laser treatment of odontological conditions. In: Kert J, Rose L (eds) Clinical laser therapy: low level laser therapy. Scandinavian Medical Laser Technology, Copenhagen

Cicero T J 1974 The effects of alpha-adrenergic blocking agents on narcotic-induced analgesia. Archives of International Pharmacodynamics 208: 5–13

Corti L, Sorce P, Pignataro M et al 1988 Low-power laser in antalgic therapy: clinical experiences. Lasers in Medical Science, Abstracts Issue, July 1988: 297

Czopf J, Czeh I, Santa P et al 1987 Laser evoked neurogram. Neuroscience Suppl 22: S547

D'Armour F E, Smith D 1941 A method for determining loss of pain sensation. Journal of Pharmacology and Experimental Therapeutics 72: 74–79

Devor M 1990 What's in a beam for pain therapy? Pain 43: 139

Dubenko E G, Zhuk A A, Safronov B G et al 1976 Experience with lasers of low intensity radiation in the clinic of nervous diseases. Vrachebnoe Delo 114–119

Earle K M, Carpenter S, Roessmann U et al 1965 Central nervous system effects of laser radiation. Federation Proceedings of the American Society for Experimental Biology, Suppl. 14: S129–S139

England S, Farrell A J, Coppock J S et al 1989 Low-power laser therapy of shoulder tendonitis. Scandinavian Journal of Rheumatology 18: 427–431

Emmanoulidis O, Diamantopoulos C 1986 CW IR low-power laser application significantly accelerates chronic pain relief rehabilitation of professional athletes. A double blind study. Lasers in Surgery and Medicine 6: 173

Evans F J 1974 The placebo response in pain reduction. In: Bonica J J (ed) Advances in neurology: International symposium on pain. Raven Press, New York

Fork R L 1971 Laser stimulation of nerve cells in Aplysia. Science 171: 907–908

Fox J L, Hayes J R, Stein M N et al 1967 Experimental cranial and vascular studies of the effects of pulsed and continuous wave laser radiation. Journal of Neurosurgery 27: 126–137

Friedman L M, Furberg C D, DeMets D L 1983 Fundamentals of clinical trials. John Wright, Boston

Galperti G, Fava G, Martino G et al 1987 He–Ne laser. Breast cancer: pain therapy in post surgery. Lasers in Surgery and Medicine 7: 79

Gartner C H, Becker M, Dusoir T 1987 Pain control in spondylarthritis with infrared laser. Lasers in Surgery and Medicine 7: 79

Glykofridis S, Diamantopoulos C 1987 Comparison between laser acupuncture and physiotherapy. Acupuncture in Medicine 4: 6–9

Goldman J A, Chiapella J, Casey H et al 1980 Laser therapy of rheumatoid arthritis. Lasers in Surgery and Medicine 1: 93–101

Greathouse D G, Currier D P, Gilmore R L 1985 Effects of clinical infra-red laser on superficial radial nerve conduction. Physical Therapy 65: 1184–1187

Gussetti P, Moroso P, Palazzo C et al 1986 Calcific shoulder joint periarthritis. Disappearance of calcifications after laser therapy. Radiologia Medica 72: 934–936

Haker E 1991 Lateral epicondylalgia (tennis elbow): a diagnostic and therapeutic challenge. PhD thesis, Karolinska Institute, Stockholm

Haker E, Lundeberg T 1990 Laser treatment applied to acupuncture points in lateral humeral epicondylalgia. A double blind study. Pain 43: 243–248

Hansen H J, Thoroe U 1990 Low-power laser biostimulation of chronic oro-facial pain. A double-blind placebo controlled cross-over study in 40 patients. Pain 43: 169–180

Harazaki M, Isshikii Y, Nojima K et al 1990 A survey on the pain relief effect following the application of soft laser in orthodontic surgical patients. Laser Therapy 2: 45

Hayes J R, Fox J L, Stein M N 1967 The effects of laser irradiation on brain tissue. I. Preliminary studies. Journal of Neuropathy and Experimental Neurology 26: 250–258

Hong J N, Kim T H, Lim S D 1990 Clinical trial of low reactive level laser therapy in 20 patients with post herpetic neuralgia. Laser Therapy 2: 167–170

Huskisson E C 1983 Visual analogue scales. In: Melzack R (ed) Pain measurement and assessment. Raven Press, New York

Iversen S D, Ivsersen L L 1981 Behavioral pharmacology, 2nd edn. Oxford University Press, New York

Jacob J J C, Ramabadran K 1978 Enhancement of a nociceptive reaction by opioid antagonists in mice. British Journal of Pharmacology 64: 91–98

Jarvis D, Maciver M B, Tanelian D L 1990 Electrophysiologic recording and thermodynamic modeling demonstrate that Helium–Neon laser irradiation does not affect peripheral Aδ- or C-fiber nociceptors. Pain 43: 235–242

Jensen H, Harreby M, Kjer J 1987 Is infra-red laser effective in painful arthrosis of the knee? Ugeskr Laeger 149: 3104–3106

Johnston M I, Ashton C H, Bousfield D R et al 1989 Analgesic effects of different frequencies of transcutaneous electrical nerve stimulation on cold-induced pain in normal subjects. Pain 39: 231–236

Kamikawa K, Kyoto J 1985 Double blind experiences with mid-lasers in Japan. International Congress Laser Medicine Surgery. Monduzzi Editore, Bologna

Kats A G, Belostotskava I, Malomud Z P et al 1985 Remote results of the complex treatment of chronic sialadenitis with the use of helium–neon lasers. Vestnik Khirurgii Imeni II Grekova 135: P39–P42

Keele C A, Armstrong D 1964 Substances producing pain and itch. Edward Arnold, London

Kemmotsu O, Kaseno S, Furimodo H et al 1990 LLLT in pain attenuation: current experience in the pain clinic at Hokkaido University Hospital. Laser Therapy 2: 18

Kert J, Rose L 1989 Clinical laser therapy: low level laser therapy. Scandinavian Medical Laser Technology, Copenhagen

King C E, Clelland J A, Knowles C J et al 1990 Effect of Helium–Neon laser auriculotherapy on experimental pain threshold. Physical Therapy 70: 24–30

Kitchen S S, Partridge C J 1991 A review of low level laser therapy. Physiotherapy 77: 168–173

Klumpp D, Zimmerman M 1980 Irreversible differential block of A- and C- fibres following local nerve heating in the cat. Journal of Physiology 298: 471–482

Kovacs E 1987 Use of a continuously operating low capacity He–Ne laser in ambulatory oral surgery. Fogorvosi Szemle 80: 257–261

Kreczi T, Klinger D 1986 A comparison of laser acupuncture versus placebo in radicular and pseudoradicular pain syndromes as recorded by subjective responses of pain. International Journal of Acupuncture and Electrotherapeutics Research 11: 207–216

Kumar P S, Jayakumar C S, Kenworthy J et al 1988 A comparative study of low level laser therapy and conventional physiotherapy for treatment of inversion injuries of the ankle. Lasers in Medical Science, Abstracts Issue, July 1988: 298

Li X H 1990 Laser in the department of traumatology. With a report of 60 cases of soft tissue injury. Laser Therapy 2: 119–122

Lin S-F, Wesselmann U, Rymer W Z 1990 Pulsed laser radiation effects on the distribution of conduction velocities in sciatic nerve of the rat. In: Joffe S N, Atsumi K (ed) Laser surgery: advanced characterisation, therapeutics, and systems II. Progress in Biomedical Optics, SPIE Volume 1200, International Society for Optical Engineering

Liss L, Roppel R 1966 Histopathology of laser produced lesions in cat brains. Neurology 16: 783–790

Lombard A, Rossetti V, Cassone M C 1990 Neurotransmitter content and enzyme activity variations in rat brain following in vivo He–Ne laser irradiation. Proceedings, Round Table on Basic and Applied Research in Photobiology and Photomedicine, Bari, Italy, November 10th–11th

Lonauer G 1986 Controlled double blind study on the efficacy of He–Ne laser beams versus He–Ne plus infra-red laser beams in the therapy of activated osteoarthritis of finger joints. Lasers in Surgery and Medicine 6: 172

Lukashevich I G 1985 Use of a helium–neon laser in facial pains. Stomatologiia 64: 29–31

Lundeberg T, Zhou J 1988 Low-power laser irradiation does not affect the generation of signals in a sensory receptor. American Journal Chinese Medicine 16: 87–91

Lundeberg T, Haker E, Thomas M 1987a Effects of laser versus placebo in tennis elbow. Scandinavian Journal of Rehabilitation Medicine 19: 135–138

Lundeberg T, Hode L, Zhou J 1987b A comparative study of the pain-relieving effect of laser treatment and acupuncture. Acta Physiologica Scandanavica 131: 161–162

Lundeberg T, Hode L, Zhou J 1988 Effect of low-power laser irradiation on nociceptive cells in Hirudo medicinalis. International Journal of Acupuncture and Electrotherapeutics Research 13: 99–104

Lupyr V M, Sergienko N G 1986 Cholinesterase and norepinephrine activity under the laser irradiation of acupuncture points. Fiziologicheskii Zhurnal 32: 297–303

Ma D M, Liveson J A 1983 Nerve conduction handbook. F A Davis, Philadelphia

McKibben L S 1988 Renervation of denervated tissue following low level laser irradiation. In: Ohshiro T, Calderhead R G (ed) Low level laser therapy: a practical introduction. Wiley, Chichester

McKibben L S 1991 Personal communication

McKibben L S, Downie R 1990 Treatment of postherpetic pain using a 904 nm low energy infrared laser. Laser Therapy 2: 20

Maeda T, Ohshiro T 1990 Diode laser restores normal condition to bradykinin-altered rat neural cells: a controlled in vivo study. Lasers in Surgery and Medicine Suppl 2: 13

Mannheimer J S, Lampe G N 1984 Clinical transcutaneous electrical nerve stimulation. F A Davis, Philadelphia

Martino G, Fava G, Galperti G et al 1987 CO_2 laser therapy for women with mastalgia. Lasers in Surgery and Medicine 7: 78

Max M B, Portenoy R K, Laska E M 1991 The design of analgesic clinical trials. Raven Press, New York

Mayordomo M M, Failde J M G, Cabrero M V et al 1985 Laser in painful processes of locomotor system: our experience. International Congress on Laser in Medicine and Surgery. Monduzzi Editore, Bologna

Melzack R 1975 The McGill Pain Questionnaire: major properties and scoring methods. Pain 1: 277–299

Melzack R, Wall P 1989 The challenge of pain, 2nd edn. Penguin, Harmondsworth

Merskey H 1979 Pain terms: a list with definitions and notes on usage. Recommended by the IASP Subcommittee on Taxonomy. Pain 6: 249–252

Mester A F, Mester A R 1987 Biotherapy 3 and Argon ion, He–Ne, ruby lasers. Comparative study of their biostimulative effects. Abstracts, Fifth Annual Congress, 28–30 January 1987. British Medical Laser Association

Mezawa S, Iwata K, Naito K et al 1988 The possible analgesic effect of soft-laser irradiation on heat nociceptors in the cat tongue. Archives of Oral Biology 33: 693–694

Milani L, Roccia L 1982 Neuroreflexotherapy of facial vascular pains with soft-laser (He–Ne). Minerva Medica 73: 715–723

Mizokami T, Yoshii N, Ushikubo Y et al 1990 Effect of diode laser for pain: a clinical study on different pain types. Laser Therapy 2: 171–174

Moore K C, Hira N, Kumar P S et al 1988a A double blind crossover trial of low level laser therapy in the treatment of post herpetic neuralgia. Lasers in Medical Science, Abstracts Issue, July 1988: 301

Moore K C, Hira N, Broome I J et al 1988b A double blind trial of low level laser therapy in the relief of postoperative pain following a)herniography and b) cholecystectomy. Lasers in Medical Science, Abstracts Issue, July 1988: 300

Moore K C, Hira N, Broome I J et al 1990 A double blind trial of LLLT in the relief of post operative pain following cholecystectomy: a pilot study. Laser Therapy 2: 23

Morselli M, Soragni O, Anselmi C et al 1985a Very low energy-density treatments by CO_2 laser in sports medicine. Lasers in Surgery and Medicine 5: 150

Morselli M, Soragni O, Lupia B P 1985b Effects of very low energy-density treatment of joint pain by CO_2 laser. Lasers in Surgery and Medicine 5: 149

Nanjin C, Minbing D, Caijye L et al 1990 Studies of effect of He–Ne laser treatment of herpes zoster and its pathogenesis. Laser Therapy 2: 21

Obata J, Yanase M, Honmura A 1990 Evaluation of acute pain relief effects of low-power laser therapy on rheumatoid arthritis by thermography. Laser Therapy 2: 28

Ohshiro T 1988 Thermographic analysis and evaluation of pain attenuation with the GaAlAs LLLT laser system. In: Ohshiro T, Calderhead RG (ed) Low level laser therapy: a practical introduction. Wiley, Chichester

Ohshiro T 1990 Editorial: safety first. Laser Therapy 2: 51–52

Ohshiro T, Calderhead R G 1988 Low level laser therapy: a practical introduction. Wiley, Chichester

Olson J E, Schimmerling W, Tobias C A 1981 Laser action spectrum of reduced excitability in nerve cells. Brain Research 204: 436–440

Palmgren N, Jensen G F, Kaae K et al 1989 Low-power laser in rheumatoid arthritis. Lasers in Medical Science 4: 193–196

Pocock S J 1987 Clinical trials: a practical approach. Wiley, Chichester

Ponnudurai R N, Zbuzek V K, Wu W 1987 Hypoalgesic effect of laser photobiostimulation shown by rat tail flick test. International Journal of Acupuncture and Electrotherapeutics Research 12: 93–100

Ponnudurai R N, Zbuzek V K, Niu H-L et al 1988 Laser photobiostimulation-induced hypoalgesia in rats is not naloxone reversible. International Journal of Acupuncture and Electrotherapeutics Research 13: 109–117

Rochkind S, Nissan M, Barr-Nea L et al 1987 Response of peripheral nerve to He–Ne laser: experimental studies. Lasers in Surgery and Medicine 7: 441–443

Rochkind S, Nissan M, Lubart R et al 1988 The in vivo nerve response to direct low-energy laser irradiation. Acta Neurochirurgica 94: 74–77

Roumeliotis D, Emmanouilidis O, Diamantopoulos C 1987 C.W. 820 nm 15 mW, 4 J/cm^2, laser diode application in sports injuries. A double blind study. Abstracts, Fifth Annual Congress, 28–30 January 1987. British Medical Laser Association

Rusakov D A 1987 The effect of spinal cord irradiation by the low-intensity laser on the characteristics of synaptic transmission in the dorsal horn. Neurofiziologiia 19: 545–548

Rusakov D A, Klering P G 1986 Structural and functional changes in spinal cord neurons after low-intensity laser irradiation. Radiobiologia 28: 130–133

Rusakov D A, Klering P G, Savich V I 1987 Morphometrical differences of normal and low-intensity laser irradiated spinal neurons of cat. Neirofiziologiia 19: 844–847

Seibert D D, Gould W R 1984 The effect of laser stimulation on burning pain threshold. Physical Therapy 64: 746

Seitz L, Kleinkort J A 1986 Low-power laser: its applications in physical therapy. In: Michlovitz S L, Wolf S L (ed) Thermal agents in rehabilitation. F A Davis, Philadelphia

Shiroto C, Sato K 1990a Retrospective study with analysis of effectiveness of GaAlAs diode laser in the therapy of chronic pain. Laser Therapy 2: 25

Shiroto C, Sato K 1990b Psychomatic effects following LLLT with a GaAlAs diode laser in the therapy of chronic pain. Laser Therapy 2: 25

Shiroto C, Ono K, Ohshiro T 1986 Laser stimulation therapy using a diode laser: 1600 patients. Lasers in Surgery and Medicine 6: 172–173

Shiroto C, Ono K, Ohshiro T 1989 Retrospective study of diode laser therapy for pain attenuation in 3635 patients: detailed analysis by questionnaire. Laser Therapy 1: 41–48

Siebert W, Siechert N, Siebert B et al 1987 What is the efficacy of 'soft' and 'mid' lasers in therapy of tendinopathies? Archives of Orthopaedic and Traumatic Surgery 106: 358–363

Simunovic Z 1987 Application of He–Ne laser therapy in major and minor oral surgery. Lasers in Surgery and Medicine 7: 125

Snyder-Mackler L 1990 Personal Communication

Snyder-Mackler L, Bork C E 1988 Effect of Helium–Neon laser irradiation on peripheral sensory nerve latency. Physical Therapy 68: 223–225

Soroka N F 1989 The laser therapy of rheumatoid arthritis. Teraperticheskii Arkhiv 61: 124–127

Terashima H, Okajima K, Motegi M 1990 Low level laser irradiation for lateral humeral epicondylitis and De Quervain's disease. Laser Therapy 2: 27

Ternovoy K S 1984a Analgesic laser therapy of patients with postraumatic and involuntional lesions of the weightbearing locomotor apparatus. Ortopediia Travmatologiia I Protezirovani 7: 1–7

Ternovoy K S 1984b Use of the helium–neon laser in diseases and sequelae of injuries of the musculoskeletal system. Vrachebnoe Delo 2: 46–51

Torebjork H E, Vallbo A B, Ochoa J L 1987 Intraneural microstimulation in man: its relation to specificity of tactile sensations. Brain 110: 1509–1529

Trelles M A, Mayayo E, Miro L et al 1989 The action of Low reactive Level Laser Therapy (LLLT) on mast cells: a possible pain relief mechanism examined. Laser Therapy 1: 27–30

Trelles M A, Rigau J, Calderhead RG et al 1990 Treatment of knee osteoarthritis with an infrared diode laser. Laser Therapy 2: 26

Vidovich D, Olson D R 1987 Neodymium YAG laser stimulation as a treatment modality in acute and chronic pain syndromes and in rheumatoid arthritis. Lasers in Surgery and Medicine 7: 79

Vierck C J, Hooper B Y, Franzen O et al 1982 Behavioural analysis of CNS pathways and transmitter systems involved in conduction and inhibition of pain sensations and reactions in primates. In: Sprague J, Epstein A (ed) Progress in psychobiology and physiological psychology. Academic Press, New York

Vizi E S, Mester E, Tisza S et al 1977 Acetylcholine effects of laser irradiation to Auerbach plexus in guinea pig ilium. Journal of Neural Transmission 40: 305–308

Walker J B 1983 Relief from chronic pain by low-power laser irradiation. Neuroscience Letters 43: 339–344

Walker J B 1985 Temporary suppression of clonus in humans by brief photobiostimulation. Brain Research 340: 109–113

Walker J B 1987 Treatment of human neurological problems by laser photostimulation. United States Patent 4 671 285, June 9

Walker J B 1988 Low-level laser therapy for pain management: a review of the literature and underlying mechanisms. In: Ohshiro T, Calderhead RG (ed) Low level laser therapy: a practical introduction. Wiley, Chichester

Walker J B, Akhanjee L K 1985 Laser induced somatosensory evoked potential: evidence of photosensitivity in peripheral nerves. Brain Research 344: 281–285

Walker J B, Katz R L 1979 Neural plasticity and analgesia: aspects of the same phenomenon? Lancet ii: 1309

Walker J B, Akhanjee L K, Cooney M M 1986 Laser therapy for pain of rheumatoid arthritis. Lasers in Surgery and Medicine 6: 171

Walker J B, Akhanjee L K, Cooney M M et al 1987a Laser therapy for pain of rheumatoid arthritis. Clinical Journal of Pain 3: 54–59

Walker J B, Akhanjee L K, Cooney M M 1987b Laser therapy for pain of trigeminal neuralgia. Pain 29: 585

Walsh D 1991 Nociceptive pathways – relevance to the physiotherapist. Physiotherapy 77: 317–321

Waylonis G W, Wilkie S, O'Toole D et al 1988 Chronic myofascial pain: management by low output helium-neon laser therapy. Archives of Physical Medicine and Rehabilitation 69: 1017–1020

Wesselmann U, Rymer W Z, Lin S-F 1990 Effect of pulsed infrared lasers on neural conduction and axoplasmic transport in sensory nerves. In: Joffe S N, Atsumi K (ed) Laser surgery: advanced characterisation, therapeutics, and systems II. Progress in Biomedical Optics, SPIE Volume 1200, International Society for Optical Engineering

Wilder-Smith P 1988 The soft laser: therapeutic tool or popular placebo? Oral Surgery Oral Medicine Oral Pathology 66: 654–658

Williams P L, Warwick R, Dyson M et al 1989 Gray's anatomy, 37th edn. Churchill Livingstone, Edinburgh

Willner R, Abeles M, Myerson G et al 1985 Low-power infrared laser biostimulation of chronic osteoarthritis in hand. Lasers in Surgery and Medicine 5: 149–150

Wolff B B 1983 Laboratory methods of pain measurement. In: Melzack R (ed) Pain measurement and assessment. Raven Press, New York

Woofle G, McDonald A D 1944 The evaluation of the analgesic action of pethidine (Demerol). Journal of Pharmacology and Experimental Therapeutics 80: 300–307

Woolley-Hart A 1988 A handbook for low-power lasers and their medical application. East Asia, London

Wu W 1983 Recent advances in laser puncture. In: Atsumi K (ed) New frontiers in laser medicine and surgery. Elsevier, Amsterdam

Wu W-H, Ponnudurai R, Katz J et al 1987 Failure to confirm report of light-evoked response of peripheral nerve to low-power Helium–Neon laser light stimulus. Brain Research 401: 407–408

Yakovenko I, Simoonova T 1985 Use of laser radiation in the treatment of patients with rheumatoid arthritis. Vrachebnoe Delo 2: 78–80

Yew D T, Chan Y-W 1977 The influence of laser on the brains of neonatal mice. Archives d'anatomie microscopique 66: 229–234

Zarkovic N, Manev H, Pericic D et al 1989 Effect of semiconductor GaAs laser irradiation on pain perception in mice. Lasers in Surgery and Medicine 9: 63–66

Zhang S, Jinhe Q, Minlei Z 1986 Electrocardiogram effects following He–Ne laser irradiation of 'Neiguan' in cats. Chen Tzu Yen Chiu 11: 60–65

Zhou Yo Cheng 1984 An advanced clinical trial with laser acupuncture anaesthesia for minor operations in the oromaxillo–facial region. Lasers in Surgery and Medicine 4: 297–303

Zhou Yo Cheng 1987 Facial cosmetic surgery under laser acupuncture anesthesia. Lasers in Surgery and Medicine 7: 94

Zhou Yo Cheng 1988 Laser acupuncture anaesthesia. In: Ohshiro T, Calderhead R G (ed) Low level laser therapy: a practical introduction. Wiley, Chichester.

Zhu L, Li C, Ji C et al 1990 The effect of laser irradiation on arthritis in rats. Pain (Suppl) 5: S385

Zynanova T N, Lavrova V M, Pikulev A T et al 1987 Catecholamine content and acetylcholinesterase activity in rat brain affected by laser radiation. Radiobiologica 227: 94–97

7. Principles and practice of laser treatment

INTRODUCTION

This chapter outlines the principles and practical aspects of laser treatment in physiotherapeutic practice. While it might be tempting to regard and to read it in isolation, the practical material as presented here is firmly based upon the biophysical principles of therapeutic lasers and upon current research findings as presented in preceding chapters. To this end, it is recommended that readers at least familiarise themselves with the material presented in earlier chapters before proceeding further.

The chapter begins with an outline of the general principles of sound clinical laser therapy practice in laser therapy, followed by an overview of various laser treatments. As the treatment of open wounds is the primary indication for low-intensity laser therapy, such lesions are considered first, followed by a synopsis of recommended treatments for a range of musculoskeletal disorders for which laser therapy may be of potential clinical benefit. These are presented here by site, i.e. head and neck, trunk, upper limb, and lower limb. Finally, after an overview of other potential applications for laser treatment, the chapter concludes with a number of short case histories by way of illustration of the potential clinical benefits of low-intensity laser therapy.

General comments

As outlined in earlier chapters, therapeutic laser equipment should be regularly examined by a competent person and routinely checked by the operator(s), in the first instance to preserve the safety of patients and equally to ensure that the apparatus delivers treatments which are within accepted tolerances/specifications. Inherent in this is ensuring that the area reserved for laser treatment (usually in the form of a screened cubicle) is kept tidy and well organised with the treatment unit arranged so that its controls are easily accessible to the operator, and with its control display within visible range. For the larger therapeutic systems, the provision of a wheeled trolley will usually be required, so that the unit may be more easily transported and optimally positioned for use.

As the flex connecting the treatment probe to the base unit is the most easily and thus most frequently damaged component of therapeutic laser systems, care should be taken in positioning the patient and arranging the treatment area so that flexes are not unduly stretched during treatment. This most commonly happens when the operator, through poor preparation, chooses to leave the base unit on a low stool or on the floor, positions the patient at some distance from the base unit and then proceeds with treatment by pulling the probe to the limit of the connecting flex.

Importance of thorough examination and diagnosis

While low-intensity laser therapy may be regarded in some circles as a magical electrotherapeutic panacea, it can in no way compensate for poor clinical skills. Most importantly, the primary importance of thorough clinical examination and diagnosis remains. The results achieved with any treatment depend upon these basic clinical skills, and this holds equally for laser therapy. Indeed, the potential for good localised therapeutic effects with laser therapy can be severely compromised if the modality is applied indiscriminately to generalised areas of pain/tenderness/swelling without adequate examination directed at localising the site of the lesion or complaint. To this end good surface anatomy skills are an essential prerequisite to good laser treatments, as they are vital for the accurate targeting of such structures as nerve roots, peripheral nerve trunks and lymph vessels.

A note on skin preparation

While not absolutely essential in every case, preparation of the skin to remove surface lipids, sebum etc. can be necessary where the patient's skin type or personal hygiene mean that treatment may be compromised due to the reflectance and/or attenuation that may occur at the treatment diode/tissue interface. Where indicated, skin preparation will usually take the form of cleaning the area with an antiseptic or alcohol wipe or by washing the area with soap and thoroughly rinsing and drying afterwards. Apart from optimising the conditions for laser treatment, cleaning the patient's skin before each laser application will also help keep the treatment unit clean.

GENERAL PRINCIPLES OF CLINICAL PRACTICE

Choice of therapeutic laser system

In the first instance, considerable care should be given to the selection of the most appropriate treatment system, given the intended applications for the unit. For therapists primarily involved in the treatment of sports injuries, this may mean the acquisition of a portable system which works from a rechargeable power pack. For those intending to use the unit primarily for the treatment of large open wounds, a multisource diode array (possibly operating at a range of wavelengths) or scanning unit may be more appropriate. Furthermore, it is also important to note here that the trend in therapeutic systems over recent years has tended to be towards the use of diode-based units producing increasingly higher radiant power outputs; the standard diode supplied with most units is now typically at least 30 mW.

Contact technique

For the delivery of optimum laser treatment using diode-based treatment systems, or indeed where fibreoptic delivery devices are used in conjunction with He–Ne laser systems, the use of contact technique whenever possible is essential. The reasons for the use and advantages of contact technique are essentially as follows (Fig. 7.1):

1. The maximisation of power density/irradiance on the target tissue, given the divergence of most therapeutic systems and the predictions of the inverse square law (see p. 36)

2. Reflection is minimised where the skin barrier is distended at the tip of the treatment probe, thus more light energy (essentially the number of photons) is delivered to the target tissue

3. Given the exponential attenuation of laser radiation in tissue and

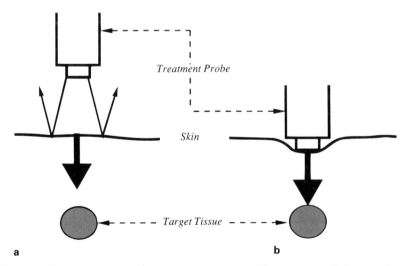

Fig. 7.1 Non-contact versus in-contact treatment. **a.** Non-contact technique produces greater reflection and lower irradiance. **b.** In-contact technique maximises irradiance at the tissue surface and at the target tissue.

the small penetration depths at the wavelengths commonly used in treatment, the depression of tissue between the treatment head and the target tissue helps to minimise attenuation of the beam, and also reduces the perfusion of the tissue. Such decrease in blood perfusion in the treatment area effectively increases the amount of radiation delivered to the underlying tissue, as haemoglobin is a potent chromophore within the red and near infra-red wavelength bands.

The only exception to this is the case of open wounds, where patient comfort and aseptic considerations will invariably exclude the possibility of treatment in-contact. However, some clinicians have used proprietary disposable film (clingfilm) pulled over the end of the treatment probe to enable the in-contact laser treatment of wounds with apparent success. Where non-contact treatment technique is used, it is imperative that the treatment head is kept stationary over the target area of tissue, with the distance between the tip of the treatment unit and the tissue being kept as small as possible (<0.5 cm).

For standard in-contact technique, the treatment probe should be held firmly and perpendicular to the target tissue, with the tip pressed into the skin (see Fig. 7.1). The amount of pressure used by the operator (and thus the depth to which the treatment probe is pressed) will primarily depend upon the depth/site of the target tissue; however the tenderness of the area of tissue to which the probe is applied will also obviously be a consideration for the therapist.

Manual stimulation during in-contact treatments

The potential therapeutic benefit of manual manipulation of the laser probe during treatment should not be overlooked. Pressure applied through the probe during laser irradiation of such clinically significant areas as acupuncture points or painful musculoskeletal trigger points effectively provides an 'acupressure'-type treatment in parallel with the laser treatment, the therapeutic benefits of each complementing the other. The most commonly used and recommended type of manipulation involves brisk pecking of the tissue with the treatment probe in a manner not unlike that used during some needle acupuncture treatments.

Non-contact technique

As already indicated above, where non-contact technique is employed in the treatment of open wounds, the distance between the treatment head and the target tissue should be kept to a minimum. In addition, careful attention should be paid to maintaining the probe perpendicular to the site of irradiation and keeping the area of irradiation as constant as possible. This is usually achieved for practical purposes by supporting the hand in which the treatment probe is held; where the larger heavier multidiode 'cluster' units are used, such support is essential. In addition to supporting the hand, some manufacturers supply stands with flexible arms in which the treatment unit can be mounted for such non-contact treatments.

Manual scanning

In a similar fashion to that produced by purpose built devices, the output of a therapeutic unit may be manually scanned across an area of target tissue where non-contact technique is used (see 'Treatment of wounds' below). While the area of irradiation will obviously be (deliberately) varied during such treatments, care should be taken to keep the treatment probe at right angles to the target tissue and to standardise the rate of movement of the beam imprint across the tissue to deliver an effective and equivalent treatment to all areas of the wound or lesion.

Effective therapeutic dosage

The difficulty in deciding upon what represents an effective dosage for a given condition should be apparent from the reviews presented in previous chapters; results from the work completed to date are unclear in this respect. In general, however, poor results, whether found in routine clinical practice or in research trials, are typically associated with the use of inappropriately low dosages. Nonetheless, the situation is not as simple as it might first appear, as some practitioners and researchers have reported considerable success using regimes based upon relatively low dosages. One explanation for these apparent conflicting observations lies in the so-called Arndt–Schultz law of photobiological activation (Fig. 7.2; see Ohshiro & Calderhead 1988). This essentially predicts that:

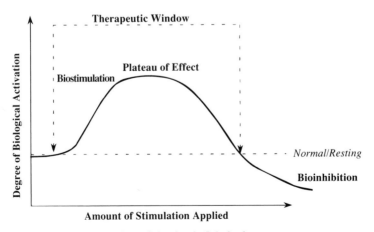

Fig. 7.2   Schematic representation of the Arndt–Schultz law.

1. a threshold amount of stimulation (in this case: dosage of laser) is required to demonstrate an effect or enhanced activation of the biological system or process under consideration
2. a dosage-dependent effect will be demonstrated at relatively low dosages above threshold, so that increasing dosage will increase the degree of activation of the biological system or process
3. immediately above these relatively low levels of stimulation (laser dosage) a plateau effect will be observed. Hence many workers in the field sometimes argue that it is for all practical purposes impossible to overdose with laser treatment
4. at the highest dosage levels, there is an *inhibitory* effect upon the given biological process or system.

The Arndt–Schultz law thus provides a useful theoretical basis to explain the varying photobiostimulatory *and* photobioinhibitory effects observed in the laboratory; however it also goes some way to accounting for the apparently conflicting results that are sometimes achieved with low-intensity laser therapy. Unfortunately, while the general operation of the law may be adequately described schematically in Figure 7.2, the precise relationship(s) existing for the treatment of those conditions encountered in clinical practice is as yet unclear.

LASER TREATMENT OF WOUNDS

General

Laser therapy can be an effective therapeutic modality in the management of a range of wounds of various aetiologies. Apart from burns, gun shot, stab and surgical wounds, including skin graft donor areas, such distressing and chronic conditions as diabetic ulcers, pressure sores and venous leg ulcers can also benefit significantly from laser treatment. Initiation of laser treatment at the earliest possible opportunity is essential to minimise patient suffering and to maximise the potential benefit. Timing and frequency of treatment seem to be less critical: in the early stages laser may be used twice per day without danger of overtreatment. In this, liaison with the rest of the health care team can ensure that provision of laser treatment is synchronised with changes of dressing and other ward or wound management routine. In particular, treatment should usually only be carried out after the wound has been cleaned/desloughed, as the presence of such slough will significantly attenuate the laser beam.

Treatment techniques

Laser treatment of wounds (and indeed conditions that may be usefully regarded as 'closed' wounds such as bruising/haematoma etc.) can be considered in two stages. For the first stage, contact technique is used

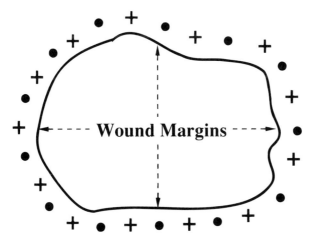

Fig. 7.3 Treatment of wounds: Phase I. Treatment of wound margins (see text for further details).

to treat a series of points around the whole wound margin, approximately 1 cm from the edge of the wound, using a standard dosage (Fig. 7.3). For this an initial dosage of 0.5–1 J/point or approximately 4–8 J/cm² is usually sufficient with which to begin treatment. Laser treatments at 2 cm intervals around the edge of the wound will usually be sufficient, with alternation of the position of points between treatment sessions (Fig. 7.3). While the primary aim of such treatment is to accelerate margination and eventually wound closure (see p. 106), promotion of increased blood flow to the wound area as well as angiogenesis are also important objectives.

As already indicated, during this first stage of wound treatment contact technique is used; for this a light but firm pressure is required to maintain adequate contact of the treatment head. Excessive/deep pressure for such laser treatments is unnecessary and will usually not be well tolerated by the patient.

During the second stage of treatment, the wound bed is treated using non-contact technique. For this a number of devices can be employed to simplify treatment including scanning devices, multisource 'cluster' treatment units and flexible arms to support and maintain the position of the treatment head and thus the area of irradiation.

Treatment devices for non-contact treatment of wounds

Scanning devices

While these represent a potentially useful means of uniformly irradiating the relatively large areas of wound bed which are typically found when treating lesions such as sacral pressure sores and venous ulcers, they

have as yet achieved only limited popularity in routine clinical practice
(p. 51). Typically used in conjunction with He–Ne units, where scanning devices are employed in the laser treatment of wound lesions, the
unit requires careful positioning prior to commencement of scanning to
ensure that all areas of the wound bed receive equivalent dosages of
irradiation during treatment. Additionally, the spot area, scanning rate
and time of irradiation need to be carefully monitored to estimate the
energy dosage applied to the wound during such treatments as accurately
as possible.

Multisource 'cluster' units

These units, although typically hand-held and thus not ideal in every
respect, represent a good means of irradiating a sizable area of wound
simultaneously. As with any treatment unit used in the non-contact mode,
cluster heads should be held as close as possible to the target tissue.
However, with such cluster treatment heads, the relatively large area of
the face of the unit may mean that some compromise may have to be
made in the treatment of inaccessible or especially deep areas of the
wound. In particular, supplementary treatment may need to be applied
directly to the relevant areas using a single diode treatment probe (see
Fig. 7.4).

Flexible support arms

These can be useful in providing a base upon which the treatment probe

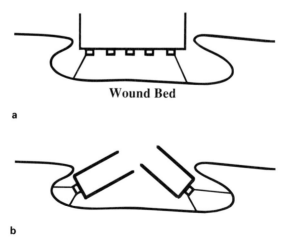

Wound Bed

a

b

Fig. 7.4 Treatment of wounds: Phase II. Treatment of wound bed with 'cluster' units.
a. Cluster head is used to treat main area of wound bed. **b.** Single probe(s) is used to
treat any recessed areas (e.g. sinus).

to be used can be fixed so that the area of irradiation remains constant. While it may seem practical to mount a (single) diode treatment probe in such a device at some distance from the wound in order to provide a sufficient size of beam imprint to cover the whole area of the wound, this solution to the problem of treating large areas of tissue is less than ideal where the wound is relatively large. This is due to the gaussian nature of the beam imprint (p. 40), the variance in irradiance of which is accentuated with increasing distances between the treatment head and target tissue. Consequently where treating wounds of relatively large area from a single fixed point, the majority of radiation would be delivered to the centre of the wound and comparatively little to the periphery of the wound.

It is therefore recommended that where such flexible arms are used, a latticework of points is targeted across the area of the wound bed, with the probe fixed by the arm at no more than 1 cm from the irradiated tissue. Under such circumstances, these arms simply provide a steadier option than manual 'gridding' as outlined below.

Manual treatment techniques

These consist of variations of two distinct techniques: manual scanning and 'gridding'.

Manual scanning

This is essentially a manual version of what can be achieved using the purpose built scanning devices outlined above. However, as scanning of the laser radiation in this case is achieved by the motion of the operator's hand, considerable care is required to ensure that a reasonably uniform dosage is delivered to all areas of the wound. For this, a steady slow movement of the treatment probe back and forth across the surface of the wound is required, the operator taking care to maintain a standard distance (<0.5–1 cm) between the tip of the probe and the surface of the wound bed. A pattern for the manual scanning treatment of a wound is suggested in Figure 7.5.

When manual scanning is employed, the calculation of dosage becomes less accurate. Where care is taken to provide a uniform irradiation to cover the whole surface of the wound, the total average radiant exposure can be estimated by dividing the product of the machine's output (in watts or milliwatts) and time of irradiation in seconds by the area of the wound in square centimetres. This latter can be best estimated by using manual tracing techniques and graph paper. For the initial or early stages of treatment an initial radiant exposure of no less than 1.5 J/cm^2 is recommended. The radiant exposure having been decided upon, the

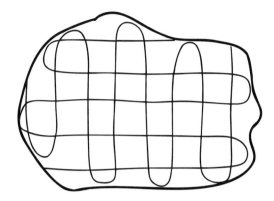

Fig. 7.5 Treatment of wounds: Phase II. Manual scanning treatment of wound bed with single probe.

size (i.e. surface area) of the wound to be treated will essentially determine treatment/irradiation time. For example, given a wound area of 10 cm^2, and a treatment unit with a radiant power output of 30 mW, a total irradiation time of 500 s (8 min 20 s) would be required to administer an *average* dosage of 1.5 J/cm^2 across the whole area of the wound.

Given the considerable practical difficulties in administering such a non-contact laser treatment for over 8 min, the considerable attraction of cluster units becomes apparent. Using a hypothetical 'cluster' unit with an average irradiance of 40 mW/cm^2, and a suitable array with a sufficient number of diodes to cover the whole area of the wound bed, an equivalent treatment in terms of average radiant exposure could be administered in just under 38 s.

'Gridding'

A more practical and usually less time-consuming alternative to manual scanning is the use of a grid technique. For this, the area of the wound bed is visualised as being covered with a gridwork of squares measuring 1 cm × 1 cm as depicted diagrammatically in Figure 7.6. Using the grid as reference, treatment is then applied systematically to each square using a single diode or fibreoptic applicator from a distance of no more than ~0.5–1 cm.

For such treatments of the wound bed, an energy density of 1.5–2.5 J/cm^2 (in each irradiated grid square) is recommended as a minimum for the early stages of wound management. Given a 30 mW unit for this type of treatment, the treatment probe would be used to irradiate each square for a total of 50 s to deliver 1.5 J/cm^2 in non-contact mode. Where time is limited, the grid can be visualised as a draught- or chequerboard and irradiation on subsequent treatment sessions alternated between

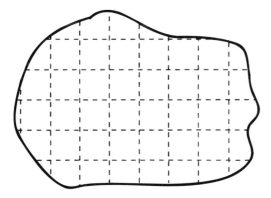

Fig. 7.6 Treatment of wounds: Phase II. 'Gridding' for treatment of wound bed with single probe. Laser treatment probe is applied to boxes described by grid.

'black' and 'white' squares. Under such circumstances, as only half the squares are irradiated during any one session, it is recommended that the frequency of laser treatment is increased.

While gridding represents a less laborious method of treating large areas of wound than manual scanning, there are some practical problems in standardising the grid for any patient. For this, some therapists have found acetate sheets or clear plastic panels marked with a custom grid to be useful, especially as they can be used as a 'stencil' to mark the intact skin surrounding the wound margins. Acetate sheets have the further advantage that, for a particular patient, the area of the wound can be marked on the sheet and thus the acetate also forms a useful record of treatment efficacy. Where clear plastic panels have been used, the squares in the grids can be drilled for the tip of the treatment probe and the panel used as a 'stencil' for treatment. While not suitable for use in all cases, these customised panels can form a useful and inexpensive means of standardising such treatments; especially as the panel can be relatively easily cleaned after each laser treatment.

A note on supplementary treatment of the lymphatic system

In addition to the direct irradiation of the margins and bed of the wound, it has also been claimed that therapeutic laser units can also be used to stimulate the functioning of the lymphatic system and thus improve the rate of wound healing. Although not widely used for such treatments, at least in the British Isles, the reported clinical successes in Japan (Ohshiro 1991) and positive results from in vitro cellular research would suggest this as a potentially effective method of treatment in the management of chronic wounds.

For these treatments, the laser is used to irradiate the main lymphatic vessels and nodes associated with the site of the wound or lesion. Thus for the lower limb, the laser would be applied to the lymph nodes in the ipsilateral groin area and at a few points along the course of the main vessels serving these nodes. Contact technique using a firm pressure is necessary if such treatments are to be successful and energy densities of around 3–5 J/cm²; it is further recommended that treatment of the lymph nodes and vessels is completed before irradiation of the wound. It should also be stressed that even where the lymph nodes are found to be swollen, the athermic nature of laser treatment means that the treatment is safe and can be delivered with confidence. Where the therapist is in any doubt, a test dosage of 1 J/cm² can be applied and the condition monitored over the subsequent 24 hours.

Recommended treatment parameters

Dosage/energy density

The difficulties inherent in recommending treatment parameters for any laser treatment have already been identified. However, based upon research findings and clinical experiences to date, it is recommended that in-contact treatments of wound margins should usually be initiated using energy densities of no less than ~4 J/cm² or about 0.5 J/point. Where wound closure progresses well, it should not normally be necessary to consider increasing the dosage. However, where the rate healing is poor or reaches a plateau, dosage can be increased and the effect monitored. Under such circumstances, healing may be enhanced with dosages of up to 12 J/cm². While there is little evidence to suggest that dosages above this value applied in contact with intact skin will adversely affect the rate of healing or indeed cause any serious side effects, the practical constraints (not least of which is the time of treatment) inherent in increasing the dosage above this value exclude unlimited progression of treatment.

In contrast, there is some evidence to suggest that the application of dosages of over 3–4 J/cm² *directly to the wound bed* may well inhibit the overall progression of wound healing. Consequently, such treatment is usually commenced with dosages of not less than ~1.5 J/cm² and progressed, where healing is considered to be slow, to dosages of up to 4 J/cm² maximum. Where only minimal or marginal effects are produced with such dosages, it is unlikely that laser therapy will be indicated for the particular patient.

Pulse repetition rate

While excellent clinical results can and have been achieved using continuous wave units for the treatment of wounds, where pulsed output units have been employed, the majority of cellular and clinical reports to date have tended to use relatively high pulse repetition rates (~1000 Hz/ 1 kHz or higher) with apparent success (see Ch. 5). To this end, a sizable percentage of therapists would instigate treatment of wounds (especially where these are chronic) using pulse repetition rates in the kilohertz range. Alternatively, where a range of pulse repetition rates are available on the unit used for treatment, the total treatment time can be apportioned so that (for example) half the treatment is given at a 'high' pulse repetition rate (e.g. 1 kHz) and the remainder at a 'low' pulse repetition rate (e.g. 70 Hz). The reasoning behind such a treatment approach is that it should take advantage of any pulsing-frequency-specific effects that may occur during treatment. The latter regime of treatment can also prove useful where the healing process has apparently reached a standstill after a number of successful laser treatments. This approach may additionally be advantageous when using those units where the choice is simply between continuous wave and pulsed output.

Frequency of treatment

In the early stages of treatment, daily irradiation is recommended; however twice- and thrice-daily treatments have also been used without adversely affecting therapeutic benefit. Where improvement has been established, frequency of treatment can usually be reduced to irradiation on alternate days, or to irradiation on several days per week. In such cases, it is important to monitor and re-assess the progression of wound healing while reducing the frequency of treatment.

Combination treatment for infected wounds

As already outlined above, some planning will usually be necessary to ensure the synchronisation of laser therapy with other wound management strategies such as wound dressing and cleaning. Desloughing of badly infected wounds is essential to ensure the maximum benefit from laser treatment, as non-viable debris and slough act as undesirable attenuators for the incident radiation. While some therapists have expressed concern over the potential photobiostimulatory effects of laser upon the wound infection, particularly given Karu's findings in *Escherichia coli* (see Ch. 5), there is little evidence to suggest that this represents a genuine problem in clinical practice. Rather, the possibility that laser treatment acts to enhance the patient's host response would appear to be more likely and is reflected in therapists' reported experiences in such cases (Baxter et al 1991).

Where infection is present at the wound site and appears to be affecting laser treatment or the wound healing process, laser can usefully be used in combination with Kromayer ultra-violet therapy. In such cases, the wound is prepared using standard aseptic technique as for routine

Kromayer treatment. Once the latter has been completed, laser therapy can be used. With the Kromayer being used just prior to any laser treatment, the bactericidal effects of the ultra-violet irradiation effectively neutralise any potential for laser photobiostimulation of infection(s) at the wound site.

LASER TREATMENT OF MUSCULOSKELETAL DISORDERS

Principles and methods of application

Before considering laser treatments for specific musculoskeletal conditions, it is useful to outline first the methods of application of laser irradiation in the physiotherapeutic management of such conditions. It should be stressed from the outset that, unless there are exceptional circumstances to contraindicate such use, laser therapy should always be applied in contact for best results.

In general, laser can be applied in any combination to the following:

1. directly to the site of the lesion
2. to any painful trigger points or tender points that may be present
3. to nerve roots and/or superficial nerve trunks
4. to acupuncture points or auricular acupuncture points.

These will each be considered briefly before proceeding further; however it should be remembered that in routine clinical practice, laser is rarely applied in isolation. In this respect laser therapy represents an ideal combination therapy which can be used in parallel to almost any other physiotherapeutic modality.

While the sequence of therapy is usually immaterial, several points need to be made with regard to combination treatments. In the first instance, where manipulative therapy is to be used with laser irradiation, it is usual to complete manipulative procedures before applying laser. In this way, the analgesic effects of laser cannot confound the assessment procedures used during the manipulative therapy. Furthermore, where phonophoresis/sonophoresis is used, it is recommended that laser is applied first. This avoids the possibility of undesired photochemical reactions with the anti-inflammatory agent in the upper layers of the dermis where the concentrations of the applied agent are likely to be very high immediately after phonophoresis.

Lastly, if laser therapy is to be used in combination with cryotherapy or other thermal modalities, the sequence of application of laser irradiation and heat or cold treatments needs to be carefully considered as this will profoundly affect the effectiveness of treatment. In those cases where cryotherapy is applied first, the resultant vasoconstriction in the superficial tissues will significantly reduce the amount of blood (and in turn the number of chromophores) within the treatment area prior to irradiation. Application of cryotherapy in this way just prior to laser application can significantly enhance the *localised* effects of laser therapy and effectively increase the depth of penetration of laser irradiation. In contrast, where modalities producing significant heating of the tissues (e.g. hot packs, infra-red therapy, short wave diathermy etc.) are used prior to laser irradiation, depth of penetration and the localisation of laser treatment effect are consequently reduced. It is therefore recommended that where these are to be used in combination with laser therapy, cryotherapy is applied *before*, and thermal modalities *after* laser treatment.

Direct application to the site of the lesion

For this, direct irradiation of the lesion is performed using contact technique. The degree of pressure applied will vary depending upon the site of the lesion (especially the depth) and the tenderness of the area to be irradiated. Apart from the pressure applied during laser treatment, the other factor critical to the success of laser treatment is the angle of application. The therapist should ensure that in all cases the laser treatment probe is applied so that the emitted radiation is appropriately directed to target the desired tissue area (Fig. 7.7). For the treatment of larger areas of tissue, e.g. large haematoma or muscle tears, some variation of the gridding technique already described above for the treatment of open wounds will be necessary to ensure that a standardised treatment is applied to the whole lesion. Alternatively, an in-contact version of the previously described manual scanning technique can be used. For this only a gentle pressure, sufficient to maintain contact between the treatment probe and the skin, is used. As with manual scanning treatments, to ensure a standardised dosage is delivered to all portions of the target tissue, care is required in moving the treatment probe across the whole area at a steady, constant speed.

Laser trigger point therapy

Trigger point therapy using a variety of physical and pharmacological

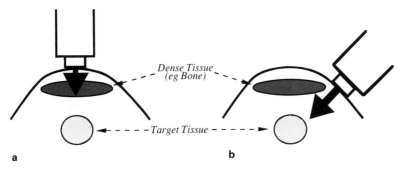

Fig. 7.7 Inaccessible structures: care in directing probe head results in more effective treatment.

agents is a well established method of treatment in physical medicine. Painful trigger points/areas are located in the affected muscles using deep manual palpation directed across the relevant muscle fibres; once identified in this way, the trigger points can be relatively easily treated with injections of analgesics, metal acupuncture needles, electrical stimulation, ultrasound and simple manual pressure. A comprehensive account of the principles and practice of trigger point therapy is provided by Baldry (1989).

Where trigger points are found to be present, therapeutic laser devices can provide a useful and effective means of treatment without recourse to invasive techniques. For trigger point therapy, a single diode treatment probe is recommended and is typically used to deliver an initial energy dosage of 1 J or ~8 J/cm^2 per point for a standard treatment. While a deep, firm pressure is essential for such trigger point treatments, the amount of pressure applied should be tempered by the patient's pain report. Once the point has been treated in this way, it is re-palpated to assess the effect of treatment and a second and third dose are applied if this is considered necessary. The treatment reaction in such cases is immediate, with decreased sensitivity being demonstrated when the irradiated point is re-palpated. If the sensitivity of the treated points is not found to be significantly reduced after three or four such applications (approximately < 30 J/cm^2), laser trigger point therapy should be discontinued in favour of needles or some alternative form of treatment.

Laser acupuncture and auricular acupuncture

Acupuncture in its traditional form is based upon the stimulation of well defined points on the body by the insertion of metal needles. Such needling is considered necessary to redress the balance of *yin* and *yang* and the flow of *chi* or energy, which in classical acupuncture theory is considered to be disrupted when the individual suffers disease. This form of therapy predates modern medicine by several thousand years and has recently found increasing acceptance in the West, at least as an effective analgesic modality. Auricular acupuncture is a therapeutic approach based upon stimulation of key points on the ear, mainly with short metal needles and electrical currents.

For some acupuncture treatments, lasers have been found to be an effective alternative to metal needles. Indeed in China and Japan this represents the most popular method of laser application. While they are currently not common applications for lasers in physiotherapy, at least in the British Isles, laser acupuncture and laser auricular acupuncture have been used successfully by some physiotherapists in the management of various types of acute, but more commonly chronic, pain.

During such treatments, the precepts of traditional acupuncture are unvaried, laser irradiation merely being applied to the appropriate acupoints in preference to metal needles. For traditional acupuncture (whether needle or laser) to be used successfully in clinical practice, a thorough knowledge of acupuncture theory and sufficient supervised clinical tuition is necessary. While an introduction to acupuncture is beyond the scope of the current text, MacDonald's overview of the analgesic application of acupuncture represents a useful starting point for the interested reader (MacDonald 1989).

Application to nerve roots and trunks

Where the reduction of pain or of muscle spasm is an important objective of laser treatment, the use of therapeutic laser devices to irradiate the skin overlying the appropriate nerve roots represents a useful adjunct to direct application of the device over the site of the lesion or pain. This is particularly so where the pain is diagnosed as being referred from structures in or around the spine, or such involvement is suspected as contributing to the patient's reported pain. Similarly, laser irradiation at sites where major nerve trunks pass superficially beneath the skin can also be a useful treatment technique not only for pain reported within the sensory distribution of the nerve, but also other neurological symptoms such as tingling and paraesthesiae (see 'Case history 1' below). Careful examination and palpation to correctly identify the appropriate site for laser application are essential when treating neural structures if the treatment is to be effective. It is recommended that dosages for such treatments should be commenced at 1–3 J/point or 8–24 J/cm^2.

It should be noted that for the comprehensive laser treatment of a given condition, the above strategies can most usefully be used in combination to enhance the effectiveness of laser treatment. Thus for a painful shoulder injury laser therapy could be used:

1. to treat the injury and site of pain directly
2. to de-activate any trigger points identified (e.g. in the trapezius muscles)
3. to treat the relevant acupuncture points
4. to irradiate the ipsilateral cervical nerve roots.

A note on reported sensations as a result of laser treatment

In a number of cases, patients will report a sensation as a result of laser irradiation. Usually described as feelings of warmth, tingling, sharp pricking or needling, these reports should be taken as an indication that laser irradiation at the site currently under treatment has been successful and that no further treatment is necessary. It is important to stress that these reports do not imply that anything untoward has occurred as a consequence of laser treatment nor, as is commonly assumed by the uninitiated, that some form of dangerous 'overtreatment' has occurred.

Conditions

These are considered here, first in general terms and then some specific examples are overviewed by anatomical site.

Haematoma/bruising

These are treated in much the same way as already described above for open wounds; however in this case contact technique is used throughout. For the treatment of the margins of the area of haematoma, laser treatment using a single diode probe is delivered at ~2 cm intervals as previously described above (p. 193) using an initial dosage of 0.5–1 J/point or 4–8 J/cm². However, for the irradiation of the haematoma, a slightly higher average dosage is recommended. Using a multisource cluster array or a single probe on a series of gridded points, an energy density of around 6–8 J/cm² is recommended as a useful starting point. The reason for the use of such comparatively higher dosages when treating these lesions is that in these cases, irradiation is being delivered through intact/ unbroken skin which acts as a potent attenuator of incident radiation; furthermore the high concentration of red blood cells in the area of the lesion acts as a pool of attenuators to absorb the incident laser radiation. Alternatively, the in-contact 'sweeping' technique as already described above can be used; this technique is, however, liable to be inappropriate where the haematoma or bruising is deep-seated. In all such cases, laser treatment should be instigated as soon as possible after injury and repeated as often as is practical and necessary throughout the acute stage (see 'Case history 2' below).

Muscle tears and injuries

Apart from accelerating the repair process, and thus speeding the onset of functional recovery, laser therapy can also be effective in reducing the associated muscular pain and the risks of hypertrophic scar formation and chronic inflammatory reactions. In the acute stage after injury, i.e. where haematoma is present, this is treated as already described above. Laser therapy is then continued, in combination with manual massage techniques as indicated, at dosages of between 1–4 J/point or 8–32 J/cm². In all such cases, it is imperative that careful examination and assessment is completed to accurately localise the muscle injury and thus identify the site for irradiation.

In those cases where excessive scar formation has become a problem in the later stages of repair, laser can usefully be used in parallel to deep friction techniques to break up the scar tissue. Where used in this way, manual frictions are performed and laser therapy is applied immediately afterwards. While the size of the tissue area to be irradiated will obviously vary depending upon the extent of the lesion itself, in order to be effective laser must be applied comprehensively to the whole area and at the margins, using a relatively high dosage of approximately 12–20 J/cm^2. At such dosages, not only will re-healing be accelerated, but the likelihood of further hypertrophic scarring will be minimised.

Tendinitis/tenosynovitis/tendinopathies

For such conditions, therapeutic laser can be an effective and practical choice of treatment, especially when used to complement ultrasound treatment. Laser irradiation should usually be applied to the most sensitive areas of the tendon on palpation, as well as to the area of tendon immediately above and below the site of tenderness or pain, using a single diode probe and energy densities of *at least* 0.5 J/point or 4 J/cm^2. When treating tendons, the operator should ensure that the tendon is placed on a slight (pain-free) stretch and that all aspects of the tendon are irradiated by directing the laser at a range of angles for treatment (Fig. 7.8).

Ligament strains

Ligament strains can be found to respond well to laser treatment, especially if treatment is initiated early. With the relevant joint appropriately positioned, laser may be applied, usually using a single probe, with a firm but comfortable pressure and energy densities of at least 1 J/point

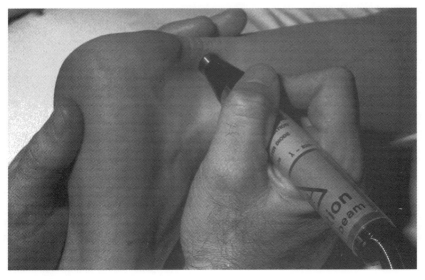

a

Fig. 7.8a,b,c. Laser treatment of achilles tendinitis.

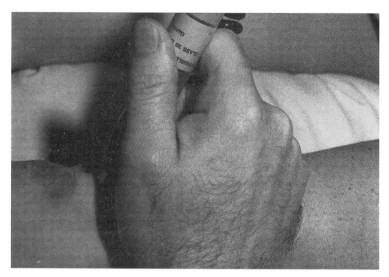

b

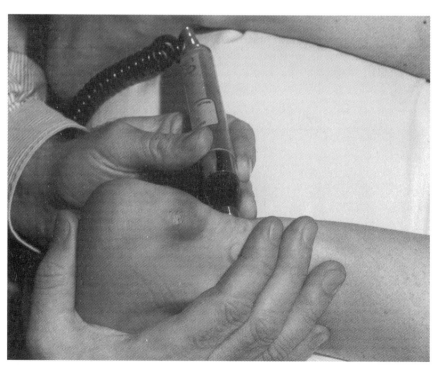

c

or 8 J/cm². In the early stages of treatment, daily irradiation is recommended. As ligament injuries tend to take a relatively long time to resolve, laser therapy can offer significant advantages in terms of reducing the duration of rehabilitation in the case of athletes or where serious ligament injury has occurred. However, the consequence of this is that application of laser therapy may be required over an extended period. In such circumstances, the frequency of treatment during the latter stages of rehabilitation should be carefully considered and decreased where practical.

Bursitis

While inflamed bursae are ideal candidates for laser treatment, their anatomical site(s) deep to structures such as tendons or heads of muscles makes their treatment somewhat problematic. In order to be successful, the treatment probe must be applied with sufficient pressure to allow the delivery of an effective therapeutic irradiance (and thus dosage) to the affected bursa. In such cases, the energy densities required tend to be relatively higher than for other treatments: typically in the range 10–30 J/cm² depending upon the site of the lesion.

Arthralgia/arthropathies/arthroses

Joint pain of various aetiologies can be effectively treated with laser therapy. In addition, a range of arthroses would also seem to respond favourably to laser treatment, resulting in decreased pain, increased range of movement and enhanced functional recovery. For laser to be effective in such cases, care should be taken to ensure that the laser is applied systematically and in a comprehensive manner over the full extent of the joint margins and as much of the joint surfaces and capsule as is possible and practical depending upon the patient's available range of movement. To accomplish a thorough laser treatment of a given joint, it is usually necessary to re-position the joint several times during treatment to allow the operator access with the laser treatment probe (Fig. 7.9). Typical starting dosages for such treatments are within the range 1–4 J/point or 8–32 J/cm².

Conditions by anatomical site

Head and neck

Laser treatments for conditions affecting sites in the head and neck are summarised in Figure 7.10 and in outline below. With all treatments in this region, care must be taken to avoid accident intrabeam viewing by the patient; however, even in those situations where goggles are not worn, such danger is negligible where in-contact technique is used.

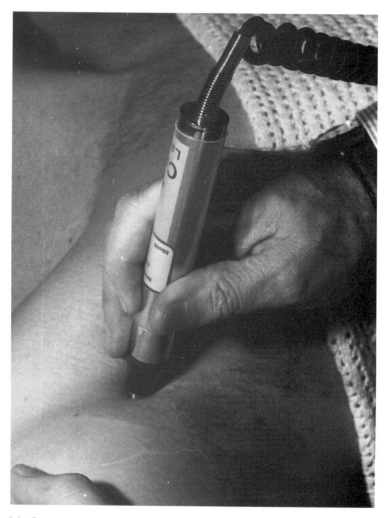

Fig. 7.9 Laser treatment of shoulder joint.

Headaches. Where headaches are reported by the patient, these can be treated by direct irradiation of the site of the pain using a gridding technique and dosages of 1–2 J/point or 8–16 J/cm². Alternatively, and depending upon the suspected underlying cause(s) of the pain, trigger points can be treated as already described above along with the relevant cervical nerve roots.

Trigeminal neuralgia. Direct treatment of the trigeminal nerve is recommended with dosages of at least 2 J or 8 J/cm² per irradiated point.

Temporomandibular joint (TMJ) pain. Laser is applied with a

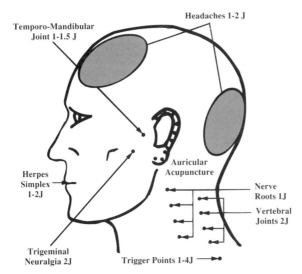

Fig. 7.10 Summary of recommended treatments: head and neck (figures in joules are per point irradiated).

medium pressure to a cluster of points around and over the affected joint. Some care is required to ensure that the probe is appropriately angled for treatment of the joint; dosages for such treatment should be initiated with energy densities of approximately 8–12 J/cm² per point of treatment.

Neck pain/whiplash, etc. As has already been stressed earlier in this chapter, where laser therapy is used in the management of neck pain/ whiplash etc., any manipulative therapy which is to be used should be completed before laser irradiation is commenced. For laser therapy to be successful in such cases, comprehensive irradiation of all affected cervical nerve roots and any painful musculoskeletal trigger points in the manner already described above is essential. Where pain is referred into the shoulder or arm, irradiation of nerve roots and trigger points should also be coupled with treatment of the appropriate nerves in the arm and possibly over Erb's point to target the main elements of the brachial plexus.

In cases where degenerative changes of the joints of the cervical spine are suspected as contributing to the patient's pain report, these should also be treated with laser, using initial dosages of no less than 2 J/point or 16 J/cm².

In all cases of laser treatment of the cervical spine, the patient should be closely monitored by the operator throughout treatment as emesis and dizziness are (rarely but) sometimes reported by patients. In such cases, laser therapy should be discontinued immediately and only recommenced at a new site once these unpleasant symptoms have passed.

Trunk

Back pain. The basic tenets for successful laser therapy for the management of pain in the upper or lower back are as already described above for neck pain. Where necessary, comprehensive treatment will include the irradiation of the costovertebral joints at the appropriate/affected levels.

Costochondritis/costochondral pain. Laser therapy is an ideal modality for the management of such conditions. For each affected joint, laser should be applied at least on three points around the joint: directly (perpendicularly) on to the joint; just above the joint with the laser treatment probe directed obliquely downwards to target the superior aspect of the joint; and below the joint with the laser beam directed upwards to target the inferior aspect of the joint. Treatment should usually be initiated at dosages of 1–2 J/point (8–16 J/cm^2).

Upper limb (Fig. 7.11)

Capsulitis of the gleno-humeral joint. Along with manipulative and exercise therapy, laser therapy should be applied at frequent intervals in the early stages of rehabilitation to a grid of points in the axilla at dosages of no less than 1 J/point. While laser therapy can offer spectacular results in terms of reduction of pain and stiffness, it should be

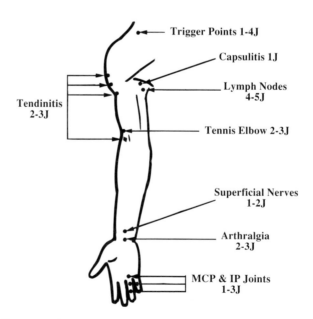

Fig. 7.11 Summary of recommended treatments: upper limb (figures in joules are per point irradiated).

understood that this does not avoid the need for active exercise of the joint in the rehabilitation of such patients.

Supraspinatus/infraspinatus tendinitis. Where these are found to be tender on palpation and resisted exercise causes pain around the insertion of these tendons, therapeutic laser on clusters of points around the tender/painful areas at initial dosages of no less than 2–3 J/point or 16–24 J/cm² can yield significant therapeutic benefits.

Lateral epicondylalgia (tennis elbow). Where laser therapy is to be used for this condition, best results are achieved by concentrating the laser treatment at relatively high dosages to the most sensitive/tender areas upon palpation of the common extensor origin/lateral epicondyle, rather than to the whole area at a comparatively lower dosage. Typical initial dosages should be in the range of 2–3 J/point or 16–24 J/cm².

Lower limb

Recommended laser treatments for the lower limb are summarised in Figure 7.12.

Groin strain/pains. Laser therapy represents an ideal choice for the treatment of lesions in this area, due to the athermic nature of the modality as well as the ability to accurately target treatment on the desired site. For such treatments, a single diode probe is most practical, and should be applied with a firm but comfortable pressure. For the treatment of

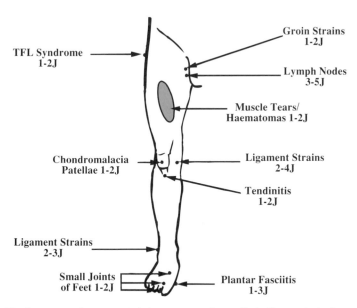

Fig. 7.12 Summary of recommended treatments: lower limb (figures in joules are per point irradiated).

lesions in this area, irradiation should begin with energy densities of at least 1 J/point or 8 J/cm² and progressed as required.

Tensor fascia lata syndrome. Laser therapy may be applied to the most painful areas of the muscle on palpation. A medium pressure is usually sufficient for such treatments and energy densities of at least 1–2 J/point or 8–16 J/cm².

Chondromalacia patellae. In such cases, laser therapy can offer results which are quite superior to those achieved with other modalities. However, if laser therapy is to be used successfully, the therapist must ensure that care is taken to move the patella away from the joint (either laterally or medially) and apply the laser probe to the retropatellar surface using a firm but comfortable pressure (Fig. 7.13). With laser treatment comprehensively applied in this manner using dosages of at least 1 J/point or 8 J/cm² patients will usually report significant improvements by the third treatment session, even in long-standing cases of the complaint.

Achilles tendinitis. With thorough and comprehensive treatment of all aspects of the tendon, laser treatment using initial dosages of at least

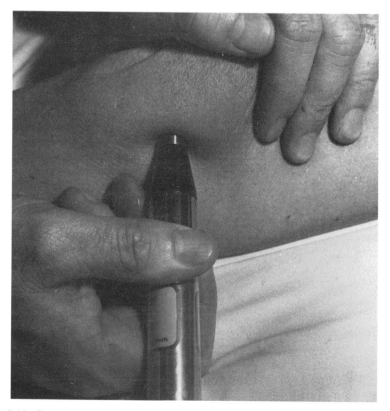

Fig. 7.13 Laser treatment of chondromalacia patella.

1–2 J/point or 8–16 J/cm^2 can prove useful in the management of this condition.

OTHER CONDITIONS

Apart from those conditions already discussed above, laser therapy can be used with good results with three other main indications: acne, herpes simplex and herpes zoster.

Acne vulgaris

In such cases, particularly where the condition is in an advanced stage, laser therapy used either in isolation or in combination with ultra-violet therapy can represent a useful means of physiotherapeutic management. Where possible, in-contact technique employing only a light pressure should be used on the most prominent lesions (pustules etc.) and the treatment head should be cleaned with a sterile wipe between treatments. Dosages for such treatments should be initiated at 0.5 J/point or 4 J/cm^2 and progressed as required.

Herpes simplex ('cold sores') and herpes zoster

While it is not considered likely that low-intensity laser therapy can act as some form of 'magic bullet' or antiviral agent for the treatment of herpes simplex or zoster, the experience of many clinicians and researchers would indicate that therapeutic laser, used at the appropriate irradiation parameters, may be able to accelerate the pathogenesis of these conditions. Used at 1–2 J/point directly on to the lesions, laser would seem to enhance the host response and thus speed the resolution of the viral infection. Furthermore, and perhaps most importantly, the systematic laser treatment of herpes zoster would also seem to reduce the incidence of postherpetic neuralgia in the patients so treated. Given the suffering associated with postherpetic neuralgia and the intractable nature of this distressing condition, therapeutic laser would seem to offer significant advantages in the early treatment of herpes zoster.

CASE HISTORIES

The following five case histories are included to illustrate the potential benefits of therapeutic laser in routine clinical practice. It should be stressed that these are not exhaustive nor are the treatments employed in each individual case designed to be prescriptive. In each case the salient history and examination findings are presented, followed by a summary of the treatment regime employed as well as an overview of treatment outcome.

Case history 1

History

This 45-year-old, right-handed male presented with a complaint of persistent paraesthesia and associated (slight) muscle weakness in the left forearm and hand. He had been the victim of an assault several months prior to his first attendance and had injured his left arm in trying to defend himself against the assailant. While the arm had been painful for a few days after the incident, this initial 'aching, deep pain' had passed, leaving a troublesome constant paraesthesia which had persisted to the date of the first appointment. There was apparently little that the patient could do to ease his symptoms.

Examination

No obvious signs of injury were found, nor was there any neurological deficit apart from what appeared to be a slight decrease in grip strength on the left side. The neck was examined and found to be clear. The patient did, however, report some increase in his symptoms upon deep pressure over the median nerve at the elbow. The patient indicated that his symptoms affected an area of his left palm and fingers within the sensory innervation of the median and the radial nerves. There were no other relevant findings.

Treatment

Laser therapy was applied in isolation to the median nerve at the wrist and at the elbow, and to the superficial radial nerve in the forearm. A total of six points were treated on the course of the median nerve: three points at the level of the wrist and three at the elbow, the points being approximately 0.5 cm apart. For the superficial radial nerve five similarly spaced points were treated. The unit used for these treatments was an 830 nm GaAlAs diode laser (CB Medico, Denmark) with a radiant power output of 30 mW and a spot size of ~0.1 cm^2. At each point 30 s of laser treatment was used, delivering 0.9 J/point or ~9 J/cm^2.

Treatment outcome

After the first treatment as described above, the patient returned 72 hours later for a second appointment. At this stage, the patient reported that he had already noticed an improvement in his symptoms: the paraesthesia was only intermittently present and he seemed to have lost the feeling of weakness in his (left-handed) grip. After the third treatment, some 8 days after his first attendance, the patient's symptoms had completely disappeared. A further review was completed a week after this third treatment, during which the patient had maintained his previously reported improvement.

Case history 2

History

This 28-year-old man reported for treatment some 2 hours after sustaining an injury to the muscles of his low back during a rugby football match. During a scrum, several players collapsed on top of the patient as he fell to the ground. His main complaint at this time was severe acute pain in the muscles of the lower back.

Examination

The patient had no neurological signs or symptoms, nor any referred pain. All lumbar movements were restricted to a greater or lesser degree and the lumbar paraspinal muscles were found to have increased tone. A large bruise (~100 cm^2) was already obvious over the lumbar spine, extending from the level of the second to the fifth lumbar vertebra. This area, together with a surrounding border of about 4 cm wide, was painful to the touch. The only other relevant finding was a tenderness to deep palpation in the patient's right buttock. This appeared to be unrelated to his pain report.

Treatment

Laser treatment was applied in isolation during the patient's first attendance, with therapeutic ultrasound being applied during the second and third attendances. The bruising on the patient's lower back was treated using a multiwavelength/multidiode array (Omega Laser Systems, London) containing 31 laser and superluminous diodes operating at wavelengths of 660–950 nm and an average irradiance of 44 mW/cm^2 across the 12 cm^2 face of the 'cluster' array. Applied to the lesion for a total of 8 min at a pulse repetition rate of 16 Hz, this gave an average energy density of 21 J/cm^2 across the lesion. Apart from this, a single laser diode operating at 820 nm and with an output of 40 mW at 16 Hz was used to irradiate 20 points around the edges of the bruising at intervals of ~2 cm for a total of 30 s per point. Used in this way, 1.2 J/point or 9.6 J/cm^2 was delivered to each of these points on the edge of the lesion. Because of the presence of tenderness in the right buttock, the cluster unit was used to give a further dosage (as described above) to this area.

Treatment outcome

By the second treatment session after 24 hours, the bruising on the patient's lumbar spine had faded to a yellow-orange colour and the patient reported an almost complete remission of symptoms. Lumbar movements were full or almost full and he reported no pain over the lumbar area. This area was however still tender to deep touch. By far the most spectacular results were found at the point where the right buttock had been treated with laser; here the whole area had turned a dark purple colour as the bruising had come to the surface. As on the first attendance, the area was tender only to deep palpation.

Laser treatment as already described was applied on two further occasions over the ensuing week, by which stage the patient's symptoms had completely resolved and the bruising had largely disappeared. The patient played rugby for his club the following week.

Case history 3

History

This 48-year-old housewife attended for treatment complaining of intractable neck and shoulder pain as a result of injuries she had sustained in a road traffic accident some 12 months previously. Symptoms were present over the area of her neck and shoulders only as a mild dull ache accompanied by some stiffness of neck movements first thing upon rising, but gradually increased in intensity over the course of her waking hours so that by evening she was in quite severe pain. Rest seemed to be the only means of limiting the pain.

At the time of her first attendance she had been treated by her GP with a variety of drugs, most notably non-steroidal anti-inflammatory drugs (NSAIDs) and codeine. On her GP's advice she had also attended a chiropractor on several occasions, but complained that the treatments had been 'too rough' and she had therefore discontinued attendance. Despite such treatments, the patient reported no significant diminution of symptoms, which she complained severely affected her social and family life and limited the amount of housework she could complete. There were no significant changes on X-ray examination apart from (?) degenerative changes at the level of C6/C7. At the time of her first visit, she had had one appointment with a consultant orthopaedic surgeon and was waiting to be called for a review.

Examination

The patient indicated the pain to be primarily located centrally over the area of C3–C7. These vertebrae were painful on central postero–anterior palpation using small amplitude movements, and also unilateral palpation on both sides. All cervical movements were restricted to a greater or lesser degree, with rotation to both sides and lateral flexion to the left being the most affected. In addition, the patient also demonstrated numerous tender and several trigger points in both trapezii. The trigger points were exquisitely painful and produced tears from the patient on deep palpation.

Treatment

A combination of treatments were used with this patient. A small, battery-powered transcutaneous electrical nerve stimulation (TENS) unit was supplied for home use after its operation had been properly demonstrated to the patient. Gentle cervical mobilisation was used in the early stages of rehabilitation, primarily to correct the decreased range of movement in the cervical spine. For the tender and trigger points a combination of needle and laser trigger point therapy was employed. Laser treatment consisted of 30 s irradiation per point with an 830 nm continuous wave source operating at a radiant power output of 40 mW (Asah Medico, Denmark) to give a dosage of 1.2 J/point or approximately 9.6 J/cm^2. Laser trigger point therapy was used in the early stages of treatment, as the patient was squeamish: fine disposable needles were used only on the more intractable *trigger* points.

Treatment outcome

Initially this patient progressed quickly with treatment and achieved almost full range of cervical movements within three treatment sessions. The home use of her TENS units coupled with a programme of gentle home exercises for her neck ensured that the patient's pain was adequately managed and that she actively maintained the enhanced range of movement that she had achieved in treatment. However, her trigger points proved to be more resilient to treatment, regardless of either laser or needle treatment. At the 12th such treatment session, the patient reported a severe exacerbation of symptoms in the right trapezius after a combined use of laser and needle trigger point therapy. This excessive treatment reaction lasted for some 36 hours, after which the symptoms in her right trapezius completely resolved. A review after a further 6 weeks confirmed that the patient's symptoms had not returned.

Case history 4

History

This 62-year-old gentleman reported for treatment complaining of 'heat' in his right quadriceps muscle and nocturnal pains which awakened him if he turned onto his right side. Being slightly overweight, the patient reported that he had been concerned about his personal fitness and in an effort to start a programme of aerobic exercise had apparently 'pulled a muscle' when attempting an uphill run. Advised by an unqualified practitioner to rest and apply embrocation rubs, the patient noticed some slight improvement in symptoms in the leg in the short term. However, he complained of a persistent dull ache in the leg, which worsened with use. Furthermore, he was particularly concerned about the heat in the right quadriceps muscle, particularly in the lateralis muscle.

Examination

There were no obvious signs of bruising or swelling. Resisted knee extension caused an increase in the patient's reported 'dull ache'. Some tender areas were also identifiable in the vastus lateralis muscle and over the common peroneal nerve at the fibular head; however the major finding was an obvious increase in skin temperature in the patient's right upper leg with the lateralis muscle being the worst affected. Over the whole of the quadriceps muscle, this difference was approximately 2–3°C compared to the unaffected limb.

Treatment

Laser therapy was used in isolation during the patient's first attendance on a grid of points across the lateralis muscle. An 830 nm continuous-wave diode unit (CB Medico, Denmark) was used to treat a total of some 30 points across the muscle with a dosage of 0.9 J/point or ~9 J/cm^2. After the first such treatment, the patient reported an 'unbelievable' improvement in symptoms, especially with respect to 'heat' in the limb and nocturnal pain. On examination during the second attendance, the temperature difference between the two lower limbs had disappeared; however the previously identified tender areas were slightly more painful on palpation. On this and two subsequent occasions, TENS was applied to the common peroneal nerve at the knee and laser to the tender areas, at the dosages already specified.

Treatment outcome

As already indicated, after the first treatment the temperature of the patient's right limb normalised. After two further sessions over the next 10 days, using combined TENS and laser treatments, the tender areas on the lateralis muscle subsided and the patient reported that he was able to sleep perfectly soundly for the first time in the several months since the initial injury. A fourth combined treatment was given after which the patient was discharged with no further symptoms.

Case history 5

History

This 36-year-old lady reported constant crippling pain in her right wrist for a 3-week period after carrying several heavy objects. The patient reported that this was unaccustomed exercise and that the wrist had felt weak immediately afterwards. This weakness had persisted, and furthermore a 'constant aching pain' had also developed, which became 'sharp' when the wrist was stressed, especially in extension. The lady was right-handed. No other treatment had been received as the patient said that she was afraid of doctors.

Examination

There were no obvious signs of swelling nor of bruising. The right wrist was considerably weaker than the contralateral limb, particularly in extension. Pain was exacerbated by resisted extension and flexion of the wrist and by passive extension at the end of range. There were no neurological signs nor symptoms.

Treatment

Treatment was provided on one occasion. An 830 nm continuous-wave diode laser (Lasotronic, Switzerland) with a radiant power output of 30 mW was used with a deep pressure to deliver 1.0 J or ~10 J/cm^2 to six points on the anterior aspect of the wrist. The patient reported at the conclusion of the laser treatment that the wrist felt hot and that the pain had increased.

Treatment outcome

This patient did not return for a second treatment. When contacted, she reported that the pain had disappeared apart from some slight pain on full extension of the wrist, and that the wrist felt strong again; indeed since the day after her (solitary) treatment she found she could carry objects in her right hand without hesitation or reservation.

SUMMARY OF KEY POINTS

1. Thorough examination and diagnosis are essential to the provision of effective laser therapy treatments.
2. Where possible, in-contact treatment technique should always be used. This enhances the efficacy of laser treatment by maximising power and energy densities, reducing reflection and approximating the treatment probe with the target tissue.
3. Non-contact treatment will usually be necessary during the treatment of open wounds. In such cases, the distance between the laser probe and the wound bed should where possible never exceed 0.5–1 cm.
4. The problem of defining effective therapeutic dosage remains.

The Arndt–Schultz law proposes a threshold dosage level before biostimulation is observed and the possibility of bioinhibition as well as biostimulation. This might go some way to explaining the apparently contradictory results in clinical practice and in research reports.

5. For the laser therapy of open wounds, treatment is carried out in two stages: the wound margins using in-contact laser treatment and the wound bed using non-contact technique. For the latter, manual scanning of the treatment head across the wound bed may be used as an alternative to multidiode arrays or scanning devices to irradiate extensive areas of wound. Where only mono- or single-diode treatment units are available, 'gridding' technique is used to standardise the laser treatment.

6. Wounds may be irradiated several times per day in the early stages of treatment without apparent risk of overtreatment. However there is evidence to suggest that energy densities of over 4 J/cm^2 delivered directly to the wound bed may have an inhibitory effect upon wound healing processes.

7. Where infected wounds are to be treated, there is little evidence to suggest that the laser therapy might stimulate the infection. However, ultra-violet therapy can be effectively used in parallel to routine laser treatment in such cases where this is considered to be indicated.

8. In the laser treatment of various musculoskeletal disorders, laser may be applied directly to the site of the lesion, to any trigger or tender points present, to nerve roots and superficial nerve trunks, and to acupuncture or auricular acupuncture points as an alternative to metal needles.

9. A wide variety of musculoskeletal problems can be effectively treated with low-intensity laser therapy, including haematoma, muscle tears, ligament strains and tendinopathies.

10. Low-intensity laser therapy may also be indicated in the physiotherapeutic management of acne vulgaris, herpes simplex and herpes zoster.

REFERENCES

Baldry P E 1989 Acupuncture, trigger points and musculoskeletal pain. Churchill Livingstone, Edinburgh
Baxter G D, Bell A J, Allen M et al 1991 Low level laser therapy. Current clinical practice in Northern Ireland. Physiotherapy 77: 171–178
MacDonald A J R 1989 Acupuncture analgesia and therapy. In: Wall P D, Melzack R (eds) Textbook of pain, 2nd edn. Churchill Livingstone, Edinburgh, pp 906–919
Ohshiro T 1991 Low reactive-level laser therapy: practical application. Wiley, Chichester
Ohshiro T, Calderhead R G 1988 Low level laser therapy: a practical introduction. Wiley, Chichester

8. Current developments and future directions

INTRODUCTION

It has already been indicated in earlier chapters that the majority of publications within the field of low-intensity laser therapy have been published in Russian or eastern European journals. This chapter will therefore start by focussing on some of this vast body of otherwise inaccessible literature in an effort to provide the reader with an overview of the work completed to date within these countries. The chapter concludes by providing the reader with an update on some selected areas of ongoing and recently published work at the two main research centres in the UK, i.e. the Tissue Repair Research Unit at Guy's Hospital in London and the Laser Research Group at the University of Ulster, and indicating possible future directions in technical developments, research and clinical practice.

RUSSIAN AND EASTERN EUROPEAN LITERATURE: AN OVERVIEW

It is an unfortunate fact that the breadth and significance of the clinical and research reports emanating from the countries of the former Soviet Union remain unrecognised and in some cases unknown, even to a large percentage of the researchers within the field of low-intensity laser therapy. The reasons for this have already been outlined in Chapter 1, but essentially the current situation is due to the difficulty for Anglophone researchers and clinicians in translating and understanding such research reports, which are often published without English abstracts. Furthermore, until relatively recently, few Russian or eastern European scientists or clinicians had the opportunity or means to present research reports at scientific meetings in the West. In an effort to redress this, the following will provide an outline of some of the most interesting findings published to date.

While it has already been outlined in previous chapters, and will become apparent to the reader from the following overview, it is important to stress again here the enormous differences in clinical practice and experience with low-intensity laser devices. Indeed, this applies equally to a number of other electrotherapeutic modalities such as ultrasound which, for example, has been used in conjunction with surgical lasers at high intensities to cause cavitation in suppurating cysts (Yaremchuk et al 1982). Part of the reason for these differences is that low-intensity laser therapy in these countries is largely the preserve of physicians, and especially surgeons, who have been able to be innovative in their laser practice and have trialled novel treatment applications. In this, particular success has been achieved where quartz/fibreoptic laser applicators have been used in conjunction with suitably constructed endoscopes to target otherwise inaccessible tissues and lesions. Using such an approach, some groups have been able to successfully manage conditions such as duodenal ulcers conservatively with low-intensity laser therapy (e.g. Dotsenko et al 1985), or to treat the circulating blood cells with laser by means of optical fibres inserted intravascularly (Zemskov et al 1985).

Apart from such applications based upon the use of fibreoptic delivery systems, the main application for laser devices would seem to be as an alternative to metal needles for the purposes of acupuncture treatment (e.g. Faradzhev & Rakcheev 1984).

Cellular effects and wound healing

Various aspects of laser's effects upon the wound healing process have been investigated in the laboratory, at the cellular and whole animal level, as well as in the clinical setting. In vitro work is well established at a number of centres; particularly noteworthy is Karu's group in Moscow, the work of which has been outlined in Chapter 5. Cellular research papers emanating from other centres have included studies on the radioprotective effects of laser (Voskanyan et al 1985) as well as an interesting report from Moroz (1983) at the Medical Institute of Lvov of altered ionic balances of potassium and sodium in irradiated erthrocytes in vitro. In the Moroz study, these changes were further found to be dosage-dependent, with a threshold of effect at 0.6 J/cm^2 of He–Ne laser exposure.

Animal studies have typically been completed on small, loose-skinned rodents (e.g. rats) and have used experimental wounds to study various aspects of laser-mediated modulation of wound healing (e.g. Chesnokova et al 1983). In a number of cases, investigators have combined observations on animals with parallel investigations on human patients or, interestingly, have used basic research on cells or animals to direct investigations in humans. A good example of this approach is Sarkisian's report of investigations on the potential positive therapeutic effects of laser upon haemopoietic cells in irradiated experimental animals and patients treated with laser for arthritis or gastric ulcers (Sarkisian 1979); further examples are outlined elsewhere.

In the clinical setting a relatively early study by Kovinsky and colleagues at Kazah University Hospital found laser irradiation to be an effective modality in the treatment of both superficial and deep burns in 36 patients (Kovinsky et al 1974). Apart from apparently increased rates of healing, in terms of increased granulation and re-epithelialisation, this group also found that microflora disappeared from the wound much more quickly as a result of laser irradiation. This report is thus interesting from two aspects: in the first instance it is one of the few reports on the successful use of laser therapy in the treatment of burns, and secondly it reports a potentially useful means of wound infection control by laser irradiation, most likely through photobiostimulation of the host response.

Professor Zhukov and his group at the Department of Hospital Surgery of the Kuibishev Medical Institute in Moscow have reported considerable success in the treatment of post-thrombophlebitic oedema and ulcers in the lower limbs of 91 patients using a He–Ne laser (Zhukov et al 1979). For these treatments, this group used a defocussing unit on the end of the laser to produce a spot of some 6 cm diameter. In those patients with oedema ($n = 37$), a dosage of $0.1 \, J/cm^2$ was applied for a total of 20 treatments, while in the group with ulcers a slightly higher radiant exposure of $0.16 \, J/cm^2$ was applied on a total of 30 occasions. Despite the use of such relatively low energy densities, this group reported the laser therapy to be effective in all the patients so treated in terms of a range of objective measures including thermography, transcapillary exchange and, perhaps most importantly, length of hospitalisation, in many cases being reduced by a factor of two to three.

Finally, Professor Burgudjieva and colleagues have reported considerable success in the use of laser therapy for the treatment of complicated postoperative wounds in obstetrics and gynaecology; they have further demonstrated a cellular basis for their clinical observations and successes (Burgudjieva et al 1985a, b). Interestingly, apart from accelerated wound healing and reduction in necrotic tissue, this group also reported decreases in bacterial wound infections as a result of laser treatment (Burgudjieva et al 1985a).

Dermatology

Low-intensity laser therapy has apparently been used to treat a range of conditions in dermatology in Russia and eastern Europe. Psoriasis is one such condition which has apparently been treated with some success; Rakcheev and colleagues have reported positive clinical effects in 50 patients, particularly in terms of reduced periods of exacerbations, accompanied by parallel photobiostimulative effects at cellular level upon the immune and kallikrein–kinin systems (Rakcheev et al 1986). In patients with neurodermatitis, laser treatment has been found to accelerate recovery, apparently through the photobiostimulation of neutrophilic leukocytes which demonstrate secondary dysfunction in such patients (Karagezyan et al 1986).

Such findings in patients have been corroborated by positive results in a variety of animal studies, for example using experimental dermatitis. Persina & Rakcheev at the Central Research Institute for Skin and Venereal Diseases of the Ministry of Health in Moscow found that in cases of dinitrochlorobenzene-induced dermatitis in guinea-pig skin, irradiation using irradiances of 8–10 mW/cm² stimulated the activity of cells in the epidermis and dermis as well as capillary transport within the area of dermatitis (Persina & Rakcheev 1984).

Urology and nephrology

Interesting results in the laser treatment of acute epididymitis have been reported by Professor Miroshnikov and colleagues at the Leningrad Medical Institute of Paediatrics. Using a He–Ne source at relatively low (unspecified) intensities applied directly to the scrotum, this group found an immediate reduction in the pain, swelling and pyrexia which are usually associated with the condition. The reduction in these symptoms was apparently so pronounced that many patients who had suffered from insomnia because of the pain, swelling and general discomfort associated with the condition would commonly fall asleep after the first laser treatment. Apart from what this group considers to be an acceleration in the resolution of the acute inflammatory phase of the condition, they also found that laser treatment reduced the necessity for surgical intervention to less than 10% of cases. Encouraged by their early results in 117 men, this group hoped that the long-term benefits of laser treatment would match those observed in the acute stage; in particular that such laser treatment would reduce the incidence of infertility in these patients (Miroshnikov & Reznikov 1989a, b).

This group has also investigated the efficacy of He–Ne laser irradiation in the treatment of 32 cases of chronic intractable urethritis (18F:14M). Using a quartz fibreoptic applicator to deliver a radiant output of approximately 12 mW through a customised catheter, treatments were performed daily for a total period of between 10 and 14 consecutive days. In 25 of these patients, such laser therapy produced reductions in pain, discharge and improvements in microscopic investigations of the urethritis especially as regards the number of leukocytes (Miroshnikov et al 1989).

In assessing the potential applications of low-intensity laser therapy in nephrology, Epishin (1980) found in studies using experimental injuries to the kidneys of rats ($n = 269$), daily He–Ne laser radiation (radiant power output = 21 mW; energy dosage = 3.78 J) applied over the lumbar region of such injured animals accelerated the re-absorption of the pararenal haematoma and the healing of the damaged kidney. No negative effects were noted upon kidney function, blood composition or coagulation. Based upon these positive results in experimental animals, laser therapy was subsequently trialled in the treatment of 32 patients suffering subcapsular and superficial ruptures of the kidney with similarly positive results (Epishin 1980); in these patients the irradiation regime was identical to that used in the experimental animals, with the laser being applied to the most painful areas of the lumbar region daily for 3–12 days.

In these patients, the positive effects of laser radiation were accompanied by decreased pain report, all patients in this trial apparently reporting pain relief by the 10th treatment, and accelerated restoration of normal blood and urine profiles; particularly in the latter case in terms of haematuria and proteinuria. Similar effects were not observed in 37 control patients who received conservative nursing care but did not receive laser irradiation. Based upon these positive experiences with the He–Ne laser, Epishin recommended low-intensity laser treatment as an effective means of conservative treatment for cases of kidney rupture (Epishin 1980).

Apart from the direct application of laser to the lesion or site of pain as in the Epishin study outlined above, a large proportion of the papers published by clinical researchers in Russia and eastern Europe have been based upon the use of the laser as an alternative to needles for acupuncture treatments. Noteworthy in this respect is a study by Mandzhgaladze, working at Professor Kintraya's centre in Tbilisi in Georgia (see 'Obstetrics and Gynaecology' below) who used a He–Ne source (of unspecified power output) for the laser acupuncture treatment of pregnancy-associated nephropathy with essential hypertension (Mandzhgaladze 1985). For the 238 patients included in this study, laser acupuncture treatments were performed using a fibreoptic applicator to the MC6, E36 and C7 points bilaterally for between 10–15 s/point under carefully controlled conditions, either in isolation or in addition to routine (hypotensive) drug management.

After two to three laser acupuncture treatments, this author noted a marked hypotensive effect in most patients and an apparent normalisation of renal function; extensive blood and urine screening of treated patients showed parallel improvements in a range of correlative indicators including decreased acidosis and proteinuria. According to Mandzhgaladze, the significant hypotensive effects of laser acupuncture demonstrated in this study, coupled with simplicity of such treatment and the decreased need for pharmacological intervention in pregnancy, indicates laser acupuncture as a treatment of first choice in these patients.

Obstetrics and gynaecology

In gynaecology, the apparent efficacy of He–Ne laser in the management of endocervicitis and chronic adnexitis has been reported by Kintraya and colleagues at the Institute of Science and Research of Perinatal Medicine, Midwifery and Gynaecology in Tbilisi, Georgia. In their experience, the use of fibreoptic delivery systems to apply laser irradiation directly to the cervix at dosages of ~2.4 J per application for a total course of 9–15 treatments produced a good resolution of the condition including reduction of pain and markedly improved rates of healing in 68 (i.e. 85%) of the 80 women so treated (Kintraya et al 1985). These results are particularly important in that the female patients so success-fully treated with laser had already been treated by a variety of other means, with little apparent success; furthermore relapse at follow up (> 18 months) was only observed in 2 patients.

Similarly encouraging results with the use of low-intensity laser in gynaecology, in this case over a 7-year period, have also been reported by a group at the State Institute of Oncology and the Institute of Technology in Medcor in Hungary (Kovach et al 1981). Using a 5 mW He–Ne source to deliver 1 J/cm^2 to the vaginal uterus, this group has re-ported effective recovery in the laser treatment of 100 cases of ectropion epithelialisation of the neck of the uterus (Kovach et al 1981). In such cases leukorrhoea is typically present, along with the dysplasia of the uterine epithelium; ultimately cancer can also result in a small number of cases.

After between 15 and 20 laser treatments, these investigators found that the accompanying leukorrhoea had disappeared in almost 90% of the women so treated. Furthermore, by the 35th laser treatment, the ectropion epithelium had been replaced by normal flat epithelium. The follow up on these patients treated by Kovach's group shows that 15 went on to give birth to apparently healthy babies. Of these 15 women, 6 suffered relapse but the majority of these were successfully managed with further laser treatment (Kovach et al 1981).

A rather unusual application for low-intensity laser was assessed by Ordzhonikidze and colleagues working with Professor Kintraya's group in Tbilisi (see above). Using a 15 mW He–Ne laser source and irra-diance levels of ~19 mW/cm^2, this group found that applications at ini-tial dosages of 1–1.5 min (i.e. 1.14–1.71 J/cm^2) to cracked and painful nipples in nursing mothers ($n = 100$) was an effective treatment in terms of such indicators as pain reduction, enhanced healing and lactation (Ordzhonikidze et al 1983). In 94% of the women so treated, complete recovery was noted; the normal routine of natural breast feeding being resumed in all cases. Furthermore, this group found that the psychologi-cal state of women in the laser-treated group was much superior to that observed in the parallel controls ($n = 100$) who received only standard conservative treatment measures (Ordzhonikidze et al 1983).

Otorhinolaryngology

A number of groups have apparently used laser therapy successfully in otorhinolaryngology, including Bikabaeva & Sharipov at the Medical Institute of Bashkiria (Bikabaeva & Sharipov 1986), Pluzhnikov's group in Leningrad (Pluzhnikov et al 1986) and Timirgaleev and colleagues at the Moscow Otorhinolaryngology Institute (Timirgaleev et al 1986).

Bikabaeva & Sharipov reported their experiences in the combined treatment of 87 ozaena patients with the use of a 10 mW He–Ne laser source applied to the nasal cavities via a fibreoptic applicator. With 3 min of such treatment on a total of between eight and 12 occasions, this group found improvements in a range of indicators of clinical efficacy, including rheorhinograph and rhinoencephalograph measurements as well as increased moistening of the nasal cavity, improvement in olifaction and reduction in the number of associated painful lesions (Bikabaeva & Sharipov 1986).

In the treatment of various inflammatory conditions affecting the clinoid bone sinuses ($n = 54$), Pluzhnikov et al found that a 10 mW He–Ne laser source applied through a fibre optic for a total of 2–3 min per treatment produced considerable improvements in a range of indicators including decreases in reported headaches, reduction in the quantity of discharges as well as visible improvements in the X-ray records, in some cases after only 2–3 treatments (Pluzhnikov et al 1986). This group also apparently found that the length of treatment course required to successfully resolve the condition was determined by the severity and chronicity of the inflammatory reaction being treated.

Timirgaleev's group treated a range of conditions affecting the middle and inner ear including purulent tubo-otitis ($n = 24$), chronic mesotympanitis ($n = 10$) and eustachitis ($n = 6$), using a He–Ne laser (~15 mW) and quartz fibreoptic applicator together with appropriate endoscopic devices (and local anaesthesia) to insert the end of the applicator into the auditory canal in the upper throat. With 5–10 min of such treatment at estimated irradiances of 0.8–5 mW/cm^2 applied on between five and ten occasions, these workers found improvements in a range of subjective and objective indicators of inflammation affecting the middle ear and auditory canal. Most importantly, the hearing of patients treated with laser improved by between 10–50 dB. Similar improvements were not observed by this group in matched controls (Timirgaleev et al 1986).

The last two groups also reported finding significant changes in the cellularity of irradiated tissues (epithelial tissues or mucous membranes), or of the exudate. Such changes included reductions in the levels of neutrophil leukocytes and damaged cells, together with parallel increases in the numbers of healthy flat epithelial cells (Pluzhnikov et al 1986, Timirgaleev et al 1986). Similar cellular correlates of laser photobiostimulation in both humans and experimental animals have consistently been found by other groups working within this field (e.g. Tulebaev et al 1989).

Rheumatology

The treatment of various types of arthritic condition has been a popular application for low-intensity laser in a number of centres, principally in

Russia, where such application is well supported by positive results from a number of experimental studies on animals (e.g. Muldiyarov & Tsirko 1983) and biochemical studies in laser-treated patients (e.g. Shutova & Pshetakovsky 1980).

Professor Bisyarina and colleagues working at the Department of Paediatric Medicine at the Omsk Medical Institute have reported marked therapeutic benefits as a result of He–Ne laser treatment of the joints of children ($n = 26$) suffering from rheumatoid arthritis (Bisyarina et al 1982). For the purposes of this trial, a 5 mW He–Ne source was used in addition to routine drug therapy to treat the two most swollen joints in each patient, with energy dosages of 0.3 J per treated point; while these authors do not specify how many points were treated on each joint, they do indicate in their report that acupuncture points were used. The group varied the length of the course of treatment, so that patients were allocated to two groups: the first received a total of five laser treatments, the second received double this number (i.e. ten).

On the basis of such treatments, Bisyarina and co-workers reported marked reductions in pain, inflammation, early morning stiffness, drug intake (particularly corticosteroids) and various indices of joint dysfunction, coupled with significant reductions or normalisations in a range of immunobiochemical indices which this group used as correlates of clinical efficacy. Furthermore, although these authors report that no significant recovery of joint function was observed in the worst cases treated, i.e. chronically affected patients showing fibrous changes and the most intense exacerbations, the best overall results were apparently seen in patients with the oligoarthritic form of the disease.

In contrast to the majority of studies in this area, which have concentrated on assessing the efficacy of laser therapy in isolation for the management of rheumatoid arthritis, at least one group has assessed the effect of laser therapy used in conjunction with immunomodulating drugs in the treatment of rheumatoid patients (Yarema et al 1987). The drug used in this trial was levamisole, which is typically prescribed as an antiworm treatment, at least in the West, in this case 150 mg being taken orally by patients for up to 2 months on a daily basis. Laser treatment was also provided daily, using a He–Ne source with a 25 mW radiant power output and an average irradiance on the target tissue of 1.2 mW/cm² to treat all the affected joints for a total of between 25 and 30 treatments. The dosage of laser given was apparently initiated at just under 0.04 J/cm² and progressed daily to up to 0.4 J/cm² in the case of the knee joints. While these dosages might appear to be rather on the low side, it must be appreciated that in this case the investigators were interested in the *combined* effect of laser radiation with the immunomodulating drug used here. Of the 104 patients recruited for the purposes of this trial, some received only laser therapy *or* levamisole in isolation, while the remainder received both therapies; furthermore, controls were apparently also recruited to provide baseline data.

Results showed a significantly better therapeutic effect in the combined treatment group compared the other groups used in this trial, measured in terms of joint pain, early morning stiffness and range of movement; improvements were also seen in various biochemical correlates of clinical efficacy including lymphocyte and immunoglobulin counts (Yarema et al 1987).

Trials have also compared the efficacy of laser therapy applied directly to the affected joints with laser acupuncture treatments: for example Matulis and co-workers have reported their experiences in the treatment of 245 patients suffering from a range of arthritic conditions, including osteoarthritis and psoriatic arthritis as well as rheumatoid arthritis (Matulis et al 1983). Using a range of clinical and laboratory indicators of treatment efficacy which included thermographic assessment and radionucleotide investigations of synovium biopsies, this group saw a significant benefit as a result of laser treatment, but furthermore also found that the results with combined use of laser therapy and laser acupuncture were superior to either used in isolation. Interestingly, in this study the patients suffering from psoriatic arthritis were also given parallel psoralen/UVA (PUVA) treatment with no apparent need to reduce the dosage of He–Ne laser due to the psoralen-induced photosensitivity in these patients.

Summary

Given the breadth and extent of the Russian and eastern European literature on low-intensity laser, an entire book could easily be devoted to its review. In the absence of such a book, the studies reviewed here have outlined the generally positive experiences of clinicians and researchers in Eastern Europe in the use and investigation of low-intensity laser therapy at the clinical, physiological and cellular levels. However it is fair to point out that many of the studies suffer from the same shortcomings as the English language publications within this field. Regardless of this criticism, the extent and scope of the published database in areas such as obstetrics and gynaecology or rheumatology would indicate these for future controlled investigations in the laboratory as well as in the clinical setting.

RECENT RESEARCH FINDINGS: THE UK PERSPECTIVE

The last several years have seen intensive investigation of the cellular and physiological effects of low-intensity laser irradiation and assessment of the potential clinical applications of laser therapy at a number of centres worldwide: e.g. Basford's group at the Mayo Clinic in the USA and Ohshiro and colleagues in Tokoyo in Japan. In the UK, these research efforts have been concentrated at two main centres: the Tissue Repair Research Unit at Guy's Hospital in London and the University of Ulster. For the purposes of the current text, the salient findings of these two groups are considered here in some detail.

Tissue Repair Research Unit, United Medical and Dental Schools, Guy's and St Thomas' Hospitals

This unit, headed by Dr Mary Dyson, is without doubt the best-known laser research group within the British Isles, if not the world. The main thrust of work of this group has been in the investigation of the photobiostimulative effects of laser upon wound healing at the cellular level, principally using macrophage-like cell lines because of the key role these play in the wound healing process (see Ch. 5). However, this group has also published a number of important papers based upon controlled research on animals, the earliest of which (Dyson & Young 1986) demonstrated an increase in wound contraction and cellularity in a murine model as a result of low-intensity laser irradiation (904/632 nm; 4.5 mW/cm²; pulsed at 700 Hz or 1200 Hz). The group has more recently studied the effects of laser irradiation upon the healthy growth plate in rats (Cheetham et al 1992). This investigation, using an 820 nm diode source to apply energy densities of 5 J/cm² to one of the animals' knee joints thrice weekly for a total of between six and 12 occasions, showed no significant effects upon the histology of the irradiated healthy growth plate compared to sham-irradiated controls or the (unirradiated) contralateral joints. These findings would suggest that the danger of adversely affecting the healthy growth plate in humans is slight.

Despite these interesting and important findings in animals, this group is best known for its various studies on the macrophage-like cell line U-937, most of which have already been considered in earlier chapters, in particular Chapter 5. Using this particular cell line, and the growth-factor-dependent murine fibroblast cell line 3T3, the group has demonstrated a number of important relationships at the cellular level:

1. The wavelength-specific nature of photobiomodulative effects (Young et al 1989). In this study, supernatant from U-937 cells irradiated with 660, 820 and 870 nm light was found to stimulate proliferation of 3T3 cell cultures; in contrast, inhibitory effects were noted at 880 nm.

2. The dosage responsiveness of photobiomodulative effects (Bolton et al 1990). For this study a 660 nm non-coherent source with a fixed irradiance of 120 mW/cm² was used to deliver a range of radiant exposures from 2.4–9.6 J/cm². Proliferation assessed as outlined above was increased in most groups of cells, with the greatest effect being seen at 7.2 J/cm²; the least effective dosage was the highest used in this study, i.e. 9.6 J/cm².

3. The critical importance of irradiance (Bolton et al 1991) and polarisation (Bolton et al 1992). Using a total of four groups mixed between two dosage levels (2.4 J/cm^2 and 7.2 J/cm^2) and two irradiance levels 400 mW/cm^2 and 800 mW/cm^2), the former study found the higher irradiance produced the greatest (significant) proliferative effect at the lower radiant exposure; in contrast, the reverse was found at 7.2 J/cm^2. In the latter, more recently published study, the relative effects of irradiation at two levels of polarisation were assessed upon cellular proliferation in the manner already described. This study found the greatest stimulatory effect at the higher level of polarisation.

These findings are particularly important in the absence of similar, systematic controlled studies in the clinical setting to investigate such effects and relationships. Apart from the above, this group has also investigated the mechanism of action of the observed photobiomodulative effects. To this end the ability of supernatant from irradiated U-937 cells to modulate the proliferation of unirradiated 3T3 cells would suggest that growth factor release plays a major part in the photobiomodulation of wound healing processes (e.g. Bolton et al 1992). Furthermore, studies at this centre on calcium uptake by U-937 cells would suggest that laser-mediated effects upon cellular membranes play an important role as another putative underlying mechanism of action of laser photobiomodulation (Young et al 1990).

Apart from ongoing research using the U-937 cell line, current studies at this centre have focussed on the effects of laser upon keratinocytes, demonstrating 904 nm laser-mediated biostimulative effects with dosages as low as 0.25 J/cm^2 (Steinlechner & Dyson 1993). This represents an interesting extension of the existing work of this small but productive group.

University of Ulster

Background

This university has been extensively involved in investigating the cellular, physiological and clinical effects of low-intensity laser irradiation since 1987. A major impetus for the expansion of the research effort at this centre was the formation of a 'Laser Research Group' within the University's Biomedical Sciences Research Centre in conjunction with the Department of Occupational Therapy and Physiotherapy under the direction of Dr Jim Allen. What is unique about this particular grouping is that it combines expertise in such areas as laser physics, biochemistry, cell biology, immunology, neurophysiology and pharmacology with the clinical skills and expertise of the chartered physiotherapists working within the group. More recently, the group has expanded somewhat in terms of size and scope, its areas of interest now including electrostimulation analgesia.

Laser research carried out to date within the centre can be considered under four main headings:

1. Cellular studies based upon established and explanted cell-lines
2. Studies of the physiological effects of low-intensity laser upon blood flow and, most importantly, neural function
3. Laboratory-based studies of the putative hypoalgesic effects of low-intensity laser therapy in humans and, more recently, in animals
4. Small-scale, controlled investigations of the efficacy of low-intensity laser therapy in the clinical setting.

Results to date in all these areas have been encouraging and are considered below in more detail.

Cellular studies

Studies to date have focussed on the photobiomodulative effects of laser irradiation upon the macrophage-like cell line U937, the fibroblast cell line 3T3 and the human myeloid cell line HL60. In addition, the RIE-1 cells have been used as a growth-factor-dependent cell line to assess the photobiomodulative effects of laser irradiation upon the other cells identified. The results of these studies, which have been reported in outline in Chapter 5, have consistently demonstrated a threshold of effect at radiant exposures of ~1 J/cm^2, followed by a marginal (i.e. non-significant) photostimulative effect at radiant exposures up to and including 7.2 J/cm^2. Beyond these levels of exposure (7.2 J/cm^2), a dosage-dependent laser-mediated photobioinhibitive effect has been noted, at least in terms of tritiated thymidine incorporation (Shields et al 1993).

Apart from such consistent demonstration of the predictions of the Arndt–Schultz law, the cellular studies at Ulster have also aimed to establish the mechanism of the observed laser-mediated effects (which is usually assessed in this laboratory by tritiated thymidine incorporation). To date, results based upon measurement of the effects of growth factor release after laser irradiation upon second (unirradiated) groups of the growth-factor-dependent cell-line RIE-1 would suggest that growth factor release by irradiated cells is one mechanism of the observed photobiostimulative effects of lasers upon wounds. Furthermore, similar effects have been noted after irradiation of circulating blood mononuclear leukocytes with equivalent energy densities (Shields et al 1992).

Neurophysiological studies

As already indicated above, these have focussed largely on the neurophysiological effects of low-intensity laser irradiation in healthy human volunteers. For this work, a variety of techniques have been used including evoked potential recordings, nerve conduction studies and microneurography. Antidromic nerve conduction studies in the median nerve have shown significant increases in conduction latencies as a result of 830 nm laser irradiation on the skin at ten points (1.2J/point; ~9.6 J/cm^2) over the course of the nerve between the stimulating and recording electrodes at the elbow and second digit respectively (Baxter 1991). These laser-mediated effects were further found to be long lasting and well localised to the ipsilateral side (Baxter 1991).

These studies have been further extended in an effort to establish quantitatively the putative dosage and pulsing frequency dependency of such laser-mediated effects. Using the median nerve again, a dosage-dependent laser-mediated effect has been noted on nerve conduction latencies (Lowe et al 1992). At relatively low dosages (1.5–6 J/cm^2) only the lowest of the energy densities produced a significant increase in conduction latency; despite this, results for the other two energy densities used in this particular study showed some small laser-mediated effect.

Preliminary results from a separate study based upon the use of relatively higher dosages (9–24 J/cm^2) show that the tendency for laser irradiation to increase conduction latency (i.e. slow conduction of the compound action potential) is reversed at the higher energy densities (Lowe et al 1993). This is in keeping with results from parallel studies by Basford's group at the Mayo Clinic, which has reported significant laser-mediated decreases in conduction latencies as a result of laser irradiation at 12 J/cm^2 (Basford et al 1992). However, the situation would appear to be anything but simple; parallel studies at Ulster carried out on the superficial radial nerve using a pulsed-output 820 nm unit (Omega Universal Technologies, London) to irradiate over the course of the nerve at five points (9.6 J/cm^2) between stimulating and recording electrodes have shown that only the highest pulse repetition rate used (5000 Hz/5 kHz) produced any significant effect upon conduction latency, while lower pulsing rates (16 Hz and 73 Hz) demonstrated a tendency towards such an effect (Walsh et al 1992).

These studies have been complemented by evoked potential investigations, using electrodes to record from Erb's point and from the scalp. By employing such techniques, it has been found that irradiation over the course of the median nerve produces a significant increase in evoked potential latency at Erb's point of the order of magnitude found in the median nerve (Mohktar et al 1991). However, preliminary results from the cerebral evoked potential studies fail to demonstrate any similar laser-mediated effect.

Microneurography is an invasive neurophysiological recording technique that relies upon the use of fine tungsten microelectrodes to selectively record the activity from individual nerve axons in peripheral nerve trunks. This technique has been employed at this centre to investigate the potential neurophysiological effects of laser irradiation upon various individual classes of afferent (Baxter et al 1992a). To date, simultaneous recording from a range of afferents and efferents of various diameters has shown no direct effect in terms of evoked activity as a result of laser irradiation at energy densities of up to 33.6 J/cm^2 (pulse repetition rate = 5000 Hz/5 kHz). Furthermore, irradiation of various types of large-diameter afferents and efferents (including muscle efferents, mechano-receptors and muscle receptors) at these intensities apparently produced no changes in responses to standardised stimuli designed to elicit maximum activity from the relevant fibre. However, in all the small diameter unmyelinated fibres (e.g. nociceptors) studied to date, laser irradiation at these dosages produced an obvious decrease in elicited activity to standardised stimuli (Baxter et al 1992a).

Apart from these studies in humans, this centre has also carried out neurophysiological investigations on the isolated frog sciatic nerve to assess the potential neurophysiological effects of *direct* laser irradiation (2.38/3.57 J; 820 nm; pulsed at 5 kHz; Walsh et al 1993). These studies, performed under carefully controlled and monitored conditions, have demonstrated significant increases in nerve conduction latencies in response to such laser irradiation at the lower dosage level used (2.38 J) but not at the higher level (3.57 J). These results would indicate that the effects observed in vivo were produced as a result of the *direct* effect of laser radiation and that the type of relationship observed in vivo, i.e. significant increases in latency at the lowest energy densities, also holds in vitro.

To date this has represented the most intensively investigated area at Ulster, and this work has produced some interesting findings which provide further evidence of the potential neurophysiological effects of laser radiation when applied at the appropriate irradiation parameters.

Blood flow

A number of clinical and research reports have noted apparent increases in cutaneous and deep blood flow as a result of laser irradiation, or suggested such putative laser-mediated alterations in blood flow as a mechanism of action of some other clinical or physiological effect. Early studies at this centre therefore centred on the use of so-called *strain gauge plethysmography* to assess the potential of laser irradiation to alter deep blood flow in the lower limb. In such studies, a sphygmomanometer cuff applied to the upper part of the lower limb is used to occlude venous outflow at regular predetermined intervals, while a strain gauge wrapped around the bulk of the calf records the change in girth and thus (indirectly) volume during venous occlusion. As the change in limb volume reflects the arterial inflow in such circumstances, the strain gauge provides a means of measurement of blood flow.

To date experiments under controlled conditions on healthy human volunteers have been completed in the short and long term (24 min and 40 min respectively) using a 31 diode multiwavelength array to assess the potential effects of radiant exposures of 15.9–52.8 J/cm^2 applied to the lateral aspect of the bulk of the triceps surae. With irradiance fixed at

44 mW/cm^2, very high and low pulse repetition rates (5 kHz and 2.28 Hz respectively) have been found to produce no significant changes in deep blood flow in either the short or long term. In contrast, the same intensity and dosage of radiation pulsed at 36.48 Hz has consistently been shown to produce a significant decrease in blood flow in both the short and long term (Martin et al 1991). It would thus appear that pulse repetition rate may be a critical parameter as far as some laser-mediated physiological effects are concerned. Furthermore, it would also seem that the popularly cited rule of thumb that lower pulse repetition rates should be used in the laser treatment of acute conditions, while higher repetition rates (e.g. in the kilohertz range) should be reserved for the treatment of chronic conditions, does at least have some validity given these findings.

Experimental pain

Several experimental models of pain in humans have been used at this centre in the investigation of the putative hypoalgesic effects of low-intensity laser therapy. These have included mechanically induced pain, experimental ischaemic pain and intraneural microstimulation-evoked pain. The variation of the submaximal effort tourniquet technique used at this centre to induce ischaemic pain experimentally in the upper limb has successfully demonstrated the hypoalgesic efficacy of laser irradiation of ipsilateral Erb's point and the cervical nerve roots (Baxter et al 1991; Mokhtar et al 1992a). These studies were based upon the use of a multisource, multiwavelength array (660–950 nm) with a relatively high total radiant output (532 mW) to deliver over 30 J/cm^2 during the 12 min course of the experiment. In each case, laser treatment demonstrated significant hypoalgesic effects in terms of both visual analogue scale (VAS) and McGill Pain Questionnaire (MPQ) scores which were used in these experiments to measure 'current pain intensity' and 'worst pain experienced' respectively.

   This pain model has also been used to assess the possible significance of pulse repetition rate in the observed laser-mediated hypoalgesia, with irradiance and radiant exposure standardised at the values already given above (Mokhtar et al 1992b). For this last experiment, laser and monochromatic light irradiation pulsed at 16 Hz was compared to that pulsed at 73 Hz. These values were selected on the basis of research carried out on animals (see p. 159) which had suggested that lower pulsing rates produce a short-duration hypoalgesia of rapid onset while, in contrast, medium pulsing repetition rates (~70 Hz) produce a longer-duration hypoalgesic effect but with an extended latency to onset. The findings in this human study would support those reported in animals, with the 16 Hz pulsing repetition rate demonstrating the superior effect over the 12 min period of the ischaemic test in terms of both VAS and MPQ scores (Mokhtar et al 1992b).

Intraneural microstimulation is essentially a development of the micro-neurographic technique already described above, in which the fine tungsten microelectrodes normally used for recording are used to selectively stimulate impaled afferents or efferents with electrical stimuli. Where nociceptors are adequately identified, intraneural microstimulation can be used to produce a selective, purely nociceptor-evoked pain. Using such *intraneural microstimulation-evoked pain*, it has been possible to investigate the effect of 820 nm laser irradiation upon pain threshold. With a pulse repetition rate of 16 Hz and radiant exposures/energy densities of 16.8–33.6 J/cm^2 applied directly to the skin over the nerve just proximal to the insertion site of the microelectrode, it has been found that pain threshold increases by the order of 7–11% as a result of laser irradiation (Baxter et al 1992b).

Clinical studies

The results obtained in the work outlined above have been used in the formulation of irradiation protocols for several placebo-controlled, double-blind randomised clinical trials which are already under way at a number of centres in Northern Ireland. These include trials on the clinical efficacy of low-intensity laser therapy in the management of:

1. chronic unhealed sacral pressure sores, in conjunction with Coleraine Hospital
2. painful rheumatoid feet, in conjunction with the Northern Ireland School of Podiatric Medicine
3. herpes zoster, in conjunction with a number of centres, including Coleraine Hospital.

It is anticipated that results from these clinical trials will be available in the not too distant future, so that the experimental work of the group will be complemented by data obtained under carefully controlled and blinded conditions.

Recent results

More recent studies at this university have included some preliminary assessment of the potential cytotoxic and mutagenic effects of laser using comet assay techniques as well as investigations of the comparative cellular effects of laser and ionising (X-ray) radiation. In an extension of the work already described above upon experimental ischaemic pain, preliminary investigations are already under way to assess the usefulness of a standardised technique for the induction of delayed onset muscle soreness in healthy human volunteers as a means of assessing the potential hypoalgesic effects of laser therapy in cases of myogenic pain.

Finally, a relatively new development for this institution has been the completion of animal studies using hotplate techniques to further investigate and characterise the hypoalgesic effects of laser. While this work is still in its infancy, preliminary findings would suggest a small but significant hypoalgesic effect of such irradiation at dosages between 1 J/cm^2 and 6 J/cm^2 applied directly to the animals' skulls, demonstrated under this experimental paradigm by increased latency to paw licking by animals exposed to the hotplate technique. Furthermore, this effect would appear to be naloxone-reversible, which would indicate that at the irradiation parameters used here the observed hypoalgesia was opiate-mediated (Wedlock et al 1993).

TECHNOLOGICAL DEVELOPMENTS AND FUTURE DIRECTIONS

Technological developments

As this book goes to press, the laser industry has undergone radical upheavals. To a large degree this has been due to the recent economic climate, the result of which is that several of the major manufacturers of therapeutic devices in Europe have ceased trading, leaving many clinicians with no service back-up for their apparatus. The emergence of at least one commercial enterprise specialising in the servicing, repair and reconditioning of therapeutic laser apparatus (see Appendix II) therefore represents a welcome addition to the marketplace, at least in the UK.

Among the devices currently on the market, the salient trends in therapeutic laser manufacture and application in recent years have been:

1. The recent availability of diode lasers with increasingly higher radiant power outputs; treatment probes with average radiant outputs approaching 500 mW are now available as prototype units.

2. The wider availability of so-called 'cluster' units, ranging from multisource, monowavelength units based upon three or four laser diodes to multiwavelength arrays incorporating over 50 laser and superluminous diodes.

3. The development of so-called superpulsing or enhanced superpulsing regimens – diode treatment units which can be driven from standard base units to take advantage of putative pulsing-frequency-specific effects at the biological and clinical levels.

4. The introduction of superfine fibreoptics to simplify the laser treatment of sutured vascular structures and such conditions as urethritis, as is commonly practised in the countries of the former Soviet Union (see above).

Future directions?

It may seem ill-advised to identify potential future applications of therapeutic laser when so much of current practice remains at worst contentious and at best unsubstantiated by research findings. However, new applications are continually being trialled and innovative research continues apace. Apart from those already identified elsewhere in this book, two areas are worthy of particular mention in this respect as a suitable conclusion to the current text.

In the first instance, the search (involving at least one manufacturer) continues for suitable photosensitising agents to allow the laser systems currently used for low-intensity laser therapy to be applied to photodynamic therapy (PDT) applications for the selective destruction of carcinomas (see Ch. 1). If successful, this would allow the simplification of such treatments for cancer, as such a development would dispense with the need for high-power, class 4 lasers with their attendant problems, not least in terms of safety requirements.

The other area in which laser therapy may yet find considerable application is in the treatment of neural lesions. Previous chapters have mentioned the findings of several groups investigating laser-mediated acceleration of experimental neural lesions in animals, in particular Rochkind's group at Tel-Aviv University in Israel (e.g. Rochkind et al 1992). Recently, this group has reported results of its preliminary findings in patients suffering from a range of neural lesions, including severe spinal cord and cauda equina lesions, where conservative interventions have been unsuccessfully tried (Rochkind & Ouaknine 1992). Based upon this latter report, it would seem that laser therapy applied at apparently high dosages directly over the site of the spinal cord lesion produces marked neurological improvement, suggesting that therapy in such cases may promote neural function and repair and prevent extensive degenerative changes. If this is found to be the case, and laser treatment can produce convincing clinical improvements in such patients, the potential implications for the future management and rehabilitation of these conditions, and for the acceptance of low-intensity laser therapy in the West, are enormous.

SUMMARY OF KEY POINTS

1. Research reports emanating from Russia and eastern Europe testify to the acceptance and wide clinical usage of low-intensity laser therapy at a range of centres and in a variety of specialties including rheumatology, urology and nephrology as well as obstetrics and gynaecology.
2. Recent research at the Tissue Repair Research Unit at Guy's Hospital in London has provided useful evidence at the cellular level for such phenomena and relationships as wavelength specificity, dosage dependency and the potential relevance of polarisation.
3. Research at the University of Ulster spans investigations of the

cellular, physiological and clinical effects of therapeutic lasers. Recent findings have included pulse repetition rate specificity in laser-mediated neurophysiological and hypoalgesic effects.

4. Recent technological developments have included the distribution of promotion of units based upon increasingly higher-powered diodes and the development of so-called superpulsed or enhanced superpulsed units.

5. Future directions in this field may include the development of units and drugs which would allow therapeutic units to be used for PDT application and the use of laser therapy for the treatment of spinal cord lesions.

REFERENCES

Basford J R, Hallman H O, Matsumato J Y et al 1992 Effects of 830 nm continuous wave laser diode radiation on median nerve function in normal subjects. Abstracts 'London Laser 1992', Second Meeting of the International Laser Therapy Association: 28

Baxter G D 1991 Low level laser therapy: current clinical practice, analgesic and neurophysiological effects. DPhil Thesis, University of Ulster

Baxter G D, Mokhtar B, Allen J M et al 1991 Effect of laser irradiation of ipsilateral Erb's point upon tourniquet-induced ischaemic pain: a single blind study. Lasers in Surgery and Medicine (Suppl) 3: 11

Baxter G D, Walsh D M, Wright A et al 1992a A microneurographic investigation of the neurophysiological effects of low intensity laser. Abstracts 'London Laser 1992', Second Meeting of the International Laser Therapy Association: 30

Baxter G D, Walsh D M, Allen J M 1992b The effect of laser upon intraneural microstimulation (INMS) evoked pain. Lasers in Surgery and Medicine (Suppl) 4: 11

Bikabaeva A I, Sharipov R A 1986 Combined treatment of ozena patients with low-energy laser radiation. Vestnik Otorinolaringologii (3): 59–61

Bisyarina V P, Savitskay V Ja, Verimeevich L I et al 1982 Laser in multiple modality treatment of children with rheumatoid arthritis. Pediatriia (3): 57–58

Bolton P A, Young S R, Dyson M 1990 Macrophage responsiveness to light therapy – a dose response study. Laser Therapy 2: 101–106

Bolton P A, Young S R, Dyson M 1991 Macrophage responsiveness to light therapy with varying power and energy densities. Laser Therapy 3: 105–111

Bolton P A, Dyson M, Young S R 1992 The effect of polarised light on the release of growth factors from the U-937 macrophage-like cell line. Laser Therapy 4: 33–42

Burgudjieva T, Katranushkova N, Blazeva P 1985a Laser therapy of complicated wounds after obstetric and gynaecological operations. Akushevstvo I Ginekologiia (6): 60–69

Burgudjieva T, Bradinska A, Prancev N 1985b Histological and histochemical changes occuring under the action of helium–neon laser in complicated wounds. Akushevstvo I Ginekologiia (6): 69–75

Cheetham M J, Young S R, Dyson M 1992 Histological effects of 820 nm laser irradiation on the healthy growth plate of the rat. Laser Therapy 4: 59–63

Chesnokova N P, Pronchenkova G F, Koshelev V N et al 1983 Metabolic effects of infrared laser radiation in a post-traumatic regeneration zone. Biulleten Eksperimentalnoi Biologii Meditsiny 96: 49–51

Dotsenko A P, Grubnik V V, Melnichenko Yu A M 1985 Use of the helium–neon laser in the complex treatment of duodenal ulcer. Klinicheskaia Khirurgiia (8): 21–23

Dyson M, Young S R 1986 Effect of laser therapy on wound contraction and cellularity in mice. Lasers in Medical Science 1: 125

Epishin N M 1980 The use of helium–neon emission in the treatment of injuries to the kidneys. Urologiia I Nefrologiia (4): 11–15

Faradzhev Z G, Rakcheev A P 1984 Combined treatment of patients with unilateral and linear dermatoses using laser puncture. Vestnik Dermatologiia i Venerologiia 12: 17–21

Karagezyan M A, Komissarova, Nesterova I V 1986 Correcting effect of laser therapy on functional defects of neutrophilic leukocytes in patients with neurodermatitis. Vestnik Dermatologiia I Venerologiia 1: 14–17

Kintraya P J, Bibileishvily Z A, Dzhebenava G G et al 1985 Helium–Neon laser for endocervicitis and chronic adnexitis. Akushevstvo I Ginekologiia 6: 34–35

Kovach L, Lehotsky D, Tisa Sh 1981 Laser emission stimulating influence on the processes of the vaginal part of the uterus neck. Akushevstvo I Ginekologiia 9: 50–51

Kovinsky I T, Ekimova E S, Absadikov N A 1974 The burn wound exudate in laser irradiation. Klinicheskaia Khirurgiia 112: 72–74

Lowe A S, Baxter G D, Walsh D M et al 1992 Low-intensity laser irradiation of the human median nerve: effect of energy density upon conduction and skin temperature. Abstracts 'London Laser 1992', Second Meeting of the International Laser Therapy Association: 56

Lowe A S, Baxter G D, Walsh D M et al 1993 Unpublished data

Mandzhgaladze N R 1985 Laserpuncture as a part of combined treatment for pregnancy-associated nephropathy with essential hypertension. Akushevstvo I Ginekologiia 6: 38–42

Martin D, Ravey J, McCoy P et al 1991 The effect of pulse repetition rate in low level laser therapy on human peripheral blood flow. Proceedings Book II, 11th International Congress, World Confederation for Physical Therapy: 1093–1095

Matulis A A, Vasilenkaitis V V, Raistensky I L et al 1983 Laser therapy and laserpuncture in rheumatoid arthritis, osteoarthritis deformans and psoriatic arthropathy. Terapevticheskii Arkhiv 55: 92–97

Miroshnikov B I, Reznikov L L 1989a Laser therapy peculiarities of non-specific epididymitis compared to other methods of therapy. Personal communication

Miroshnikov B I, Reznikov L L 1989b Laser therapy peculiarities of non-specific epididymitis compared to other methods of treatment. Proceedings 'Laser Technology and Laser Medicine', Habarousk: 78–80

Miroshnikov B I, Reznikov L Ja, Reznikov L L 1989 Laser therapy of residual urethritis and its after-effects. Personal communication

Mokhtar B, Baxter G D, Bell A J et al 1991 An investigation of the effect of low level laser therapy upon Erb's point somatosensory evoked potentials. Proceedings Book II, 11th International Congress, World Confederation for Physical Therapy: 756–758

Mokhtar B, Walker D, Baxter G D et al 1992a A double blind placebo controlled investigation of the hypoalgesic effects of low intensity laser irradiation of the cervical nerve roots using experimental ischaemic pain. Abstracts 'London Laser 1992', Second Meeting of the International Laser Therapy Association: 61

Mokhtar B, Callaghan G, Baxter G D et al 1992b The possible significance of pulse repetition rate in laser mediated analgesia: a double blind placebo controlled investigation using experimental ischaemic pain. Abstracts 'London Laser 1992', Second Meeting of the International Laser Therapy Association: 62

Moroz A M 1983 Na^+ and K^+-ATPase activity in erythrocytes after laser radiation. Ukrainskii Biokhimicheskii Zhurnal 55: 674–676

Muldiyarov P Ja, Tsirko V V 1983 The effect of monochromatic helium–neon laser red light on the morphology of zymosan arthritis in rats. Biulleten Eksperimentalnoi Biologiia Meditsiny 95: 104–107

Ordzhonikidze N V, Gotsadze G G, Dgebinave G G 1983 Use of the helium–neon laser in the treatment of cracks in nipples. Akushevstvo I Ginekologiia 8: 64–66

Persina I S, Rakcheev A P 1984 Effect of helium–neon laser radiation on the morphology of experimental allergic contact dermatitis. Biulleten Eksperimentalnoi Biologiia Meditsiny 97: 603–605

Pluzhnikov S N, Ivanov B S, Usanov A A et al 1986 Use of intracavity low-intensive laser therapy in the multiple treatment of inflammatory diseases of clinoid bone sinuses. Vestnik Ototrhinolaringologiia 4: 72–73

Rakcheev A P, Voloshin R N, Samsonov V A 1986 Effectiveness of low intensity laser irradiation and its influence on immune complexes, parameters of kallikrein–kinin system and sialic acids in treatment of patients with psoriasis. Vestnik Dermatologiia I Venerologiia 2: 8–10

Rochkind S, Ouaknine G E 1992 New trend in neuroscience: LLLT for treatment of severe spinal cord and cauda equina injuries and disorders. Abstracts 'London Laser 1992', Second Meeting of the International Laser Therapy Association: 73

Rochkind S, Isak A, Novikov Y et al 1992 Influence of low level laser irradiation upon acetylcholine receptor (AChR) and creatine phosphokinase (CPK) content in denervated muscle. Abstracts 'London Laser 1992', Second Meeting of the International Laser Therapy Association: 72

Sarkisian A P 1979 The effect of radiation of the helium–neon laser upon the haemopoietic system in experiment and in laser therapy of surgical diseases. Vestnik Khirurgiia 123: 65–68

Shields T D, O'Kane S, Gilmore W S et al 1992 The effect of laser irradiation upon human mononuclear leukocytes in vitro. Lasers in Surgery and Medicine (Suppl) 4: 11

Shields T D, O'Kane S, Allen J M et al 1993 The direct of 660 nm laser irradiation upon U-937 and HL-60 cell-line. Article in preparation

Shutova T V, Pshetakovsky I L 1980 The effect of laser radiation on immunological values in patients with arthroses. Vrachebnoe Delo 6: 76–79

Steinlechner C W, Dyson M 1993 The effects of low level laser therapy on the proliferation of keratinocytes in vitro. Article in preparation

Timirgaleev M H, Shuster M A, Gavrilenko S L 1986 Transtubal laser therapy of inflammatory diseases of auditory tube and middle ear. Vestnik Otorinolaringologii 1: 63–66

Tulebaev R K, Sadykov Sh B, Romanov V A et al 1989 Immune responses to laser therapy of vasomotor rhinitis. Vestnik Otorinolaringologii 1: 46–49

Voskanyan K Sh, Simonyan N V, Avakyan T sM et al 1985 Effect of helium–neon laser on X-radiation sensitivity of Escherichia coli K-12 cells. Radiobiologica 4: 557–560

Walsh D M, Baxter G D, Allen J M et al 1992 The effect of low intensity laser irradiation upon conduction and skin temperature in the superficial radial nerve. Abstracts 'London Laser 1992', Second Meeting of the International Laser Therapy Association: 83

Walsh D M, Lowe A S, Baxter G D et al 1993 An investigation of the effect of 820 nm laser irradiation upon nerve conduction in the frog sciatic nerve in vitro. Irish Journal of Medical Science: in press

Wedlock P, Shephard R, Allen J M et al 1992 Analgesia with cranial laser irradiation in rats is reversible with naloxone. Irish Journal of Medical Science: in press

Yarema N Z, Nazar P S, Zoria L V 1987 The use of immunomodulating drugs and laser therapy in the treatment of rheumatoid arthritis. Vrachebnoe Delo 4: 59–61

Yaremchuk A Ya, Korolenko V B, Stepanov Yu V 1982 Use of ultrasound and laser radiation to treat suppurating epithelial passages and cysts of the sacrococcygeal region. Vestnik Khirurgiia 128: 64–66

Young S R, Bolton P, Dyson M et al 1989 Macrophage responsiveness to light therapy. Lasers Surgery Medicine 9: 497–505

Young S R, Dyson M, Bolton P 1990 Effect of light on calcium uptake in macrophages. Laser Therapy 2: 53–57

Zeliak V L, Yurakh E M, Gereliuk et al 1985 Choice of optimum regimen of radiation in the treatment with low energy Helium–Neon laser. Vrachebnoe Delo 8: 108–110

Zemskov V S, Gamaleya N F, Makeyev A F et al 1985 Use of intravascular laser irradiation of the blood in the complex treatment of patients with obstructive jaundice and purulent cholangitis. 4: 46–48

Zhukov B N, Zolotariova A I, Musienko S M et al 1979 Use of laser therapy in some forms of post-thrombophlebitic disease of the lower extremities. Klinicheskaia Khirurgiia 7: 46–47

Appendix I. Key terminology

The following summarises and defines in outline the most important terms used in low-intensity laser therapy. The listing is not intended to be exhaustive. For further detail the reader is directed to the relevant chapters of the book.

Coherence refers to the inherent 'synchronicity' of laser radiation; such light is described as both spatially and temporally coherent, signifying that the light is monochromatic, in phase/'in step' and highly collimated

Collimation is a term which describes the high degree of 'parallelity' of laser light. **Divergence** is more commonly specified by manufacturers and researchers; this is essentially the opposite of collimation

Continuous wave describes the output of those therapeutic units where **radiant power** output is relatively constant over time

Dosage is sometimes used when describing laser therapy treatments as an alternative to either **radiant exposure** or **energy**

Energy can be thought of as the amount of work done or photons delivered by a given unit; it is measured in J and is given by multiplying the average **radiant power output** by the irradiation time in s

Energy density *see* **Radiant exposure**

Irradiance or **power density** is the incident power per unit area. It is typically specified in milliwatts per square centimetre (mW/cm^2). For the calculation of irradiance for in-contact treatments, the unit's **radiant power output** is divided by the spot size

Laser is an acronym for Light Amplification by Stimulated Emission of Radiation

Low-intensity laser therapy (LILT) is the recommended term to describe the use of laser devices as a therapeutic modality. Alternative terms such as 'cold laser therapy', 'soft laser therapy' and 'low power laser therapy' are inappropriate and misleading

Low (reactive) level laser therapy (LLLT) is an acceptable alternative to low-intensity laser therapy (LILT)

Medium is the central component of a laser device; the medium determines the wavelength(s) of light or near infra-red radiation emitted by the device

Monochromaticity literally means 'single coloured'; monochromatic light is 'practically all at one wavelength' with very narrow bandwidth

Photobioinhibition is the term used to describe the inhibitory effects of light upon biological functions (see also below)

Photobiomodulation is the correct generic term to describe the biological effects of light upon tissue, as both biostimulation and bioinhibition are each possible

Photobiostimulation is the term used to describe the stimulatory effects of light upon biological functions e.g. in clinical practice this might be various wound healing processes. The term has been inappropriately used as an alternative to more precise generic terms such as **photobiomodulation** or **low-intensity laser therapy (LILT)**

Polarisation refers to the orientation of waves of light. The clinical relevance of polarisation is not clear

Power density *see* **Irradiance**

Power output see **Radiant power output**

Pulsed output describes the output of those devices which allow the **radiant power output** to be delivered as short pulses of energy. Pulsing can be produced by chopping the output of **continuous wave** devices, modulating the diode's output or by using a diode which is inherently pulsed

Radiant exposure or **energy density** is the energy delivered per unit area. It is usually measured and specified in joules per square centimetre (J/cm^2) and is given by multiplying the **radiant power output** (in watts) by the time of irradiation (in seconds) and dividing this product by the area of irradiation (in square centimetres)

Radiant power output of a therapeutic laser unit is usually specified in milliwatts. This gives a measure of the number of photons emitted per second

Spontaneous emission of radiation occurs when an excited electron spontaneously returns to its resting level and gives off a photon of light energy as a result

Stimulated emission of radiation typically occurs when a photon of a precise quantal energy interacts with an excited atom to give rise to a second photon, which will carry exactly the same energy as the first

Superluminous diode (SLD) is a diode source, the output of which is exactly like that of a laser diode, except for the property of coherence. The clinical relevance of coherence remains a subject of ongoing debate

Wavelength is typically expressed in nanometres (nm) (or less commonly micrometres – µm) and, expressed in terms of the wave theory of light, is the distance between one positive maximum of the electromagnetic field and the next. At a given wavelength of light, all photons carry exactly the same energy.

Appendix II. Guide to commercial systems

INTRODUCTION

The following listing is by manufacturer and is provided as an overview to the range of commercial systems currently available. It should be stressed that:

1. this listing is not designed to be complete in terms of either manufacturers or of the products offered by an individual manufacturer. Further details can be obtained from the addresses given in the relevant sections
2. in general, the specifications are as supplied by the manufacturer. While the author has tested the output of many of the devices listed, the ultimate responsibility for the accuracy of the specifications given lies entirely with the manufacturer
3. the inclusion of a therapeutic device in the following listing in no way constitutes an endorsement for the product.

ASAH MEDICO

Address

Asah Medico A/S
Valseholmen 11–13
2650 Hvidovre
Denmark

Products

This firm manufactures several 'Uni-laser' units, relying on high quality laser diodes operating at 830 nm. There have been numerous enhancements to the basic system over the last few years, resulting in the current Uni-laser 201 and 301P unit; the latter comprises a rechargeable base unit which is used to power a range of probes from 30–140mW. Once only available as continuous wave output units, Asah lasers now feature a pulsing option ranging from 10–1500 Hz; however the use of pulsing options on these units reduces output power. Probes are well designed, with easy on/off control. Perhaps the most interesting feature of the 301P unit is an integral LCD display which records treatment in terms of number of points treated, total dosage in joules and treatment time in seconds; furthermore a built-in printer can provide a hard copy record of treatment for patients' records.

These are popular, easily portable units which have improved steadily over the last few years.

CB MEDICO

Address

CB Medico Ltd
4O Derngate
Northampton
England
NN1 IUH

Products

The 'CBM Master' series of laser treatment units from CB Medico comprises two units of standard design with a mains-driven base unit and flex-connected treatment probes (CBM Master 1 and 2), and a further two portable units based upon a battery pack and recharger unit (CBM Master 3 and 4; Fig. A.1). The standard probe for these units is a 30 mW/830 nm diode unit comprising a lens arrangement to focus the output and thus maximise light flux within treated tissues. In addition to the standard probe range, this manufacturer also produces a three (laser) diode multisource 'cluster' unit as well as probes specifically designed for veterinary and dental applications (Fig. A.1).

A useful feature on some of these units is that the treatment probe can only be activated when held in contact, thus making them inherently safer than the average treatment unit as the danger of intrabeam viewing is practically non-existent. Unfortunately, this feature does render the units difficult (if not impossible) to use in non-contact mode, which may serve to limit their application in the treatment of open wounds.

ENRAF NONIUS

Address

Nomeq
Pharma-plast Ltd
Steriseal Division

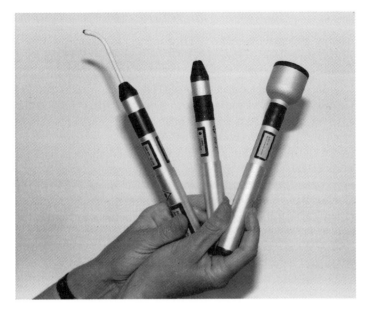

Fig. A.1 CB Medico Master Series, portable diode laser units.

Thornhill Road
REDDITCH
Worcestershire
B98 9ND

Products

Enraf Nonius produce and distribute a laser treatment system based upon the Asah range of 830 nm diode treatment probes and incorporating their own mains-powered base unit. This unit provides both continuous wave (CW) and pulsing options; however, as the CW output is 'chopped' to provide pulsing in these devices, the average radiant output in this mode is approximately 25% of that during CW operation. Treatment times need to be commensurately increased to maintain desired dosage levels. This notwithstanding, the Enraf Nonius laser system remains a popular, well designed unit.

LASER EXCHANGE/THOR LASER SYSTEMS

Address

The Laser Exchange
9 Lymington Road
LONDON
NW6 1HX

Products

The relatively recently launched Thor range of laser systems consists of a choice of three drive units (LX, PL or DD; Fig. A.2) which are each able to drive any one of a selection of five probes. All units feature a fixed selection of pulsed output (2.5–2 kHz) and so-called 100 kHz 'dual pulsing' option with fixed radiant power output; the single diode probes range in power output from 15–100 mW and the 'cluster' units feature a choice of either 19 or 69 diodes (Fig. A.2).

In addition to the Thor laser systems as outlined above, Laser Exchange also undertake testing and repair of any therapeutic laser system; they additionally offer service contracts on most of these devices. For those clinicians who have purchased systems where the original distributor is no longer supporting the system, or the manufacturer has ceased to trade, this service is indispensable.

LASOTRONIC

Address

Lasotronic AG
PO Box CH-6302
Zug
Switzerland

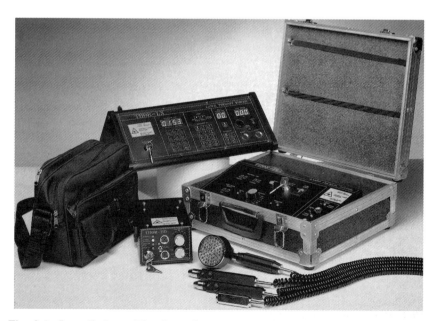

Fig. A.2 Laser Exchange/Thor Laser Systems, range of therapeutic units (reproduced with permission of Indusphoto).

Products

This well established company previously concentrated on the manufacture and distribution of He–Ne-based systems which utilised fibreoptic applicators and, most significantly, mechanical scanning devices (Fig. A.3). However, given the practically universal popularity of diode-based systems, the company has in recent years specialised in the production of pocket-sized, battery driven 830 nm laser systems. Typically these are packaged in a slimline plastic carrying case together with a power meter and a range of fibreoptic attachments for various applications, including dentistry (Fig. A.4). While these highly portable typically operate at 30 mW, the company also produces a similar unit incorporating a 670 nm diode (< 5 mW).

OMEGA LASER SYSTEMS

Address

Omega Laser Systems
211 New North Road
LONDON
N1 6UT

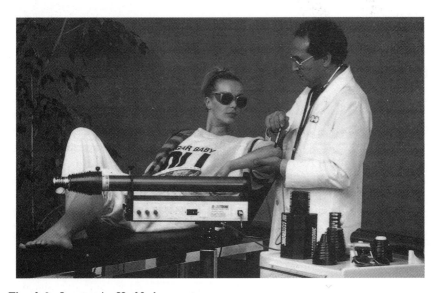

Fig. A.3 Lasotronic, He–Ne laser system.

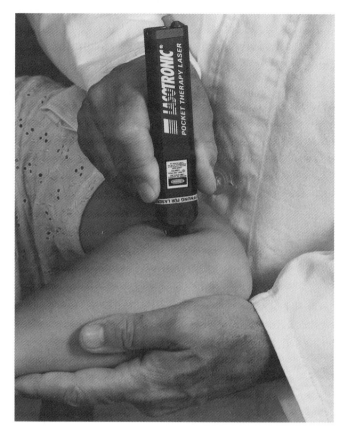

Fig. A.4   Lasotronic, portable diode unit.

Products

Omega Laser Systems (formerly Omega Universal Technologies) has been the market leader in the British Isles for a number of years. The company has achieved much of its popularity through its innovative multisource, multiwavelength 'cluster' treatment systems, usually containing 31 diodes in a single hand-held unit (Fig. A.5). In clinical terms, this much imitated unit allows for the easy treatment of relatively large areas of tissues simultaneously. The Omega base unit has been steadily improved over the last few years from an original '2000' unit, which was replaced by a more portable 'Biotherapy 3ML' unit contained in a distinctive silver photographer's box.

More recently the company has produced an upgrade known as a '2001' model base unit, the most recent version of which is microprocessor-controlled (Fig. A.6). This system incorporates a skin conductance meter

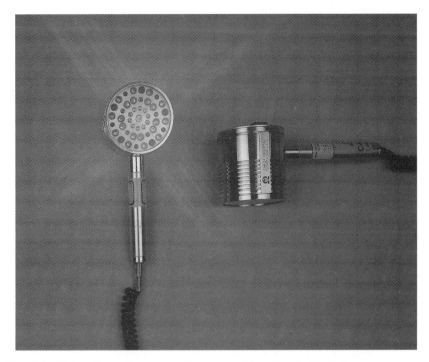

Fig. A.5   Omega Laser Systems: multisource, multiwavelength 'cluster' array.

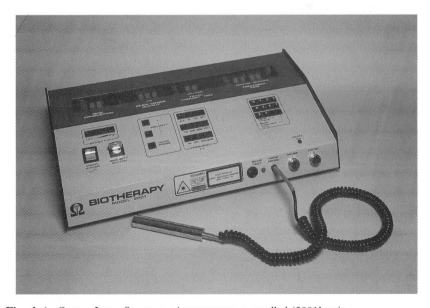

Fig. A.6   Omega Laser Systems: microprocessor controlled '2001' unit.

and the usual Omega modulated pulsed output; variation in pulse repetition rate on these does not affect power output and thus neither irradiance nor, for a given treatment time, radiant exposure. Apart from the 'cluster' units already described, the company also produces a range of single-diode treatment probes at wavelengths from 660–950 nm.

This company has maintained a vigorous research effort and has directly or indirectly been involved in research spanning the cellular, physiological and clinical levels at a range of centres worldwide for a number of years. Most recently, Omega Laser Systems have begun trials on a so-called 'super-pulsed' treatment unit combining high peak and average power output as well as a double pulsing regime with output pulsed first in the kilohertz and then the megahertz range (see Ch. 8).

SONACEL

Address

JPM Products
71 Furlong Way
Great Amwell
Nr Ware
Hertfordshire
SG12 9TE

Products

This company is already well known for its highly popular and reliable ultrasound units. More recently, the company has also been manufacturing and distributing a programmable laser therapy system known as a 'Photron'. Capable of operating either continuous wave or in pulsing mode, these units can drive up to four treatment probes simultaneously. Options for treatment attachments include single-diode 660 nm probes, distinctive hand-held 'cluster' units comprising either 16 or 17 diodes (Fig. A.7) as well as a so-called 'lamp' unit containing a supercluster of 200 diodes with a coverage of over 70 cm^2. The company also produces a flexible arm support to simplify treatment especially with the larger units. The 17-diode cluster unit is a battery-powered, hand-held unit comprising diodes operating at 660 nm, 820 nm and 950 nm and capable of being operated with any combination of these wavelengths, and in either continuous wave or pulsed (16 Hz) mode.

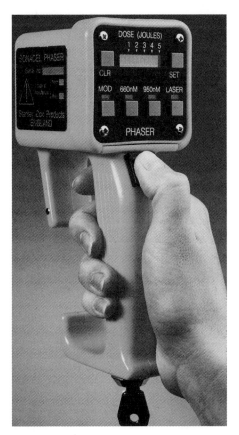

Fig. A.7 Sonacel, multiwavelength/multidiode 'cluster' unit.

Index

Absorption, 68, 69–72
  coefficient, 77
  dominant, 79–80
  incident light and, 81–83
  process of, 29–30
  scattering and, 74–75
  wavelength specificity and, 34–35
Acetylcholine (ACh), 167–168
Acne vulgaris, 213
Actinotherapy, 5–6
Acupuncture, laser, 12, 18–19, 146, 150, 190, 202–203
  analgesia and, 158, 161–162
  dentistry and, 153
  pregnancy nephropathy and, 225
  tennis elbow and, 150–151
Adnexitis, chronic, 225–226
ADP, 97, 98
Algesimetry, 143
  rating scale, 154
Amino acids, 70–71
Anaesthesia, LILT for, 153
Angiogenesis, 96, 106
Animals
  analgesia in, 17–18, 158–161
  dermatology studies in, 223–224
  hypoalgesic effects of lasers in, 237
  neurophysiological effects of lasers on, 170–174
  nociception and, 169–170
  serotinin levels in, 166–167
  wound healing in, 18, 117–127, 222
Anisotropy coefficient, 74
Ankle clonus, suppression of, 174
Argon laser, 8, 9, 170
Arndt–Schultz law, 191–192, 232
Arthritic conditions, 16, 229
Artifact, electrical, 175
ATP, 114
Attenuation, 74–75, 79

Back pain, 210, 215–216
Basement membrane reformation, 103
Basophils, 96
Beam profiles, 40, 78–83

Beer's law, 75–76
Bioenergetics of laser light, 67–88
Bioheat transfer equation, 78
Blinding, limited, 2
Blood flow, laser irradiation and, 59, 234
Bradykinin, 99, 100
Bruising, 204
Burn injuries, 123, 126, 223
  scanners for, 51
Bursitis, 207

Capsulitis of gleno-humeral joint, 210–211
Carbon dioxide laser (CO_2), 7, 8, 9
  for pain relief, 152–153, 156
Carcinomas
  animal research on, 12
  photodynamic therapy for destruction of, 11, 238
Case histories, 213–220
Cellular research, 109–117
  cell and tissue culture, 111
  cell irradiation, 111–112
  clinical situation and, 116–117
  effects and wound healing, 92–99, 222–223
  protocols, 111–113
  putative mechanisms of action, 113–116
  types of cell used, 110–111
  University of Ulster, 232
Central nervous system, 165–166, 168–169
Chalones, 102–103
Chemoattractants, 93
Chondromalacia patellae, 212
Chopped output unit, 44
Chromophores, 70, 71–72
Classification of lasers, 54–55
Cling film, use of, 64, 190
Cluster units, 52–54, 156, 194
Coagulation system and platelets, 97–99
Coherence, 36–38
Collagen, 105, 114
  He–Ne laser irradiation and, 125
  types of, 107–108
Collimation, 35–36
Commercial systems, 245–253

Compound action potential (CAP),
  increased amplitude of, 173, 174
Conduction latency, 176–177, 233, 234
Contact technique, 189–190, 192–193,
  201
  non-contact technique, 190–191, 193
Continuous wave (CW) lasers, 41, 50
Contraction, wound, 106–107
  animal, 121, 123
Contraindications to LILT, 58–62
Costochondritis/costochondral pain, 210
Cryotherapy, 200–201
CW lasers, 41, 50

Dentistry, 16–17, 153
de Quervain's disease, 150
Dermatology, 10, 223–224
DHSS regulations, 55–56
Distance of sample from irradiation
  source, 113, 130
Divergence, 35–36
Dopamine, 169
Dosage 67, 83–85, 112–113, 117, 198
  ankle clonus suppression, 174
  cluster units and, 52
  conduction latencies and, 233
  effective therapeutic, 191–192
  extrapolation of, 86–87
  manual scanning and, 195–196
  open wound, 130–131
  photosentivity and, 175
  responsiveness of photobiomodulative
    effects, 230
Duty factor (unit cycle), 45–46

Ear conditions, 227
Ectropian epithelialisation of neck of
  uterus, 226
Elastin, 108
Electrical safety of lasers, 56
Electroencephalograms, laser-mediated
  alterations in, 175–176
Electromagnetic spectrum, 24–26
Emission, laser
  mode of, 40–46
  sequence of events, 29–33
Endocervicitis, 225–226
Energy, 83–84
Energy density (radiant exposure), 79,
  84–85, 113, 198
  for open wounds, 130–131
  for pain relief, 157
Energy source, 28
Eosinophils, 96
Epididymitis, 224
Epiphyseal lines in children, treatment
  over, 61
Escherichia coli, 60, 199
Evoked potential (EP) techniques,
  174–175

Excimer lasers, 9, 10
Extracellular matrix, 104–105

Fibreoptic applicators, 49–50
  He–Ne lasers and, 222
Fibroblasts, 101, 110, 113, 115
Fibronectin, 104, 106
Fibronexus, 107
Fibroplasia, 103–106
Flexible support arms, 194–195
Fluence, 76–77
Food and Drug Administration (FDA),
  13, 17, 56, 155
Frequency, 24–26

Gallium arsenide (GaAs), 27
Gallium aluminium arsenide (GaAlAs),
  27, 112
Gate control theory, 163–164
Gaussian distribution, 78–79
Glycosaminoglycans (GAG), 104
Goggles, protective, 55, 57–58
Gonads, irradiation of, 61
Granulation tissue, 101
Gridding, 196–197
Groin strain/pains, 211–212
Growth factors
  EGF, 103
  fibroblast, 106
  GM-CSF and G-CSF, 96–97
  PDGF, 99, 103
  polypeptide, 116
  release of, 231, 232
Gynaecology, 10–11, 152, 223, 225–226
  He–Ne laser and, 130

H- and T-reflex studies, 177
Haemoglobin, 72
Haematoma, 204
Haemorrhage, areas of
  contraindication, 59–60
Hageman factor, 99
Head, 207–209
Heart disease, 61
Heart rate decreases, laser acupuncture,
  173
Heat production and diffusion during
  irradiation, 77–78
Heliotherapy, 4–5
Helium–neon (He–Ne) laser, 7, 11–13
  acetylcholine and, 168
  cell irradiation with, 112
  fibreoptic applicators and, 49–50
  production of laser radiation by, 31–32
Herpes simplex, 17, 213
Herpes zoster, 151, 213
Histamine, 91, 100, 169
Historical perspective, 3–8
HMWK (high molecular weight
  kininogen), 99

Hotplate tests, 159, 160, 237
Hyaluronic acid (HA), 104
Hypertrophic scars, 109
Hypoaesthesia, laser treatment and, 60
Hypoalgesic effects of LILT, 159, 235, 237

Infection in wounds, 60–61, 63–64
  combination treatment for, 199–200
Inflammation and immune response, 90–101
Infra-red devices, 23
International standards and regulations, 54–55
Intraneural microstimulation, 236
Intussusceptive growth, 107
Irradiance see Power density

Joint pain, 207, 208

Kallikrein, 99
Keloids, 109, 130
Keratinocytes, 231
Kromayer ultra-violet therapy, 199–200

Lasers
  applications, 8–11, 14–19
  choice, 188–189
  classification, 54–55
  components, 26–29
  development, 6–8, 11–14
  dosage see Dosage
  emission, 29–33
  history, 3–8
  light distribution see Light, laser
  maintenance, 63–64, 187–188
  mechanical structure, 28–29
  mode of emission, 40–46
  safety, 56–64
  tissue interaction with, 68–75
  treatment see Treatment
  types, 9, 49–54, 245–252
  see also Low-intensity laser therapy
Lasing medium, 26–28
Levamisole, 228
Ligament strains, 205, 207
Light, laser
  absorption see Absorption
  beam profiles, 40, 78–83
  characteristics of, 33–40
  depth of penetration, 67, 79–83, 156
  distribution, 75–78
  incident and absorbed, 81–83
  scattering, 68, 72–75
LILT see Low-intensity laser therapy
Lipoprotein composition, 124, 126
Low-intensity laser therapy (LILT), 2, 3
  applications, 14–19
  biostimulation for wound healing, 109
  contraindications, 58–62

development, 11–14
pain relief and see Pain relief
potential dangers of, 56–62
wound healing and see Wound healing
Lower limb, 211–213
Lymphatic system, laser treatment of, 126, 197–198
Lymphocytes, 96–97, 110, 115

McGill Pain Questionnaire (MPQ), 143, 235
Macrophages, 95–96, 101, 110, 116
Maintenance of lasers, 63–64, 187–188
Median nerve conduction latencies, 232–233
Melanin, 72
Meters, output, 64
Microneurography, 233–234
Modulated output units, 45
Monochromaticity and wavelength, 33–35
Monocytes, 110, 116
Monte Carlo models, 76–77
Multidiode arrays see Cluster units
Muscle tears and injuries, 204–205
Musculoskeletal disorders, 200–213
Musculoskeletal pain, 148–151
Myofibroblasts, 103–104, 105–106, 114

Naloxone, 159, 237
Nd-YAG laser, 7, 9, 10, 28
Neck pain/whiplash, 209, 216
Neoplasm, 59
Nerves
  laser application to roots and trunks, 203
Nephrology, 224
Neural lesions, 173–174, 238
Neurological effects of LILT, 162–177
  background, 162–165
  historical perspective, 165–166
  neuropharmacological effects, 166–170
  neurophysiological effects, 170–177, 232–234
Neuropraxia, reversal of, 18
Neutrophils, 92–94
Nipples, cracked and painful, 226
Nociception and peripheral
  pharmacological effects, 169–170

Obstetrics and gynaecology, 152, 223, 225–226
Ocular hazards of lasers, 56–58
Oedema formation, 16, 91–92, 223
Oncology, 8, 11
Ophthalmology, 7–8, 9–10
  contraindications to LILT, 59
Opiates, endogenous, 164–165, 168–169
Osteoarthritis, 146–147
Otorhinolaryngology, 226–227
Ozaena, 227

Pain
  experimental models of, 235–236
  neuropathic/neurogenic, 151–152
Pain relief, LILT for, 16, 139–186
  conditions treated, 144–155
  in animals, 17–18
  in dentistry, 17
  laboratory studies, 158–162
  neurological effects, 162–177
  published reports on, 140–144
  treatment parameters, 155–158
Paraesthesia, 214
Penetration, depth of, 67, 79–83, 156
Periarthritis and other arthritic conditions,
    147–148
Photobiomodulation, 14
  dosage responsiveness of, 230–231
  of wound healing see Wound healing
  wavelength-specific nature of, 230
Photobiostimulation, 14, 15
Photodynamic therapy (PDT), 11, 69,
    238
Photomedicine, 4–6
Photometer, 64
Photoreactive therapy (PRT), 11
Photosensitivity of peripheral nerves, 174,
    175
Physiotherapy, 15–16
Plastic surgery, 10
Platelets, 97–99
Polarisation, 38–39
  power density and, 231
Porphyrins, 72
Post-herpetic neuralgia (PHN), 151
Power, radiant, 39–40, 156–157
  cluster units and, 52, 53
  meters for checking, 64
Power density (irradiance), 39–40, 78, 85
  cluster units and, 52–53
  polarisation and, 231
Proliferation, cell, 113, 115, 116
Prostaglandins, 100–101
Proteoglycans, 105
Psoriasis, 6, 223
Pulse repetition rate (PRR), 45, 125, 157,
    198–199
  deep blood flow and, 235
  pain model and, 235
Pulsed output lasers, 41–46, 50, 64
  chopped, 44
  duty factor, 45–46
  fixed, 43
  modulated, 45

Radial nerve, neurophysiological testing
    on, 176–177
Radiant exposure see Energy density
Radiative transfer theory, 76
Radicular pain syndrome, 152
Reactive oxygen species (ROS), 95

Research
  cellular see Cellular research
  future directions, 237–238
  in Russia and Eastern Europe, 221–229
  in UK, 229–237
  inadequate, 2
  technological developments, 237
Respiratory tract infections in horses, 18
Rheumatoid arthritis, 144–146
Rheumatology, 227–229
Ruby laser, 7–8
  acetylcholine and, 167–168
Russian and Eastern European research
    reports, 221–229

Safety, laser
  care and maintenance, 64–65
  contraindications to use, 58–62
  electrical, 56
  environment, 63
  ocular, 56–58
  verbal warnings, 62
Scanners, 51, 193–194
  manual, 191, 195–196
Scattering, 68, 72–75
Sciatic nerve, crushed, 123–124, 126
Semiconductor systems, 13, 27, 32–33,
    50–51
Sensations and laser treatment, 203
Serotinin, 99–100, 150, 154, 165,
    166–167
Skin
  preparation, 188
  temperature increase, 217–218
  testing, 60, 62
  treatment, 63
  wounds in animals, 121, 123, 126
Skin flap survival rates (animal), 124
Soft tissue injuries, 15–16
Somatosensory evoked potential (SEP),
    176
Sports injuries, 149–151
  equipment for, 189
Strain gauge phethysmography, 234
Superluminous diodes (SLDs) 23, 37–38

Tail flick, 159
Temporomandibular joint pain,
    208–209
Tendinitis, 17, 205, 206
  Achilles, 212–213
  supraspinatus/infraspinatus, 149, 211
Tendon regeneration, 121, 126
Tennis elbow, 150, 211
TENS, 150, 217, 218
Tensile strength of irradiated wounds,
    125–126
Tensor fascia lata syndrome, 212
Terminology, 13–14, 33–46, 243–244
Thromboxane A, 97, 101

Thymidine, 232
Tissue interaction laser, 13–14, 68–75
Tissue Repair Research Unit, London,
    230–231
Treatment, 187–200
  case histories, 213–219
  choice of system, 188–189
  conditions for, 204–213
  contact technique, 189–190
  contraindications, 58–62
  devices, 193–195
  diagnosis, 188
  distance, 113
  dosage see Dosage
  frequency of, 113, 157, 199
  lymphatic system, 197–198
  musculoskeletal disorders, 200–213
  non-contact technique, 190–191
  parameters, 3, 198–199
  techniques, 192–193, 195–197
  wound see Wound healing
Trigeminal neuralgia, 151–152, 208
Trigger point therapy, 201–202
Trunk, 210

UK research, 229–238
Ulcers, 128–130, 223
Ultra-violet radiation, 5–6
U-937 cell line, 230, 231
University of Ulster research, 231–237
Upper limb, 210–211
Urethritis, 224

Urology and nephrology, 224–225

Vascular reactivity, 91
Veterinary practice, 17–18
Visual analogue scale (VAS), 128, 143,
    145, 235

Wavelength, 24–26, 112, 155–156
  penetration depth and, 80
  scattering and, 73
  specificity and absorption, 34–35
Whiplash, 209
Wound healing, 12, 15, 89–138
  angiogenesis, 106
  animal studies, 18, 117–127, 222
  cellular events and reactions, 92–99
  cellular research, 109–117, 222–223
  contraction, 106–107
  chemical mediators, 99–101
  dentistry, 16–17
  fibroplasia, 103–106
  human studies, 127–131
  inflammation, 90–101
  infection and, 60–61, 63–64
  keloids and hypertrophic scars, 109
  matrix remodelling, 107–109
  oedema formation, 91
  open, 130–131
  re-epithelialisation, 101–106
  surgical, 152
  vascular response, 91
Wrist pain, 219

BELMONT UNIVERSITY LIBRARY